Viral and Atypical Pneumonia in Adults

Editors

CHARLES S. DELA CRUZ
RICHARD G. WUNDERINK

CLINICS IN CHEST MEDICINE

www.chestmed.theclinics.com

March 2017 • Volume 38 • Number 1

ELSEVIER

1600 John F. Kennedy Boulevard ● Suite 1800 ● Philadelphia, Pennsylvania, 19103-2899

http://www.theclinics.com

CLINICS IN CHEST MEDICINE Volume 38, Number 1
March 2017 ISSN 0272-5231, ISBN-13: 978-0-323-50975-6

Editor: Katie Pfaff
Developmental Editor: Casey Potter

Clinics in Chest Medicine (ISSN 0272-5231) is published quarterly by Elsevier Inc., 360 Park Avenue South, New York, NY 10010-1710. Months of issue are March, June, September, and December. Periodicals postage paid at New York, NY and additional mailing offices. Subscription prices are $352.00 per year (domestic individuals), $652.00 per year (domestic institutions), $100.00 per year (domestic students/residents), $388.00 per year (Canadian individuals), $810.00 per year (Canadian institutions), $479.00 per year (international individuals), $810.00 per year (international institutions), and $230.00 per year (international and Canadian students/residents). International air speed delivery is included in all Clinics subscription prices. All prices are subject to change without notice. **POSTMASTER:** Send address changes to Clinics in Chest Medicine, Elsevier Health Sciences Division, Subscription Customer Service, 3251 Riverport Lane, Maryland Heights, MO 63043. **Customer Service: Telephone: 1-800-654-2452** (U.S. and Canada); **1-314-447-8871** (outside U.S. and Canada). **Fax: 1-314-447-8029. E-mail: journalscustomerservice-usa@elsevier.com (for print support); journalsonlinesupport-usa@elsevier.com (for online support).**

Reprints. For copies of 100 or more of articles in this publication, please contact the Commercial Reprints Department, Elsevier Inc., 360 Park Avenue South, New York, NY 10010-1710. Tel.: 212-633-3874; Fax: 212-633-3820; E-mail: reprints@elsevier.com.

Clinics in Chest Medicine is covered in *MEDLINE/PubMed (Index Medicus), Current Contents/Clinical Medicine, EMBASE/ Excerpta Medica, Science Citation Index,* and *ISI/BIOMED.*

Contributors

EDITORS

CHARLES S. DELA CRUZ, MD, PhD
Associate Professor, Section of Pulmonary,
Critical Care and Sleep Medicine,
Departments of Internal Medicine and
Microbial Pathogenesis, Director, Center
of Pulmonary Infection Research and
Treatment (CPIRT), Yale University, New
Haven, Connecticut

RICHARD G. WUNDERINK, MD
Professor of Medicine, Division of Pulmonary
and Critical Care, Northwestern University
Feinberg School of Medicine, Chicago, Illinois

AUTHORS

VIRGINIA BRADY, MD
Section of Pulmonary, Critical Care and Sleep
Medicine, Department of Internal Medicine,
Yale University, New Haven, Connecticut

CLEMENTE J. BRITTO, MD
Adult Cystic Fibrosis Program, Section of
Pulmonary, Critical Care and Sleep Medicine,
Department of Internal Medicine, Yale
University, New Haven, Connecticut

BIN CAO, MD
Department of Respiratory Medicine, Capital
Medical University; Lab of Clinical Microbiology
and Infectious Diseases, Centre of Respiratory
and Critical Care Medicine, China-Japan
Friendship Hospital, Beijing, China

CHARLES S. DELA CRUZ, MD, PhD
Associate Professor, Section of Pulmonary,
Critical Care and Sleep Medicine, Departments
of Internal Medicine and Microbial
Pathogenesis, Director, Center of Pulmonary
Infection Research and Treatment (CPIRT),
Yale University, New Haven, Connecticut

JANE C. DENG, MD, MS
Associate Professor, Division of Pulmonary
and Critical Care Medicine, Veterans Affairs
Healthcare System and University of Michigan,
Ann Arbor, Michigan

SCOTT E. EVANS, MD, FCCP
Division of Internal Medicine, Department
of Pulmonary Medicine, The University of
Texas MD Anderson Cancer Center,
Houston, Texas

**CLEMENTINE S. FRASER, BMBS, BSc,
MRCP**
Respiratory Sciences, National Heart and Lung
Institute, Imperial College London (St Mary's
Campus), London, United Kingdom

DAVID S. HUI, MD, FRACP, FRCP
Stanley Ho Professor of Respiratory Medicine,
Department of Medicine and Therapeutics,
Director of Stanley Ho Center for Emerging
Infectious Diseases, The Chinese University of
Hong Kong, Prince of Wales Hospital, Hong
Kong, China

MICHAEL G. ISON, MD, MS, FIDSA, FAST
Divisions of Infectious Diseases and Organ
Transplantation, Northwestern University
Feinberg School of Medicine, Chicago, Illinois

SEEMA JAIN, MD
Influenza Division, Centers for Disease Control
and Prevention, Atlanta, Georgia

AKHILESH JHA, MBBS, BSc, MRCP
Respiratory Sciences, National Heart and Lung
Institute, Imperial College London (St Mary's
Campus), London, United Kingdom

SEIWON LEE, MD
Section of Pulmonary, Critical Care and Sleep Medicine, Department of Internal Medicine, Yale University, New Haven, Connecticut

HUI LI, MD
Department of Respiratory Medicine, Capital Medical University, Beijing, China

ASHLEY LOSIER, MD
Department of Internal Medicine, Norwalk Hospital, Norwalk, Connecticut

CHAD R. MARION, DO, PhD
Section of Pulmonary, Critical Care and Sleep Medicine, Yale University School of Medicine, New Haven, Connecticut

PETER J.M. OPENSHAW, MBBS, BSc, PhD, FRCP, FMedSci
Respiratory Sciences, National Heart and Lung Institute, Imperial College London (St Mary's Campus), London, United Kingdom

JASON E. PRASSO, MD
Fellow, Division of Pulmonary and Critical Care Medicine, University of California, Los Angeles, Los Angeles, California

RAJ D. SHAH, MD
Instructor in Medicine, Division of Pulmonary and Critical Care Medicine, Northwestern University Feinberg School of Medicine, Chicago, Illinois

LOKESH SHARMA, PhD
Section of Pulmonary, Critical Care and Sleep Medicine, Yale University School of Medicine, New Haven, Connecticut

THOMAS TOLBERT, MD
Department of Internal Medicine, Yale University School of Medicine, New Haven, Connecticut

ERIK VAKIL, MD
Division of Internal Medicine, Department of Pulmonary, Critical Care and Sleep Medicine, The University of Texas Health Sciences Center, Houston, Texas

EDWARD E. WALSH, MD
Professor of Medicine, Infectious Diseases Division, Rochester General Hospital, University of Rochester School of Medicine, Rochester, New York

GRANT W. WATERER, MD, PhD
Professor of Medicine, University of Western Australia, Royal Perth Hospital, Perth, Australia; Adjunct Professor of Medicine, Northwestern University Feinberg School of Medicine, Chicago, Illinois

RICHARD G. WUNDERINK, MD
Professor of Medicine, Division of Pulmonary and Critical Care, Northwestern University Feinberg School of Medicine, Chicago, Illinois

KRISTINE M. WYLIE, PhD
Assistant Professor, Department of Pediatrics, McDonnell Genome Institute, Washington University School of Medicine, St Louis, Missouri

Contents

> The burden of pneumonia, including that due to respiratory viruses, is markedly higher in the very young (<5 years) and older adults ($\geq$50 years). Respiratory viruses substantially contribute to pneumonia in both adults and children, and when systematically tested for, are more commonly detected than bacteria in both adults and children. It is difficult to distinguish between viruses by clinical presentation, and the exact clinical implication of viral detections among patients with pneumonia depends on the pathogen detected; however, there is increasing evidence of their importance in pneumonia.

> The human respiratory tract virome is defined here as the viruses present in the human respiratory tract that can infect human cells. Sensitive, culture-independent molecular assays (polymerase chain reaction and high-throughput sequencing) reveal that in addition to common viruses that cause acute, symptomatic infections, the virome also includes viruses that do not cause clinical symptoms, have unknown pathogenic effect, or cause symptoms but are not among the most common viral respiratory tract pathogens. These molecular tools provide means for better defining the virome and studying the effects of viral infections on the dynamics of chronic lung diseases.

> The 'atypical' pathogens causing pneumonia have long been problematic for physicians because we have had to rely on serologic tests to make a diagnosis. The introduction of polymerase chain reaction techniques revolutionized the diagnosis of respiratory infections and now a new wave of technologies promising faster, cheaper, and more comprehensive testing are becoming available. This review focuses principally on the diagnosis of *Legionella*, *Mycoplasma*, and influenza infections, but also covers recent publications on the cutting edge of diagnostic tools likely to transform the field of infectious diseases over the coming decade.

> Respiratory syncytial virus (RSV) is the single most important cause of severe respiratory infection in very young infants. It has also been recently recognized as a significant cause of severe illness in elderly adults, those with underlying cardiopulmonary disease, and the immunocompromised. RSV is suspected of playing a major

role in the development of asthma. Prophylaxis in high-risk infants using a monoclonal antibody is the only effective specific therapy available but recent breakthroughs in vaccine design and antiviral drugs offer the promise of effective prophylactic and therapeutic agents against RSV.

Polymerase chain reaction–based diagnosis has become the standard for viral pneumonia and other respiratory tract infections. Expansion of respiratory viral panels (RVPs) outside of influenza and, possibly, respiratory syncytial virus has led to the ability to diagnose viral infections for which no approved specific antiviral treatment exists. Careful clinical evaluation of the patient with a positive RVP is, therefore, critical given the limited repertoire of treatments. Generic treatments with intravenous immunoglobulin, ribavirin, and interferons may benefit select severe viral pneumonia patients, whereas cidofovir has activity for severe adenoviral pneumonia.

Community-acquired pneumonia (CAP) has multiple causes and is associated with illness that requires admission to the hospital and mortality. The causes of atypical CAP include *Legionella* species, *Chlamydophila*, and *Mycoplasma*. Atypical CAP remains a diagnostic challenge and, therefore, likely is undertreated. This article reviews the advancements in the evaluation and treatment of patients and discusses current conflicts and controversies of atypical CAP.

The intermittent outbreak of pandemic influenza and emergence of novel avian influenza A virus is worldwide threat. Although most patients present with mild symptoms, some deteriorate to severe pneumonia and even death. Great progress in the understanding of the mechanism of disease pathogenesis and a series of vaccines has been promoted worldwide; however, incidence, morbidity, and mortality remains high. To step up vigilance and improve pandemic preparedness, this article elucidates the virology, epidemiology, pathogenesis, clinical characteristics, and treatment of human infections by influenza A viruses, with an emphasis on the influenza A(H1N1)pdm09, H5N1, and H7N9 subtypes.

Bats are the natural reservoirs of severe acute respiratory syndrome (SARS)-like coronaviruses (CoVs) and likely the reservoir of Middle East respiratory syndrome (MERS)-CoV. The clinical features of SARS-CoV infection and MERS-CoV infection are similar but MERS-CoV infection progresses to respiratory failure more rapidly. Although the estimated pandemic potential of MERS-CoV is lower than that of

SARS-CoV, the case fatality rate of MERS is higher. The transmission route and the possibility of other intermediary animal sources remain uncertain among many sporadic primary cases. Clinical trial options for MERS-CoV infection include monotherapy and combination therapy.

viruses, more research into the immunologic mechanisms of this disease is warranted with the hope of discovering new potential therapies.

Most viral respiratory tract infections are caused by classic respiratory viruses, including influenza, respiratory syncytial virus, human metapneumovirus, parainfluenza, rhinovirus, and adenovirus, whereas other viruses, such as herpes simplex, cytomegalovirus, and measles virus, can opportunistically affect the respiratory tract. The M2 inhibitors, amantadine and rimantadine, were historically effective for the prevention and treatment of influenza A but all circulating strains are currently resistant to these drugs. Neuraminidase inhibitors are the sole approved class of antivirals to treat influenza. Ribavirin, especially when combined with intravenous antibody, reduces morbidity and mortality among immunosuppressed patients.

Pneumonia is of great global public health importance. Viral infections play both direct and indirect parts in its cause across the globe. Influenza is a leading cause of viral pneumonia in both children and adults, and respiratory syncytial virus is increasingly recognized as causing disease at both extremes of age. Vaccination offers the best prospect for prevention but current influenza vaccines do not provide universal and durable protection, and require yearly reformulation. In the future, it is hoped that influenza vaccines will give better and universal protection, and that new vaccines can be found for other causes of viral pneumonia.

PROGRAM OBJECTIVE

The goal of the *Clinics in Chest Medicine* is to provide provide practitioners with state-of-the-art information that is clinically useful, concise, well referenced, and comprehensive.

TARGET AUDIENCE

All practicing physicians and healthcare professionals who provide patient care utilizing findings from *Chest Medicine Clinics of North America*.

LEARNING OBJECTIVES

Upon completion of this activity, participants will be able to:
1. Review pneumonia and other community respiratory viruses.
2. Discuss post-viral complications and antiviral treatments.
3. Recognize the presentation and diagnosis of atypical cases of pneumonia including Legionella, Chlamydophila and Mycoplasma Pneumonia.

ACCREDITATION

The Elsevier Office of Continuing Medical Education (EOCME) is accredited by the Accreditation Council for Continuing Medical Education (ACCME) to provide continuing medical education for physicians.

The EOCME designates this enduring material for a maximum of 15 *AMA PRA Category 1 Credit*(s)™. Physicians should claim only the credit commensurate with the extent of their participation in the activity.

All other health care professionals requesting continuing education credit for this enduring material will be issued a certificate of participation.

DISCLOSURE OF CONFLICTS OF INTEREST

The EOCME assesses conflict of interest with its instructors, faculty, planners, and other individuals who are in a position to control the content of CME activities. All relevant conflicts of interest that are identified are thoroughly vetted by EOCME for fair balance, scientific objectivity, and patient care recommendations. EOCME is committed to providing its learners with CME activities that promote improvements or quality in healthcare and not a specific proprietary business or a commercial interest.

The planning committee, staff, authors and editors listed below have identified no financial relationships or relationships to products or devices they or their spouse/life partner have with commercial interest related to the content of this CME activity:
Virginia Brady, MD; Clemente J. Britto, MD; Bin Cao, MD; Charles S. Dela Cruz, MD, PhD; Jane C. Deng, MD, MS; Anjali Fortna; Clementine S. Fraser, BMBS, BSc, MRCP; David S. Hui, MD, FRACP, FRCP; Seema Jain, MD; Akhilesh Jha, MBBS, BSc, MRCP; Seiwon Lee, MD; Hui Li, MD; Ashley Losier, MD; Chad R. Marion, DO, PhD; Palani Murugesan; Katie Pfaff; Jason E. Prasso, MD; Raj D. Shah, MD; Lokesh Sharma, PhD; Thomas Tolbert, MD; Erik Vakil, MD; Edward E. Walsh, MD; Grant W. Waterer, MD, PhD; Amy Williams; Kristine M. Wylie, PhD.

The planning committee, staff, authors and editors listed below have identified financial relationships or relationships to products or devices they or their spouse/life partner have with commercial interest related to the content of this CME activity:
Scott E. Evans, MD, FCCP has stock ownership in, and receives royalties/patents from, Pulmotect, Inc.
Michael G. Ison, MD, MS, FIDSA, FAST is a consultant/advisor for Chimerix; Celltrion Inc; Genentech, a Member of the Roche Group; MediVector, Inc; and Sequiris, and receives royalties/patents from Janssen Global Services, LLC; Chimerix; and Gilead.
Peter J.M. Openshaw, MBBS, BSc, PhD, FRCP, FMedSci is a consultant/advisor for Janssen Global Services, LLC and Mucosis, has research support from GSK group of companies; Medical Research Council UK; Wellcome Trust UK; and Mucosis.
Richard G. Wunderink, MD is a consultant/advisor for Accelerate Diagnostics, Inc and GenMark Diagnostics, Inc, and has research support form Curetis.

UNAPPROVED/OFF-LABEL USE DISCLOSURE

The EOCME requires CME faculty to disclose to the participants:
1. When products or procedures being discussed are off-label, unlabelled, experimental, and/or investigational (not US Food and Drug Administration [FDA] approved); and
2. Any limitations on the information presented, such as data that are preliminary or that represent ongoing research, interim analyses, and/or unsupported opinions. Faculty may discuss information about pharmaceutical agents that is outside of FDA-approved labelling. This information is intended solely for CME and is not intended to promote off-label use of these medications. If you have any questions, contact the medical affairs department of the manufacturer for the most recent prescribing information.

TO ENROLL

To enroll in the *Chest Medicine Clinics* Continuing Medical Education program, call customer service at 1-800-654-2452 or sign up online at http://www.theclinics.com/home/cme. The CME program is available to subscribers for an additional annual fee of USD $225.

METHOD OF PARTICIPATION

In order to claim credit, participants must complete the following:

1. Complete enrolment as indicated above.
2. Read the activity.
3. Complete the CME Test and Evaluation. Participants must achieve a score of 70% on the test. All CME Tests and Evaluations must be completed online.

CME INQUIRIES/SPECIAL NEEDS

For all CME inquiries or special needs, please contact elsevierCME@elsevier.com.

CLINICS IN CHEST MEDICINE

THE CLINICS ARE AVAILABLE ONLINE!
Access your subscription at:
www.theclinics.com

CLINICS IN CHEST MEDICINE

Preface
Respiratory Viral and Atypical Pneumonias

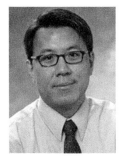   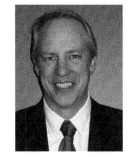

Charles S. Dela Cruz, MD, PhD   Richard G. Wunderink, MD

Editors

Respiratory viral infections continue to be a major global health problem affecting all ages. Respiratory viruses are the most commonly detected causes of community-acquired pneumonia with the incidence highest among very young children and the elderly. Molecular-based nucleic acid detection has become the standard diagnostic method for respiratory viral pathogens, having replaced older serologic and antigen–detection methods. The respiratory tract virome is becoming better defined based on culture-independent molecular assays. These methods have identified common viral pathogens as well as less common viruses with an unknown role in lung pathogenicity. This issue of *Clinics of Chest Medicine* brings together current up-to-date reviews of respiratory viral and atypical pneumonias written by experts in the field. These reviews explore multiple aspects of respiratory infection from epidemiology through specific seasonal and pandemic viruses and atypical bacteria, clinical presentation, their role in acute and chronic lung diseases, as well as treatment and prevention. The importance of respiratory syncytial virus (RSV) is highlighted as an important respiratory pathogen at both ends of the age spectrum with a general lack of awareness of RSV in adult providers. Respiratory viral infections contribute to the pathogenesis of acute lung process, such as acute respiratory distress syndrome, and chronic lung diseases, such as asthma and chronic obstructive pulmonary disease. Viruses can have particularly life-threatening adverse clinical consequences in immunocompromised patients. Nonviral atypical pneumonias, particularly *Legionella*, *Mycoplasma*, and *Chlamydophila*, which have significant overlap with viral pneumonia syndromes and are difficult to diagnose given the nonspecific nature of their presentations, are reviewed. Emerging respiratory viral pathogens that cause problems in epidemic proportions, such as pandemic influenza and coronaviruses, are discussed. Viral infections can contribute to complicated bacterial pneumonias. Current available antiviral therapies for some respiratory viral infections are described. Development of more antiviral therapies is clearly needed as well as identification of groups of patients who would have greatest benefit. Vaccination is a most effective way of preventing infection, but is only available for a limited number of respiratory pathogens with vaccine efforts for more viruses under development. The goal of this issue on respiratory viral and atypical pneumonia is to provide our current understanding of the topic and to highlight gaps of knowledge and basis for future research.

Clin Chest Med 38 (2017) xiii–xiv
http://dx.doi.org/10.1016/j.ccm.2016.12.001
0272-5231/17/© 2016 Published by Elsevier Inc.

We thank all the contributing authors for their outstanding articles.

Charles S. Dela Cruz, MD, PhD
Section of Pulmonary, Critical Care
and Sleep Medicine
Department of Internal Medicine
and Microbial Pathogenesis
Center of Pulmonary Infection Research and
Treatment
Yale University
300 Cedar Street
TAC S441-D, New Haven, CT 06513, USA

Richard G. Wunderink, MD
676 North St. Clair Street
Arkes 14-045
Chicago, IL 60611, USA

Northwestern University
Feinberg School of Medicine
McGaw Pavilion Suite M-300
240 East Huron
Chicago, IL 60611, USA

E-mail addresses:
charles.delacruz@yale.edu (C.S. Dela Cruz)
r-wunderink@northwestern.edu (R.G. Wunderink)

Epidemiology of Viral Pneumonia

Seema Jain, MD

KEYWORDS

- Respiratory viruses • Pneumonia • Epidemiology

KEY POINTS

- The burden of pneumonia, including that due to respiratory viruses, is markedly higher in the very young (<5 years) and older adults (≥50 years).
- Respiratory viruses substantially contribute to pneumonia in both adults and children, and when systematically tested for, are more commonly detected than bacteria in both adults and children.
- The most commonly detected respiratory viruses in adults and children are adenoviruses, coronaviruses, human metapneumovirus, human rhinoviruses, influenza viruses, parainfluenza viruses, and respiratory syncytial virus.
- It is difficult to distinguish between viruses by clinical presentation, and the exact clinical implication of viral detections among patients with pneumonia depends on the pathogen detected; however, there is increasing evidence of their importance in pneumonia.
- The circulation of respiratory viruses varies from region to region around the world, demonstrating seasonal variation in different parts of the world, which affects the prevalence and incidence of viral pneumonia globally.

INTRODUCTION

Worldwide, 900,000 children aged less than 5 years die from pneumonia every year.[1] Pneumonia is a leading infectious cause of hospitalization and death among US adults, resulting in more than $10 billion annual expenses.[2] Despite advances in clinical diagnostic methods, especially molecular-based methods, a cause is not always ascertained in a patient with pneumonia. Recent prospective pneumonia etiology studies have failed to detect a pathogen in greater than 50% of adults and approximately 20% of children hospitalized with pneumonia.[3–7] In these same studies, viruses were more commonly detected than bacteria in both adults and children, accounting for greater than 25% of detections in adults and greater than 70% in children.[3,7] The exact implications of viral detections among patients with pneumonia depend on the pathogen detected, but there is increasing evidence of their importance in pneumonia.[8]

US PREVALENCE/INCIDENCE

The Etiology of Pneumonia in the Community (EPIC) study was a large prospective multicenter US population-based active surveillance study in which viruses were more commonly detected than bacteria in both adults and children hospitalized with community-acquired pneumonia when systematic testing was used.[3,7] Detailed study details have been previously described,[3,7] but in brief, community-acquired pneumonia was defined as evidence of acute infection, acute respiratory illness, and radiographic evidence of pneumonia; patients with severe immunosuppression and recent hospitalization were excluded. Multiple modalities for pathogen detection of bacteria and viruses were used, including culture, polymerase chain reaction (PCR), serology, and antigen-based diagnostic assays.[3,7]

The results of the EPIC study demonstrated that prevalence and incidence of different pathogens varied by age. Among children less than 18 years

Disclaimer: The findings and conclusions in this report are those of the authors and do not necessarily represent the views of the Centers for Disease Control and Prevention.

Influenza Division, Centers for Disease Control and Prevention, 1600 Clifton Road, Atlanta, GA, 30329, USA

E-mail address: bwc8@cdc.gov

Clin Chest Med 38 (2017) 1–9

http://dx.doi.org/10.1016/j.ccm.2016.11.012

0272-5231/17/Published by Elsevier Inc.

old enrolled in the EPIC study, 70% of pneumonia hospitalizations occurred among children less than 5 years old.[7] Overall annual incidence of community-acquired pneumonia hospitalization in children was 15.7/10,000 children, and incidence was highest in children less than 2 years old (62.2/10,000 children), decreased in children 2 to 4 years old (23.8/10,000), and further decreased with increasing age. These rates were slightly lower than the 2009 national Kids' Inpatient Database, which reported 22.4 hospitalized pneumonia cases per 10,000 children less than 18 years old.[9] There are methodologic differences that likely explain these differences, including nonoverlapping years of analysis, distinctions between the populations studied, and varying case definitions, including exclusion of the severely immunocompromised in the EPIC study. Nonetheless, there were similar trends indicating that pneumonia burden is highest among the youngest children.

In the EPIC study, among 2222 children with clinical and radiographic pneumonia who had specimens available for bacterial and viral diagnostic testing, a pathogen was detected in 1802 (81%) children with one or more viruses in 1472 (66%), bacteria in 175 (8%), and both bacteria and viruses in 155 (7%). Among these 2222 children, the most commonly detected viruses were respiratory syncytial virus (RSV, 28%), human rhinoviruses (HRV, 27%), human metapneumovirus (HMPV, 13%), adenoviruses (AdV, 11%), parainfluenza 1 to 3 viruses (PIV, 7%), influenza A and B viruses (7%), and coronaviruses (CoV, 5%) (**Fig. 1**B, codetections are indicated by the lighter shading).[7] Compared with older children, RSV, AdV, and HMPV were all more commonly detected among children less than 5 years old (**Fig. 1**C). The incidence of RSV, HRV, HMPV, AdV, influenza viruses, PIV, and CoV was all higher among children less than 5 years old than among older children but was highest among children less than 2 years old.[7]

In adults enrolled in the EPIC study, overall annual incidence of community-acquired pneumonia hospitalization was 24.8/10,000 adults.[3] The overall and pathogen-specific incidences increased with age with rates highest among adults 50 years of age and older. The EPIC study rates and trends are similar to previous pneumonia etiology studies conducted in the 1990s despite methodologic differences,[10] but the EPIC study hospitalization rates were lower than more recent estimates based on hospitalization claims data likely due to certain excluded groups in the EPIC study, including those with severe immunosuppression.[11]

Among the 2259 adults enrolled in the EPIC study with clinical and radiographic pneumonia who had specimens available for bacterial and viral diagnostic testing, a pathogen was detected in 853 (38%) with one or more viruses in 530 (23%), bacteria in 247 (11%), bacteria and viruses in 59 (3%), and a fungal or mycobacterial pathogen in 17 (1%). Among the 2259 adults, the most commonly detected viruses were HRV (9%), influenza A and B viruses (6%), HMPV (4%), RSV (3%), PIV (2%), CoV (2%), and AdV (1%) (**Fig. 1**A).[3] Importantly, the incidence of pneumonia hospitalization with influenza was almost 5 times higher among adults 65 years and older than among younger adults, and the incidence of HRV was almost 10 times as high. Interestingly, the overall incidence of pneumonia hospitalization with influenza (1.5/10,000) was similar to that of pneumococcus (1.2/10,000), a well-known bacterial cause of community-acquired pneumonia.

WORLDWIDE/REGIONAL PREVALENCE, INCIDENCE, AND MORTALITIES

It is well known that respiratory viruses contribute to acute respiratory infections, including those involving the lower respiratory tract and leading to bronchiolitis, pneumonia, and other complications. Although some global estimates of respiratory virus burden have been derived, including some from low- and middle-income countries, these data remain sparse because little surveillance for respiratory viruses is systematically carried out in many countries. In addition, most surveillance and thus estimates are not specific to pneumonia, and definitions of pneumonia vary widely between studies, making comparisons difficult.

In a 2005 study, RSV was associated with 22% of acute lower respiratory infections in children less than 5 years old worldwide with 3.4 (2.8–4.3) million hospitalizations and 66,000 to 199,000 deaths; 99% of deaths occurred in developing countries.[12] Data from this same analysis demonstrated that most RSV deaths in high-income countries were in children less than 1 year old, whereas in low- and middle-income countries, these deaths extended into the second year of life.

Similar analyses have been done for the burden of influenza virus infection, again not necessarily limited to pneumonia. According to the World Health Organization (WHO), influenza occurs globally with an annual attack rate estimated at 5% to 10% in adults and 20% to 30% in children.[13] Worldwide, these annual epidemics are estimated to result in about 3 to 5 million cases of severe illness, and about 250,000 to 500,000 deaths. Although hospitalizations and deaths occur in healthy people, certain groups are at higher risk for complications, and thus, influenza vaccines are targeted for these high-risk groups, including children 6 months to 5 years old, elderly 65 years and older, people with chronic medical conditions, pregnant women, and health care workers.

As part of the Pneumonia Research for Child Health (PERCH) project, 7 low- and middle-income countries have conducted research on pneumonia etiology among children less than 5 years old. In the PERCH project, the pneumonia case-definition per the WHO definitions was of severe (lower chest-wall indrawing in a child with history of cough or difficulty breathing) or very severe (cyanosis, oxygen saturation <90%, inability to feed, head nodding, or impaired consciousness in a child with history of cough or difficulty in breathing) pneumonia. Two types of outpatient controls without pneumonia included asymptomatic children and children with upper respiratory tract infection. In a preliminary analysis from one study site in rural Kenya, respiratory viruses were detected in most (60%) children less than 5 years old with pneumonia but also in controls (47%).[14] Of the viruses detected, RSV was the most commonly detected virus in case-patients but not controls with a statistically significant association between virus detection and pneumonia hospitalization.[14]

In other pneumonia studies conducted in high-, low-, and middle-income countries, although the prevalence of specific viruses varies greatly, viruses are more commonly detected than bacteria, particularly in children. Prevalence of viruses can vary by geography and other factors, such as immunization coverage, as well as study design, including case definitions, specimen collection methods, and diagnostic tools applied; however, in most of these studies, certain viruses predominate, including RSV but also HMPV, AdV, and PIV. In a study of severe and very severe pneumonia conducted in Kenya and using multiplex PCR, a virus was detected in 56% of children less than 12 years old; RSV was most common and detected in 34% of children.[15] In a different study conducted in Mozambique, viruses were detected in 49% of children with severe pneumonia, and in this case, HRV (41%), AdV (21%), and RSV (11%) were the most common.[16] In similar studies, HMPV, AdV, PIV, and CoV combined account for 25% to 40% of pathogens detected in children when using PCR methods.[17,18] In many studies, codetections (viral and bacterial) in children with pneumonia have been demonstrated in more than one-quarter of cases.[7,14,19]

The role of viruses in adults has had increasing attention because viruses like RSV and HMPV have been commonly detected in systematic studies of hospitalized adults.[20,21] Although the same viruses that circulate in children also affect adults, the prevalence of the viruses differs between children and adults with pneumonia and also compared with data from controls. For example, HRV has been commonly detected in adult pneumonia patients, including from sterile lower respiratory tract specimens; in contrast with children, HRV is not commonly detected among adult asymptomatic controls and is often detected as the sole pathogen in adults, whereas, in children, it is often codetected.[3,4,8,22–25] Influenza viruses are a known contributor to viral pneumonia,[25] as well as a precursor to bacterial pneumonia, and are a common cause of pneumonia among persons 65 years and older. The range of other virus detections, including HMPV, RSV, PIV, CoV, and AdV, in adults with pneumonia is broad, ranging from 11% to 28% depending on the study location, design, and diagnostic tools.[4,5,17–28] Bacterial or viral codetections are less frequently detected in adults than in children.[3]

WORLDWIDE/REGIONAL SEASONALITY AND CIRCULATION PATTERNS

The circulation of respiratory viruses varies from region to region around the world and demonstrates seasonal variation in different parts of the world, which affects the prevalence and incidence of viral pneumonia globally. In the United States, similar to other Northern Hemisphere countries, there are distinct peaks and troughs for different viruses. Generally, except for the 2009 H1N1 pandemic period from 2008 to 2009, there have been very clear peaks of influenza virus circulation annually in the United States that occur in the late fall or early winter, although it is never predictable exactly when the influenza season will start, and there is also regional variation. US influenza virus circulation data are reported weekly at the national and regional level on the Centers for Disease Control and Prevention (CDC) FluView Web site: http://www.cdc.gov/flu/weekly/fluactivitysurv.htm. Similarly, influenza circulation varies worldwide and surveillance methods vary from nation to nation, but data on global influenza circulation can be accessed on the WHO FluNet Web site: http://www.who.int/influenza/gisrs_laboratory/flunet/en/. Weekly global update reports are also available here: http://www.who.int/influenza/surveillance_monitoring/updates/latest_update_GIP_surveillance/en/.

In the United States, RSV circulation usually starts in late October and lasts until late January but can shift, starting in late January and lasting until early April depending on the year and circulation of other respiratory pathogens. Like influenza viruses, there is also regional variation with an earlier season starting in Florida and lasting longer than other US regions. National and regional RSV surveillance trends can be monitored at the CDC National Respiratory and Enteric Virus Surveillance System (NREVSS) Web site: http://www.cdc.gov/surveillance/nrevss/rsv/natl-trend.

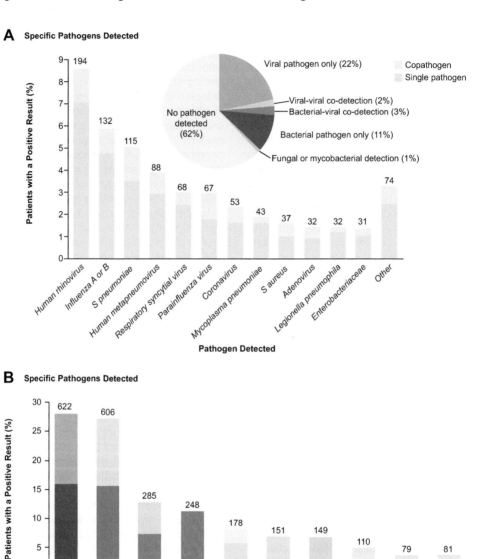

Fig. 1. (A) Numbers (above the bars) and percentages of all adults in whom a specific pathogen was detected in the adult component of the EPIC study. The proportions of viral, viral-viral, bacterial-viral, bacterial, fungal or mycobacterial pathogens detected, and no pathogen detected are shown in the pie chart. (B) Numbers (above the bars) and percentages of all children in whom a specific pathogen was detected in the pediatric component of the EPIC study. (C) Proportions of pathogens detected, according to age group in the pediatric component of the EPIC study. (From [A] Jain S, Self WH, Wunderink RG, et al. Community-acquired pneumonia requiring hospitalization among U.S. adults. N Engl J Med 2015;373:420, with permission from Massachusetts Medical Society; and [B, C] Jain S, Williams DJ, Arnold SR, et al. Community-acquired pneumonia requiring hospitalization among U.S. children. N Engl J Med 2015;372:840; with permission from Massachusetts Medical Society.)

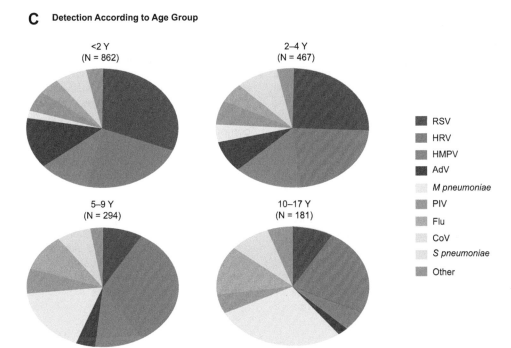

C Detection According to Age Group

<2 Y
(N = 862)

2–4 Y
(N = 467)

5–9 Y
(N = 294)

10–17 Y
(N = 181)

RSV
HRV
HMPV
AdV
M pneumoniae
PIV
Flu
CoV
S pneumoniae
Other

Fig. 1. (*continued*)

html. Through NREVSS, national and regional data are available for HMPV (http://www.cdc.gov/surveillance/nrevss/hmpv/natl-trend.html) and national data are also available for AdV (http://www.cdc.gov/surveillance/nrevss/adeno/natl-trend.html) and PIV (http://www.cdc.gov/surveillance/nrevss/human-paraflu/natl-trend.html), although specimens are not routinely tested for these viruses.

Globally, RSV surveillance efforts and methods vary from country to country. Data from 7 countries (Bangladesh, China, Egypt, Guatemala, Kenya, South Africa, and Thailand) over 8 years (2004–2012) demonstrated that RSV infection had 1 to 2 epidemic periods each year in each country; in general, seasonality patterns were similar within country but differed between countries from year to year. Likely factors affecting circulation were weather, geography, precipitation, and temperature.[29] Similar reports from tropical and subtropical areas of southern and southeastern Asia have also shown that influenza virus circulation is highly dependent on weather patterns, especially rainfall and monsoons, and affects the seasonality of influenza virus circulation regionally, which has direct implications for influenza vaccination timing in these regions.[30,31]

CLINICAL CORRELATION AND RISK FACTORS

Many pneumonia etiology studies rely on naso/oropharyngeal specimens for pathogen detection in addition to blood, serum, sputum, and urine (only in adults) because lower respiratory specimens are not practical or possible unless clinically necessary. Because most of these specimens do not come not directly from the lung, it is difficult to discern the association of a pathogen detection with pneumonia. Thus, many studies have enrolled asymptomatic controls along with pneumonia cases to help determine the possible contribution of respiratory viruses (attributable risk) to pneumonia at a population level. However, studies show variable prevalence of viruses among controls, possibly due to differences in definitions and methods for ascertainment of controls.[32] Different strategies for control enrollment may be applicable to different study objectives and settings.[32]

In the EPIC study, all pathogens except for HRV were detected in 3% or less of asymptomatic controls; HRV was detected in 17% of pediatric controls compared with 22% of children with pneumonia ($P = .04$).[7,8] In asymptomatic adult controls, only 2% had any pathogen detection, compared with 27% among the patients hospitalized with pneumonia; interestingly, HRV was rarely detected in adult controls (1%).[3,8] In the EPIC study, the attributable fraction (AF) was calculated by comparing prevalence of viruses in pneumonia cases with asymptomatic controls, and adjusting for age, enrollment month, and enrollment city. In this analysis, the AF indicated that the detection of influenza, RSV, and HMPV among all patients, both children and adults, indicated an etiologic role. However, the detections of PIV, CoV, and AdV, particularly in children, did not demonstrate high AF for pneumonia. HRV was associated with pneumonia in adults but not children.[8] The exact role of HRV in pneumonia remains unclear and controversial, even when detected as a single pathogen, particularly because HRV can shed for greater than 2 weeks after a primary infection, making its detection at time of pneumonia challenging to interpret with respect to the current clinical illness.[22–24]

Data from the EPIC study are similar to other US data from Singleton and colleagues,[33] which compared asymptomatic Alaskan children less than 3 years old from the community with children hospitalized with respiratory infections. In this study, RSV, PIV, HMPV, and influenza viruses were all significantly more common in hospitalized children than controls, but HRV, AdV, and CoV were not; interestingly, children with RSV only or HMPV only had more severe illness compared with children with the other viruses.

Data from the recent US studies, including the EPIC study, are somewhat in contrast to data from the PERCH project site in Kenya, which tested for multiple pathogens (bacteria and viruses) in children less than 5 years old with pneumonia and in comparison to community controls (who could have had an upper respiratory infection). In the Kenya site for the PERCH project, compared with controls, RSV was the only virus determined to have a statistically significant association with hospitalization.[14] The differences between the study results are likely due to variations in case and control definitions, prevalence of pathogens in the different studies, geography, and sociocultural characteristics that determine access to health care, threshold for hospitalization, and vaccination coverage for available immunizations.

In addition to nuances around etiology, the clinical spectrum of illness due to respiratory viruses is broad and encompasses asymptomatic infection, upper respiratory infection, and lower respiratory tract infection, resulting in pneumonia as well as other complications (eg, acute respiratory distress or secondary bacterial infection). Clinically, symptoms due to any specific virus infection, including in relation to pneumonia, largely overlap; thus, there are few clinical clues to distinguish between illnesses due to different pathogens. Some epidemiologic clues such as age and seasonality may be helpful. In addition, greater than 25% of children and less than 5% of adults are found to have multiple pathogens, potentially including both viruses and bacteria, and on this basis alone could be expected to have a mixed clinical presentation.[3,7]

There are some data from comparisons of patients with illness of varying severity that suggest that bacterial pneumonia contributes to more severe illness. For example, in the EPIC study, *Streptococcus pneumoniae*, *Staphylococcus aureus*, and Enterobacteriaceae combined accounted for 16% of detected pathogens among adults admitted to the intensive care unit (ICU) as compared with 6% among adults not admitted to the ICU.[3] Thus, when bacteria were detected, it was more likely in a severely ill patient. However, it is important to note that viruses were detected in 22% of adults admitted to the ICU compared with 24% not admitted to the ICU; so although there were no statistically significant differences between the severe and nonsevere groups, viral pneumonia contributed to ICU admissions, mechanical ventilation, and also death.

Influenza viruses are some of the more commonly recognized viruses that cause pneumonia and can lead to a primary viral pneumonia, secondary bacterial pneumonia, or mixed viral-bacterial pneumonia.[25,34,35] Much of the influenza-associated pneumonia literature has focused on pandemics,[36,37] including the most recent 2009 H1N1 pandemic.[38–40] During interpandemic years, influenza virus circulation varies, and thus, rates of influenza-associated pneumonia vary from year to year. Data from these reports indicate that in comparison to patients with influenza virus infection without pneumonia, patients with influenza virus infection and radiographic evidence of pneumonia have a more severe course of illness in terms of longer length of stay, ICU admission, mechanical ventilation, acute respiratory distress syndrome, sepsis, and death.[40]

Although RSV is commonly associated with bronchiolitis, it is also a well-known cause of the clinically and radiographically defined pneumonia, with RSV burden highest among children less than 2 years old. Most children are infected with RSV by 2 years of age, and the first infection, which may not confer immunity, is usually most severe. Prematurity and young age have been shown to be independent risk factors for hospitalization.[41] In countries with a high HIV prevalence, RSV-associated acute lower respiratory tract infection has led to an increased risk of hospitalization and death, and longer hospital stay in children with HIV infection compared with children without HIV infection.[42] RSV has also been shown to lead to acute respiratory infection in adults, including hospitalization, with the highest burden among adults greater than 50 years old.[20] In addition to older age, other risk factors for RSV infection in adults include immunocompromised states and chronic lung conditions.[43]

Pneumonia was reported in almost half of the children who were hospitalized with HMPV infection in one multisite study of acute respiratory illness conducted in the United States.[44] Similar to RSV, prematurity and asthma have been shown to be more frequent among hospitalized children with HMPV infection than children without HMPV infection.[44] Risk factors for HMPV infection and subsequent complications, including pneumonia and hospitalization in adults, include older age, and underlying conditions, including asthma, cancer, and chronic obstructive pulmonary disease.[21]

In addition to annual epidemics of respiratory viruses, it is important to be vigilant for new and emerging viruses that can lead to severe illness including pneumonia, hospitalization, and death. Recent examples include Severe Acute Respiratory Syndrome Coronavirus (SARS-CoV)[45] and Middle-East Respiratory Syndrome Coronavirus (MERS-CoV).[46] SARS-CoV was first recognized in China in 2002 and caused a worldwide outbreak with 8098 probable cases and 774 deaths from 2002 to 2003; however, no cases have been reported since 2004. MERS-CoV was first reported in 2012 in Saudi Arabia and has since caused outbreaks in multiple countries in the region. Most MERS cases have been in older men and those with chronic medical conditions, but all ages have been affected, including those in contact with a person who had MERS, especially health care workers.[47]

Avian influenza viruses are circulating in birds, both wild and domesticated, throughout the world. Although many viruses are considered low pathogenic avian influenza A viruses, there are highly pathogenic virus strains as well that have been detected in humans. Illness can range from mild to severe, including pneumonia, and cases are often sporadic and after contact with infected birds or their fluids; closing of live bird markets has been shown to reduce transmission. From 2003 to 2016, there have been 854 infections of avian influenza A (H5N1) virus reported to WHO, among which there were 450 (53%) deaths.[48] Human infections with avian influenza A (H7N9) virus were first reported in China in 2013.[49] Since then, there have been 798 laboratory-confirmed infections in China; most infections are sporadic with a few clusters of infection. There is no evidence of sustained human-to-human transmission.[50] Since 2014, there have also been outbreaks in North America and elsewhere among wild and domesticated birds with influenza A (H5Nx and H7N8), which are considered highly pathogenic viruses in birds, but thus far, there have not been any human cases (http://www.oie.int/en/animal-health-in-the-world/update-on-avian-influenza/2016/).

GAPS IN KNOWLEDGE ABOUT THE EPIDEMIOLOGY OF RESPIRATORY VIRUS–ASSOCIATED PNEUMONIA

Although active and systematic surveillance for all respiratory viruses has increased globally and is strongest for influenza viruses, it is still lacking throughout much of the world.[51] Many questions remain about the seasonality of influenza and other respiratory viruses in tropical countries where there is increasing evidence of year-round circulation of influenza in warmer, more humid climates.[29–31,52] Country-specific studies to better understand the contribution of viruses to pneumonia are still required, especially from low- and middle-income countries. The PERCH project will further the understanding of pneumonia in children less than 5 years old,[14] but data on older adults and pneumonia remain scant.

Country-specific data on pneumonia, from high, low, and middle income are continually needed because the prevalence of respiratory viruses varies due to seasonal and geographic differences. Incidence also varies, including by age but also due to socioeconomic and sociocultural factors. In addition, access to prevention and control methods that may be in place in some but not all countries (ie, vaccination coverage for *S pneumoniae* or *Haemophilus influenzae*, antibiotics, or antivirals) can affect the epidemiology of viral pneumonia. Risk factors for pneumonia, such as malnutrition, air pollution, tuberculosis, or coexisting malarial infection, may be more relevant in low- and middle-income countries than in more developed countries, where underlying conditions or tobacco exposure may be more prevalent among patients with pneumonia.[34,35]

In addition, most pneumonia studies have been performed in hospital settings. However, in many parts of the world, including developed and developing nations, viral pneumonia does not always result in hospitalization; deaths are missed because they occur at home.[53] Thus, more studies conducted in the community and also outpatient settings are needed to more fully understand the burden and epidemiology of respiratory viral pneumonia.

SUMMARY

The burden of pneumonia, including that due to respiratory viruses, is markedly higher in the very young (<5 years) and older adults (≥50 years). Viruses are commonly detected, and clinically, it is difficult to distinguish between viral and bacterial pneumonia for most patients at presentation. Further development of new rapid diagnostic tests that can accurately distinguish among potential pathogens is urgently needed to better inform clinical care and public health practice.[54] Treatment and vaccination are only currently available for influenza despite the high burden of RSV, HMPV, and other viruses. Development of effective vaccines and treatments for these viruses of importance could reduce the burden of pneumonia and their complications in both children and adults around the world.

REFERENCES

1. Liu L, Oza S, Hogan D, et al. Global, regional, and national causes of child mortality in 2000–13, with projections to inform post-2015 priorities: an updated systematic analysis. Lancet 2015;385:430–40.
2. Pfunter A, Wier LM, Steiner C. Costs for hospital stays in the United States, 2011 (Statistical Brief No. 168). Rockville (MD): Agency for Healthcare Research and Quality, Healthcare Cost and Utilization Project; 2013.
3. Jain S, Self WH, Wunderink R, et al. Community-acquired pneumonia requiring hospitalization among U.S. adults. N Engl J Med 2015;373:415–27.
4. Jennings LC, Anderson TP, Beynon KA, et al. Incidence and characteristics of viral community-acquired pneumonia in adults. Thorax 2008;63:42–8.
5. Johnstone J, Majumdar SR, Fox JD, et al. Viral infection in adults hospitalized with community-acquired pneumonia: prevalence, pathogens, and presentation. Chest 2008;134:1141–8.
6. Charles PGP, Whitby M, Fuller AJ, et al. The etiology of community-acquired pneumonia in Australia: why penicillin plus doxycycline or a macrolide is the most appropriate therapy. Clin Infect Dis 2008;46:1513–21.
7. Jain S, Williams DJ, Arnold SR, et al. Community-acquired pneumonia requiring hospitalization among U.S. children. N Engl J Med 2015;372:835–45.
8. Self WH, Williams DJ, Zhu Y, et al. Respiratory viral detection in children and adults: comparing asymptomatic controls and patients with community-acquired pneumonia. J Infect Dis 2016;213:584–91.
9. Lee GE, Lorch SA, Sheffler-Collins S, et al. National hospitalization trends for pediatric pneumonia and associated complications. Pediatrics 2010;126:204–13.
10. Marston BJ, Plouffe JF, File TM, et al. Incidence of community-acquired pneumonia requiring hospitalization. Arch Intern Med 1997;157:1709–18.
11. Griffin MR, Zhu Y, Moore MR, et al. U.S. hospitalization for pneumonia after a decade of pneumococcal vaccination. N Engl J Med 2013;369:155–63.
12. Nair H, Nokes DJ, Gessner BD, et al. Global burden of acute lower respiratory infections due to respiratory syncytial virus in young children: a systematic review and meta-analysis. Lancet 2010;375:1545–55.
13. World Health Organization. Influenza (Seasonal) Fact Sheet Number 211. 2014. Available at: http://www.who.int/mediacentre/factsheets/fs211/en/. Accessed September 19, 2016.
14. Hammitt LL, Kazungu S, Morpeth SC, et al. A preliminary study of pneumonia etiology among hospitalized children in Kenya. Clin Infect Dis 2012;54(S2):S190–9.
15. Berkley JA, Munywoki P, Ngama M, et al. Viral etiology of severe pneumonia among Kenyan infants and children. JAMA 2010;303:2051–7.
16. O'Callaghan-Gordo C, Bassat Q, Morais L, et al. Etiology and epidemiology of viral pneumonia among hospitalized children in rural Mozambique: a malaria endemic area with high prevalence of human immunodeficiency virus. Pediatr Infect Dis J 2011;30:39–44.
17. García- García ML, Calvo C, Pozo F, et al. Spectrum of respiratory viruses in children with community-acquired pneumonia. Pediatr Infect Dis J 2012;31:808–13.
18. Pavia AT. Viral infections of the lower respiratory tract: old viruses, new viruses, and the role of diagnosis. Clin Infect Dis 2011;52(Suppl 4):S284–9.
19. Michelow IC, Olsen K, Lozano J, et al. Epidemiology and clinical characteristics of community-acquired pneumonia in hospitalized children. Pediatrics 2004;113:701–7.
20. Falsey AR, Hennessey PA, Formica MA, et al. Respiratory syncytial virus infection in elderly and high-risk adults. N Engl J Med 2005;352:1749–59.
21. Walsh EE, Peterson DR, Falsey AR. Human metapneumovirus infections in adults: another piece of the puzzle. Arch Intern Med 2008;168:2489–96.
22. Fry AM, Lu X, Olsen SJ, et al. Human rhinovirus infections in rural Thailand: epidemiological evidence for rhinovirus as both pathogen and bystander. PLoS One 2011;6(3):e17780.
23. Karhu J, Ala-Kokko TI, Vuorinen T, et al. Lower respiratory tract virus findings in mechanically ventilated patients with severe community-acquired pneumonia. Clin Infect Dis 2014;59:62–70.
24. Ruuskanen O, Järvinen A. What is the real role of respiratory viruses in severe community-acquired pneumonia? Clin Infect Dis 2014;59:71–3.
25. Brundage JF. Interactions between influenza and bacterial respiratory pathogens: implications for pandemic preparedness. Lancet Infect Dis 2006;6:303–12.
26. Johansson N, Kalin M, Tivelhung-Lin-dell A, et al. Etiology of community-acquired pneumonia: increased microbiological yield with new diagnostic methods. Clin Infect Dis 2010;50:202–9.
27. Lieberman D, Shimoni A, Shemer-Avni Y, et al. Respiratory viruses in adults with community-acquired pneumonia. Chest 2010;138:811–6.
28. Templeton KE, Scheltinga SA, van den Beden WC, et al. Improved diagnosis of the etiology of community-acquired pneumonia with real-time polymerase chain reaction. Clin Infect Dis 2005;41:345–51.
29. Haynes AK, Manangan AP, Iwane MK, et al. RSV Circulation in 7 countries with GDD regional centers. J Infect Dis 2013;208(S3):S246–54.

30. Saha S, Chadha M, Al Mamun A, et al. Influenza seasonality and vaccination timing in tropical and subtropical areas of southern and south-eastern Asia. Bull World Health Organ 2014;92:318–30.

31. Chadha MS, Potdar VA, Saha S, et al. Dynamics of influenza seasonality at sub-regional levels in India and implications for vaccination timing. PLoS One 2015;10:e0124122.

32. Deloria-Knoll M, Feikin DR, Scott AG, et al. Identification and selection of cases and controls in the pneumonia etiology research for child health project. Clin Infect Dis 2012;54(S2):S117–23.

33. Singleton RJ, Bulkow LR, Miernyk K, et al. Viral respiratory infections in hospitalized and community control children in Alaska. J Med Virol 2010;82:1282–90.

34. Mandell LA, Wunderink RG, Anzueto A, et al. Infectious Diseases Society of America/American Thoracic Society consensus guidelines on the management of community-acquired pneumonia in adults. Clin Infect Dis 2007;44:S27–72.

35. Bradley JS, Byington CL, Shah SS, et al. The management of community-acquired pneumonia in infants and children older than 3 months of age: clinical practice guidelines by the Pediatric Infectious Diseases Society and the Infectious Diseases Society of America. Clin Infect Dis 2011;53(7):e25–76.

36. Louria DB, Blumenfield HL, Ellis JT, et al. Studies on influenza in the pandemic of 1957-1958. II. Pulmonary complications of influenza. J Clin Invest 1959;38:213–65.

37. Schwarzmann SW, Adler JL, Sullivan RJ, et al. Arch Intern Med 1971;127:1037–41.

38. Perez-Padilla R, de la Rosa-Zamboni D, Ponce de Leon S, et al. Pneumonia and respiratory failure from swine-origin influenza A (H1N1) in Mexico. N Engl J Med 2009;361:680–9.

39. Reyes S, Montull B, Martinez R, et al. Risk factors of A/H1N1 etiology in pneumonia and its impact on mortality. Respir Med 2011;105:1404–11.

40. Jain S, Benoit SR, Skarbinski J, et al. Influenza-associated pneumonia among hospitalized patients with 2009 pandemic influenza A (H1N1) virus—United States, 2009. Clin Infect Dis 2012;54(9):1221–9.

41. Hall CB, Weinberg GA, Iwane MK, et al. The burden of RSV infection in young children. N Engl J Med 2009;360:588–98.

42. Moyes J, Cohen C, Pretorius M, et al. Epidemiology of RSV-associated ALRTI hospitalizations among HIV-infected and HIV-uninfected south African children, 2010-2011. J Infect Dis 2013;208(S3):S217–26.

43. Dowell SF, Anderson LJ, Gary HE Jr, et al. RSV is an important cause of community-acquired lower respiratory infection among hospitalized adults. J Infect Dis 1996;176:456–62.

44. Edwards KM, Zhu Y, Griffin MR, et al. Burden of human metapneumovirus infection in young children. N Engl J Med 2013;368:633–43.

45. Lee N, Hui D, Wu A, et al. A major outbreak of a severe acute respiratory syndrome in Hong Kong. N Engl J Med 2003;348:1986–94.

46. Zaki AM, van Boheemen S, Bestebroer TM, et al. Isolation of a novel coronavirus from a man with pneumonia in Saudi Arabia. N Engl J Med 2012;367:1814–20.

47. Assiri A, McGeer A, Perl TM, et al. Hospital outbreak of Middle East respiratory syndrome coronavirus. N Engl J Med 2013;369(5):407–16.

48. World Health Organization. Cumulative number of confirmed human cases for avian influenza A(H5N1) reported to WHO. 2003–2016. Available at: http://www.who.int/influenza/human_animal_interface/2016_07_19_tableH5N1.pdf?ua=1. Accessed September 21, 2016.

49. Gao H, Lu HZ, Cao B, et al. Clinical findings in 111 cases of influenza A(H7N9) virus infection. N Engl J Med 2013;368:2277–85.

50. World Health Organization. Human infection with avian influenza A(H7N9) virus—China. Available at: http://www.who.int/csr/don/17-august-2016-ah7n9-china/en/. Accessed September 21, 2016.

51. Polansky LS, Outin-Blenman S, Moen AC. Improved global capacity for influenza surveillance. Emerg Infect Dis 2016;22:993–1001.

52. Hirve S, Newman LP, Paget J, et al. Influenza seasonality in the tropics and subtropics—when to vaccinate? PLoS One 2016;11(4):e0153003.

53. Nasreen S, Luby SP, Brooks WA, et al. Population-based incidence of severe acute respiratory virus infections among children aged <5 years in rural Bangladesh, June-October 2010. PLoS One 2014;9(2):e89978.

54. Caliendo AM, Gilbert DN, Ginocchio CG, et al. Better tests, better care: improved diagnostics for infectious diseases. Clin Infect Dis 2013;59:S139–70.

The Virome of the Human Respiratory Tract

Kristine M. Wylie, PhD

KEYWORDS

- Virus • Infection • Lung • Culture independent • Chronic lung disease • Diagnostics
- High-throughput sequencing

KEY POINTS

- Culture-independent molecular assays detect viral pathogens with great sensitivity and can be used to define the virome in the upper and lower respiratory tract.
- The respiratory tract virome is defined by very common pathogens (rhinoviruses, paramyxoviruses) as well as viruses that occur less frequently and those with unknown pathogenicity.
- Viruses with the potential for pathogenicity are detected in both symptomatic and asymptomatic people.
- Monitoring emerging respiratory pathogens is important, and high-throughput sequencing can be used as a tool to complement epidemiologic studies and to design diagnostics.
- In the future, comprehensive pathogen detection and host response may be coupled to create better assays for research studies and diagnostics.

INTRODUCTION

Viral infections of the respiratory tract are very common. In a recent study of 26 households in Utah that were followed weekly over 1 year, modern molecular methods were used to detect respiratory viruses in the anterior nares.[1] This study found that children less than 5 years old had about 12 viral episodes in the respiratory tract each year, whereas adults averaged about 6 per year. These numbers are higher than previous studies,[2] which is likely explained by the use of molecular assays instead of culture- and serology-based tests and the discovery of new respiratory viruses in intervening years that would not have been assessed in older studies.

Modern molecular methods for virus detection are highly sensitive and specific. Polymerase chain reaction (PCR) assays are also rapid and generally inexpensive. High-throughput nucleic acid sequencing (HTS) methods are slower but have the potential to be more comprehensive because there is no need to select specific targets beforehand, and the method can detect genomes with substantial sequence variation compared with known reference genomes (**Fig. 1**). With these tools in hand, we can begin to think about characterizing the virome of the respiratory tract, herein defined as all of the viruses in the respiratory tract that can infect and replicate in human cells, which includes known pathogens and viruses with unknown pathogenicity. We have begun to learn about the virome of the respiratory tract through studies of patients with acute infections, chronic lung diseases, and undergoing lung transplantation, among others. The author reviews some of these studies in addition to recent technological developments, which will improve characterization of the respiratory virome and diagnostics in coming years.

Disclosure: The author has nothing to disclose.
Department of Pediatrics, McDonnell Genome Institute, Washington University School of Medicine, Campus Box 8208, 660 South Euclid Avenue, St Louis, MO 63110, USA
E-mail address: kwylie@wustl.edu

Clin Chest Med 38 (2017) 11–19
http://dx.doi.org/10.1016/j.ccm.2016.11.001
0272-5231/17/© 2016 Elsevier Inc. All rights reserved.

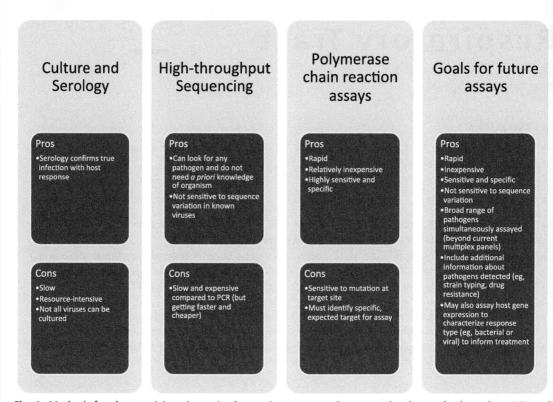

Fig. 1. Methods for characterizing viruses in the respiratory tract. Current molecular methods, such as PCR and HTS, have clear advantages over older methods (culture and serology) in terms of cost, speed, and sensitivity. Future assays for research and diagnostics will be aimed at capturing and improving on the best features of the current methods.

OVERVIEW OF THE VIROME IN THE RESPIRATORY TRACT

Defining the virome in the respiratory tract and understanding the implications of the viruses detected are significant challenges. The work is complicated by several factors. First, the lower airway is not easily accessible and sometimes requires invasive sampling. For instance, bronchoalveolar lavage samples are often only available from symptomatic individuals who are having lavage performed for diagnostic testing and not from asymptomatic controls. Second, a study of the viruses in the lungs of patients with cystic fibrosis (CF) showed that the viral populations were distinct in different regions of the lung.[3] This variation within the respiratory tract and lung means it can be difficult to get a clear, or complete, view of the virome. Third, only recently have relatively unbiased approaches to identifying viruses become available in the form of HTS assays. With that said, a great deal of progress has been made in defining the human virome in the respiratory tract (summarized in **Table 1**).

The Virome in Patients with Respiratory Tract Infections and Controls

One cost-effective approach to broadly identify viruses associated with the respiratory tract is to pool samples and screen for a comprehensive set of viruses. The downside to this approach is that one cannot determine the frequency at which any individual virus occurs among patients. However, as characterization of the respiratory tract virome using molecular methods is a relatively new area of exploration, these studies can be useful in order to determine if viruses beyond the common, known respiratory pathogens are detected.

In one study, 210 adults and children with severe lower respiratory tract infections were sampled.[4] Nasopharyngeal aspirates were collected and samples were combined, creating 13 pools of 8 to 24 samples per pool. Virus particles were enriched, and DNA and RNA viruses were assessed using HTS. Thirty-nine viral species were observed in these samples, giving a broad view of the scope of the respiratory tract virome during infection. Based on read counts, the most abundant viruses in the data set were the paramyxoviruses

Table 1
Common viruses detected in the respiratory tract virome

Virus Groups	Species or Types	References from this Review
Picornaviruses	Rhinoviruses A, B, and/or C	Lysholm et al,[4] 2012; Wang et al,[5] 2016; Jain et al,[6] 2015; Jain et al,[7] 2015; Colvin et al,[8] 2012; Wylie et al,[9] 2012; Flight et al,[13] 2014; Goffard et al,[14] 2014; Wat et al,[15] 2008; Graf et al,[24] 2016; Thorburn et al,[25] 2015; Zoll et al,[26] 2015
	Enteroviruses	Colvin et al,[8] 2012; Wylie et al,[9] 2012; Wylie et al,[22] 2015; Wylie et al,[23] 2015; Graf et al,[24] 2016; Thorburn et al,[25] 2015; Zoll et al,[26] 2015
	Parechovirus	Wylie et al,[9] 2012
Paramyxoviruses	Respiratory syncytial virus	Lysholm et al,[4] 2012; Wang et al,[5] 2016; Jain et al,[6] 2015; Jain et al,[7] 2015; Flight et al,[13] 2014; Wat et al,[15] 2008; Graf et al,[24] 2016; Thorburn et al,[25] 2015; Zoll et al,[26] 2015
	Parainfluenzaviruses 1–4	Lysholm et al,[4] 2012; Wang et al,[5] 2016; Jain et al,[6] 2015; Jain et al,[7] 2015; Colvin et al,[8] 2012; Wylie et al,[9] 2012; Flight et al,[13] 2014; Goffard et al,[14] 2014; Wat et al,[15] 2008; Graf et al,[24] 2016; Thorburn et al,[25] 2015
	Metapneumovirus	Lysholm et al,[4] 2012; Wang et al,[5] 2016; Jain et al,[6] 2015; Jain et al,[7] 2015; Colvin et al,[8] 2012; Graf et al,[24] 2016; Thorburn et al,[25] 2015; Zoll et al,[26] 2015
	Measles virus	Lysholm et al,[4] 2012; Wang et al,[5] 2016; Wylie et al,[9] 2012; Flight et al,[13] 2014; Graf et al,[24] 2016
	Pneumovirus	Wylie et al,[9] 2012
Orthomyxoviruses	Influenzavirus A, B, and/or C	Lysholm et al,[4] 2012; Wang et al,[5] 2016; Jain et al,[6] 2015; Jain et al,[7] 2015; Colvin et al,[8] 2012; Wylie et al,[9] 2012; Flight et al,[13] 2014; Goffard et al,[14] 2014; Wat et al,[15] 2008; Graf et al,[24] 2016; Thorburn et al,[25] 2015
Coronaviruses	HKU1, OC43, 229E, and/or NL63	Lysholm et al,[4] 2012; Wang et al,[5] 2016; Jain et al,[6] 2015; Jain et al,[7] 2015; Colvin et al,[8] 2012; Wylie et al,[9] 2012; Goffard et al,[14] 2014; Wat et al,[15] 2008; Graf et al,[24] 2016; Thorburn et al,[25] 2015
Adenoviruses	Adenovirus C or untyped	Lysholm et al,[4] 2012; Wang et al,[5] 2016; Jain et al,[6] 2015; Jain et al,[7] 2015; Colvin et al,[8] 2012; Wylie et al,[9] 2012; Flight et al,[13] 2014; Graf et al,[24] 2016; Thorburn et al,[25] 2015
Parvoviruses	Bocavirus or unclassified	Lysholm et al,[4] 2012; Wang et al,[5] 2016; Colvin et al,[8] 2012; Wylie et al,[9] 2012; Willner et al,[16] 2009; Young et al,[17] 2015; Graf et al,[24] 2016; Zoll et al,[26] 2015
Herpesviruses	Cytomegalovirus, Epstein-Barr virus, Roseolovirus, and/or Kaposi sarcomavirus	Wang et al,[5] 2016; Wylie et al,[9] 2012; Willner et al,[16] 2009; Young et al,[17] 2015; Graf et al,[24] 2016
Anelloviruses	Torque teno virus, torque teno midi virus, and/or torque teno mini virus or untyped	Lysholm et al,[4] 2012; Wang et al,[5] 2016; Wylie et al,[9] 2012
Papillomaviruses	Various	Wang et al,[5] 2016; Willner et al,[16] 2009; Young et al,[17] 2015
Polyomaviruses	KI and/or WU	Lysholm et al,[4] 2012; Colvin et al,[8] 2012; Wylie et al,[9] 2012

(including human respiratory syncytial virus, human metapneumovirus). Picornaviruses were the next most abundant (primarily rhinoviruses A and C). Orthomyxoviruses were the third most abundant (influenza viruses A, B, and C). There were several rare and/or unexpected viruses represented at low abundance. These viruses included bocavirus, KI polyomavirus, picobirnavirus, measles virus, and anelloviruses. In a study from China, a similar sequencing-based approach was taken to characterize the virome in children less than 6 years old with severe acute respiratory illness and 15 controls without respiratory illness.[5] Nasopharyngeal swabs were pooled into 9 pools of 15 samples each; virus particles were enriched; and HTS data were generated to assess both RNA and DNA viruses. The most highly represented viruses included the paramyxoviruses (primarily human respiratory syncytial virus), and the other common viruses detected in the study described earlier were detected. This study also detected human coronaviruses, bocaviruses, picornaviruses, influenza viruses, adenoviruses, and anelloviruses. Rare sequences included those from metapneumovirus, measles, hepatitis B and C, papillomavirus, and others. These two studies demonstrate the power of HTS compared with targeted PCR assays for defining the virome. In both studies, common and expected respiratory pathogens were detected. However, other viruses, some with unknown pathogenicity in the respiratory tract, were also detected. Detection of these viruses is valuable as we aim to fully understand the biology of the respiratory tract. Although these studies were exploratory, they raise questions about whether some of the viruses with unclear pathogenicity could be contributing to the presentation of symptoms, complicating the course of infection with other pathogens, or are biomarkers for infection or host response. These questions remain to be addressed in future studies.

The Virome in Children and Adults with Pneumonia

Viruses are clearly an important cause of pneumonia, particularly in the postpneumococcal vaccine era. A prospective multicenter study sponsored by the Centers for Disease Control and Prevention focused on the Etiology of Pneumonia in the Community (EPIC).[6,7] This study used extensive diagnostic testing (culture, serology, molecular testing) to understand the causes of pneumonia in more than 2000 adults in the United States, in the time after the implementation of the pneumococcal vaccine. In this study, a pathogen was detected in 38% of the samples. At least 1 virus was detected in 23% of the samples available for testing, and 3% had both bacterial and viral pathogens detected. Rhinoviruses and influenza viruses were the most common pathogens detected in 9% and 6% of patients, respectively. The EPIC study took a similar approach to study the cause of community-acquired pneumonia in children. Again, more than 2000 subjects were enrolled. The children were less than 18 years old, with a median age of 2 years. A microbial pathogen was detected in 81% of samples. At least one virus was detected in 66% of the samples, and both bacterial and viral pathogens were detected in 7% of the children. In children, respiratory syncytial virus, rhinovirus, metapneumovirus, and adenovirus were the most common pathogens. These studies identify viruses as key pathogens in pneumonia since the implementation of the pneumococcal vaccine. Furthermore, it is important to note that no pathogen was detected in 62% of adults and 19% of children, suggesting the possibility that pneumonia was caused by viruses not included in the set of targeted assays used in this study. Identification of the etiologic agent of pneumonia may benefit from unbiased HTS assays to detect unexpected or rare pathogens that are not be included in standard clinical testing.

The Virome in Children with Unexplained Fever and Asymptomatic Controls

In a study of children with unexplained fever, both targeted PCR assays[8] and HTS[9] were used to characterize the respiratory tract virome in individual samples from subjects. Children with fever were compared with afebrile children who were in the hospital for same-day surgery. Nasopharyngeal swabs from 75 febrile children and 116 afebrile children were tested with a panel of PCR assays that targeted common respiratory pathogens and viruses of interest, including influenza A, parainfluenza virus, metapneumovirus, rhinovirus, enterovirus, coronavirus, adenovirus, bocavirus, and the recently discovered KI and WU polyomaviruses. HTS was performed on 50 samples from febrile children and 81 samples from afebrile controls. Using sequencing, 17 viral genera were detected overall. These genera included viruses listed earlier; cytomegalovirus, parechovirus and others were detected in febrile children, whereas *Roseolovirus* was detected in nasopharyngeal swabs from both febrile and afebrile children. Although febrile children were more likely to have a virus present in the sample compared with controls, afebrile children still carried viruses asymptomatically. Rhinoviruses/enteroviruses and anelloviruses were particularly common in asymptomatic children in this study. However, anelloviruses, particularly torque teno virus, were associated with fever.[10] This study demonstrates 2 points very well. First, even with a panel of respiratory virus PCR assays that extends far beyond targets that would be used for clinical testing, additional viruses were detected in the respiratory tract only by sequencing. This finding emphasizes the potential to improve viral diagnostic testing by broadening the set of viruses evaluated. Second, viruses are commonly found in the respiratory tracts of asymptomatic children and many of these viruses have potential to cause symptomatic infection. This point means that pathogen detection may not always be enough to make a clear diagnosis. Other information may be needed, as discussed in more detail later in this review.

The Respiratory Tract Virome in Patients with Cystic Fibrosis

Although many viral infections are mild or resolve without complication in generally healthy individuals, viruses in the respiratory tract are associated with exacerbations of chronic lung diseases, including CF, chronic obstructive pulmonary disease, and asthma (reviewed in the following[11,12]). Exploration of the virome in the respiratory tracts of patients with chronic lung diseases has emphasized the prevalence of common pathogens and also further defines the scope of the respiratory tract virome.

To illustrate this point, the author discusses a few studies of the virome in patients with CF. Molecular methods of detection, specifically PCR assays, have increased the association of viral infection with pulmonary exacerbation. Incidence of viral infections in adult patients with CF was estimated at 1 to 2 viral infections per year based on a study of 100 patients who were sampled every 2 months for a year and on exacerbation.[13] Samples from the respiratory tract (sputum, nose and throat swabs) were tested using PCR assays for common respiratory pathogens, including respiratory syncytial virus, rhinovirus, influenza virus, and others. Rhinovirus and metapneumovirus were the most commonly detected viruses, accounting for 72.5% and 13.2% of virus-positive samples, respectively. Viral infection was associated with pulmonary exacerbation, with virus detected in 40% of exacerbation samples compared with 24% of samples collected on regular visits. In another study, sputum was collected from 46 adult patients and viruses were screened using PCR assays.[14] In this study, rhinoviruses and coronaviruses were the most common viruses, and

rhinoviruses were associated with exacerbation. In children with CF, exacerbation has also been associated with viral infection. In a study of 71 patients, viruses were assessed in nasal swabs using a panel of targeted PCR assays for common respiratory pathogens.[15] Viruses were detected in 46% of samples collected during exacerbation but only 17% of samples collected when asymptomatic. Influenza A, influenza B, and rhinovirus were all associated with exacerbation.

The virome of patients with CF has also been characterized using HTS. One study aimed to study the virome in sputum from 5 patients with CF and 5 healthy controls.[16] Virus particles were enriched, and DNA viruses were sequenced. This study was particularly interesting because the use of HTS instead of targeted PCR assays resulted in the detection of viruses that would not have been included in typical PCR panels evaluating respiratory viruses. In the patients with CF, reticuloendotheliosis virus, Epstein-Barr virus, human herpesvirus 6B, and human herpesvirus 8 were detected. In control patients, human papillomaviruses were detected in 2 samples. Several single-stranded DNA viruses were also detected in patients and/or controls, including geminiviruses and circoviruses. In a second study, the virome was assessed in explanted lungs from patients with CF undergoing lung transplant and lungs obtained post mortem.[3] Anelloviruses, papillomaviruses, and herpesviruses were detected; viruses were detected in distinct regions of the lung rather than diffusely throughout. These studies were valuable because many of the viruses detected were not those that would have been included in PCR screens for common respiratory pathogens, yet they may impact disease progression in the lung by creating or promoting inflammation in the respiratory tract.

The Respiratory Tract Virome after Lung Transplantation

In one study, the virome was studied in bronchoalveolar lavage and oral washes from lung transplant patients within the first year of transplant, human immunodeficiency virus (HIV) positive subjects without respiratory symptoms, and healthy volunteers.[17] Anelloviruses, papillomaviruses, and herpesviruses were detected. The striking observation in this study was that the diversity and abundance of anelloviruses was highly increased in the transplant patients compared with patients with HIV and healthy controls. This finding was true in both the lower airway lavage samples and the upper airway oral washes. Although anelloviruses are not known to be pathogenic, they seem to be a marker of immunosuppression.[18] The effects of their dysregulation on engraftment or outcome, if any, are not known at this time.

Emerging Respiratory Viruses

Since the discovery of severe acute respiratory syndrome coronavirus in 2003,[19] other novel respiratory pathogens have emerged, including coronaviruses NL63, HKU1, and MERS (reviewed in[20]) and influenza viruses H1N1 pandemic strain and H7N9.[21] In each case, the molecular tools to adequately survey the spread of the virus had to be developed. Once assays become available, the transmission of these viruses can be tracked and recommendations for protecting public health can be made. HTS assays can be useful to survey outbreaks of emerging viruses. A recent example of this occurred in the fall of 2014, when the United States experienced a widespread outbreak of enterovirus D68 in 49 states and the District of Columbia. This virus had previously been observed rarely. In multiplex PCR panels, the virus was either undetected or broadly typed only as an enterovirus/rhinovirus, which limited the study of the outbreak. Typing of the virus initially involved a labor-intensive and slow method in which an amplicon was generated and sequenced, and the sequence was compared with reference strains for typing. The genomes of the outbreak strains were sequenced[22](and also by the Centers for Disease Control and Prevention), and subsequently a highly specific molecular assay was developed in order to aid in detection and typing of the outbreak strain.[23] In this case, sequencing provided specific viral typing and allowed for genomic characterization and design of a specific laboratory developed test. This model could be useful for future outbreaks.

HIGH-THROUGHPUT SEQUENCING IN THE CLINIC
Sequencing Assays Compared with Standard Clinical Tests

The workhorses for clinical testing of respiratory viruses are multiplex PCR panels that target the most common respiratory viruses. These assays are highly sensitive and yield rapid results. However, PCR-based assays can have limitations. In most multiplex panels, the assays cannot be used to subtype viruses, identify drug-resistant alleles, or identify viruses not targeted by the panel. Evolving viruses may also mutate in the region targeted by the PCR primers and be missed by the assay. For these reasons, HTS-based assays could have a role in the clinic.

Recently, several groups have compared the results from HTS with standard clinical assays for detection of viruses in the respiratory tract. One study found that RNA sequencing and the GenMark eSensor Respiratory Virus Panel (RVP) had an 86% correlation rate on one set of 42 known positive nasopharyngeal swab samples and 93% correlation on a second set of 67 samples.[24] High-throughput RNA sequencing detected 12 viruses that were either not included in the RVP panel or whose sequence was divergent from the RVP target and, thus, not detected. Furthermore, viral subtypes were determined for influenza A (as well as identification of the oseltamivir resistance mutation), respiratory syncytial viruses, and rhinoviruses. Another study tested 89 nasopharyngeal swabs from adults with upper respiratory tract infections using reverse transcription (RT)-PCR assays for a series of common viruses, including human rhinoviruses, coronaviruses, influenza viruses and others, and by RNA sequencing.[25] The HTS assay had a sensitivity of 77% compared with the PCR assays. The viruses that were not detected by HTS had higher cycle threshold (Ct) values in the real-time RT-PCR assays, indicating there were lower levels of viral nucleic acid present in those samples. Again, HTS had the advantage of providing additional subtyping information, in this case for human enteroviruses, rhinoviruses, metapneumovirus, and respiratory syncytial virus. A third study demonstrated that HTS could be used to detect a pathogen (rhinovirus C) in a sample from a child with respiratory symptoms in which no virus had been detected by PCR.[26] Taken together, these data show that in some cases HTS could be advantageous compared with PCR assays, but sensitivity of sequencing can be a limitation.

Improving Sensitivity of High-Throughput Nucleic Acid Sequencing for Virus Detection

The studies comparing clinical tests with HTS demonstrate that sequencing can add information to clinical assays in terms of typing viruses and detecting resistance mutations. Importantly, they illustrate that viruses not included in the PCR panels are sometimes present. In each case, despite the slightly different method used for sample collection and preparation and the different patient cohorts used, sensitivity for detection was an issue. Recently 2 groups developed an approach to enrich viral nucleic acids from a comprehensive set of viruses before sequencing.[27,28] This approach uses targeted sequence capture, a hybridization-based approach for selecting targets of interest. Probes or baits are made using target sequences, and these are hybridized to the nucleic acid in the sample of interest. The baits are then captured along with the sequences that hybridized to them and washed; the result is an enrichment of the target nucleic acids in the sequencing assays. These newly developed target-based enrichment strategies do not target specific viruses or viral families that are expected to be associated with a disease, but rather they include targets for all viruses that are known to infect vertebrates, allowing for a comprehensive screen of both expected and unexpected viruses in the same assay. This kind of approach greatly improves sequencing sensitivity, with the percentage of viral reads increasing from approximately 10 to approximately 10,000 fold using targeted sequence capture compared with standard HTS.[27,28] As a result, virus targeted sequence capture may be particularly useful in helping to diagnose infections where no virus has been detected by routine methods. Failures of routine tests occur because the virus has divergent sequence from the target in the PCR panel, the virus is an emerging infectious disease, or the virus is not one of the prominent causes of respiratory infection.

Host Response to Infection

Interestingly, sensitive molecular methods currently used for diagnostics and many research studies demonstrate that viruses can frequently be detected in asymptomatic individuals. In the Utah study of 26 households mentioned earlier, bocaviruses and rhinoviruses could frequently be detected in asymptomatic children and adults.[1] A Missouri study that used both PCR assays[8] and HTS[9] demonstrated that viral nucleic acid could be detected in nasopharyngeal swabs from asymptomatic children, in particular enteroviruses/rhinoviruses. It is necessary to appreciate that the detection of viral nucleic acid with molecular methods does not necessarily indicate the virus had infected the cell and/or was successfully replicating or that symptoms are necessarily resultant from the particular virus that was detected.

Additional information regarding the host response can be used to determine whether symptoms are caused by viral or bacterial pathogens (**Fig. 2**). Using a set of 30 samples from febrile children and 22 samples from afebrile controls, Hu and colleagues[29] demonstrated that there were distinct host gene expression patterns in the blood that distinguished viral and bacterial infections; furthermore, symptomatic and asymptomatic infections could be clearly delineated. Similarly, in 118 adults with lower respiratory tract infections and 40 healthy controls, host gene expression in the blood could distinguish viral and bacterial infections with 95% sensitivity and 92% specificity.[30] Bacterial-viral coinfections could also be distinguished. Tsalik and colleagues used publicly available microarray data to develop a host gene expression classifier that could distinguish bacterial, viral, and noninfectious illnesses with 87% accuracy.[31] Both the Suarez and colleagues[30] and Tsalik and colleagues studies showed that gene expression profiling performed better than procalcitonin. In the future, one might imagine that diagnostics may couple pathogen detection with host response to provide clinicians clear results that indicate whether there is a need

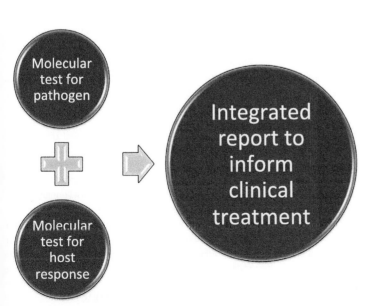

Fig. 2. Future diagnostics. In the future, respiratory tract infections may be diagnosed by merging pathogen detection (the current method for diagnostics) with host response measures that further define the cause of the symptoms (viral, bacterial, coinfections, not pathogenic). This merger will help clarify diagnoses and define appropriate treatment measures.

for antibiotics in each case. In fact, approaches that couple pathogen detection and host response are being put forth as highly effective diagnostic approach; software tools are being developed to rapidly provide reports that may in the very near future be used by clinicians for diagnostic purposes.[32]

SUMMARY

We are beginning to define the scope of the human respiratory tract virome. The prevalence of individual viruses vary from study to study (see **Table 1**), likely due to differences in seasonality of sample collection, variation in local virus circulation, and methodological choices (eg, sample type, sample preparation). The studies reviewed here demonstrate that HTS and expanded panels of PCR assays can identify rare viral pathogens that might not be included in multiplex diagnostic panels or PCR panels in which only the most common pathogens or viruses of interest are selected. The relatively unbiased sequencing approach can also reveal viruses that may not directly cause respiratory illness but whose presence may impact the trajectory of illness through mechanisms we do not yet understand. Methodological improvements to virus detection will help us better define the respiratory tract virome and monitor outbreaks. In the future, clinical tests may include both pathogen detection and an assessment of host response in order to more clearly distinguish viral and bacterial infections.

REFERENCES

1. Byington CL, Ampofo K, Stockmann C, et al. Community surveillance of respiratory viruses among families in the Utah better identification of germs-longitudinal viral epidemiology (BIG-LoVE) study. Clin Infect Dis 2015;61(8):1217–24.
2. Monto AS. Studies of the community and family: acute respiratory illness and infection. Epidemiol Rev 1994;16(2):351–73.
3. Willner D, Haynes MR, Furlan M, et al. Case studies of the spatial heterogeneity of DNA viruses in the cystic fibrosis lung. Am J Respir Cell Mol Biol 2012;46(2):127–31.
4. Lysholm F, Wetterbom A, Lindau C, et al. Characterization of the viral microbiome in patients with severe lower respiratory tract infections, using metagenomic sequencing. Highlander SK. PLoS One 2012;7(2):e30875.
5. Wang Y, Zhu N, Li Y, et al. Metagenomic analysis of viral genetic diversity in respiratory samples from children with severe acute respiratory infection in China. Clin Microbiol Infect 2016;22(5):458.e1-e9.
6. Jain S, Finelli L, CDC EPIC Study Team. Community-acquired pneumonia among U.S. children. N Engl J Med 2015;372(22):2167–8.
7. Jain S, Self WH, Wunderink RG, et al. Community-acquired pneumonia requiring hospitalization among U.S. adults. N Engl J Med 2015;373(5):415–27.
8. Colvin JM, Muenzer JT, Jaffe DM, et al. Detection of viruses in young children with fever without an apparent source. Pediatrics 2012;130(6):e1455–62.
9. Wylie KM, Mihindukulasuriya KA, Sodergren E, et al. Sequence analysis of the human virome in febrile and afebrile children. PLoS One 2012;7(6):e27735.
10. McElvania TeKippe E, Wylie KM, Deych E, et al. Increased prevalence of anellovirus in pediatric patients with fever. PLoS One 2012;7(11):e50937.
11. Hendricks MR, Bomberger JM. Digging through the obstruction: insight into the epithelial cell response to respiratory virus infection in patients with cystic fibrosis. J Virol 2016;90(9):4258–61.
12. Hewitt R, Farne H, Ritchie A, et al. The role of viral infections in exacerbations of chronic obstructive pulmonary disease and asthma. Ther Adv Respir Dis 2016;10(2):158–74.
13. Flight WG, Bright-Thomas RJ, Tilston P, et al. Incidence and clinical impact of respiratory viruses in adults with cystic fibrosis. Thorax 2014;69(3):247–53.
14. Goffard A, Lambert V, Salleron J, et al. Virus and cystic fibrosis: rhinoviruses are associated with exacerbations in adult patients. J Clin Virol 2014;60(2):147–53.
15. Wat D, Gelder C, Hibbitts S, et al. The role of respiratory viruses in cystic fibrosis. J Cyst Fibros 2008;7(4):320–8.
16. Willner D, Furlan M, Haynes M, et al. Metagenomic analysis of respiratory tract DNA viral communities in cystic fibrosis and non-cystic fibrosis individuals. PLoS One 2009;4(10):e7370.
17. Young JC, Chehoud C, Bittinger K, et al. Viral metagenomics reveal blooms of anelloviruses in the respiratory tract of lung transplant recipients. Am J Transplant 2015;15(1):200–9.
18. De Vlaminck I, Khush KK, Strehl C, et al. Temporal response of the human virome to immunosuppression and antiviral therapy. Cell 2013;155(5):1178–87.
19. Wang D, Urisman A, Liu Y-T, et al. Viral discovery and sequence recovery using DNA microarrays. PLoS Biol 2003;1(2):E2.
20. Berry M, Gamieldien J, Fielding BC. Identification of new respiratory viruses in the new millennium. Viruses 2015;7(3):996–1019.
21. Trombetta C, Piccirella S, Perini D, et al. Emerging influenza strains in the last two decades: a threat of a new pandemic? Vaccines (Basel) 2015;3(1):172–85.
22. Wylie KM, Wylie TN, Orvedahl A, et al. Genome sequence of enterovirus D68 from St Louis, Missouri, USA. Emerg Infect Dis 2015;21(1):184–6.

23. Wylie TN, Wylie KM, Buller RS, et al. Development and evaluation of an enterovirus D68 real-time reverse transcriptase PCR assay. J Clin Microbiol 2015;53(8):2641–7.

24. Graf EH, Simmon KE, Tardif KD, et al. Unbiased detection of respiratory viruses by use of RNA sequencing-based metagenomics: a systematic comparison to a commercial PCR panel. J Clin Microbiol 2016;54(4):1000–7.

25. Thorburn F, Bennett S, Modha S, et al. The use of next generation sequencing in the diagnosis and typing of respiratory infections. J Clin Virol 2015; 69:96–100.

26. Zoll J, Rahamat-Langendoen J, Ahout I, et al. Direct multiplexed whole genome sequencing of respiratory tract samples reveals full viral genomic information. J Clin Virol 2015;66:6–11.

27. Wylie TN, Wylie KM, Herter BN, et al. Enhanced virome sequencing using targeted sequence capture. Genome Res 2015;25(12):1910–20.

28. Briese T, Kapoor A, Mishra N, et al. Virome capture sequencing enables sensitive viral diagnosis and comprehensive virome analysis. MBio 2015;6(5): e01491–515.

29. Hu X, Yu J, Crosby SD, et al. Gene expression profiles in febrile children with defined viral and bacterial infection. Proc Natl Acad Sci USA 2013; 110(31):12792–7.

30. Suarez NM, Bunsow E, Falsey AR, et al. Superiority of transcriptional profiling over procalcitonin for distinguishing bacterial from viral lower respiratory tract infections in hospitalized adults. J Infect Dis 2015; 212(2):213–22.

31. Tsalik EL, Henao R, Nichols M, et al. Host gene expression classifiers diagnose acute respiratory illness etiology. Sci Transl Med 2016;8(322):322ra11.

32. Flygare S, Simmon K, Miller C, et al. Taxonomer: an interactive metagenomics analysis portal for universal pathogen detection and host mRNA expression profiling. Genome Biol 2016;17(1):111.

Diagnosing Viral and Atypical Pathogens in the Setting of Community-Acquired Pneumonia

Grant W. Waterer, MD, PhD[a,b,*]

KEYWORDS

- Pneumonia • Viral • Diagnostic • Point of care

KEY POINTS

- The concept of atypical pneumonia is outdated because clinically it is impossible to determine the pathogen.
- Nucleic acid detection is now the standard diagnostic method for all these pathogens, having replaced older serologic and antigen detection methods.
- Multiple pathogens are commonly detected in patients, particularly with *Legionella*, *Mycoplasma*, and *Chlamydia*.

INTRODUCTION

Despite many promises that molecular diagnostics would transform the management of infection, empiric therapy remains the standard of care in community-acquired pneumonia (CAP). Outside of etiologic studies, the vast majority of patients never have a pathogen diagnosed as the cause of their pneumonia. Although physicians are generally quite comfortable with empiric therapy, the need to guess and fear of missing an important pathogen inevitably leads to a broader than necessary spectrum of coverage, particularly in the setting of more severe illness.

That viruses are an important cause of pneumonia has been known since the identification of influenza in the early 1930s.[1] Despite an awareness that viruses can cause CAP, it is only recently that they have appeared as more than a footnote on the list of common pathogens. However, with modern generations of diagnostic panels, and particularly nucleic acid amplification tests, viral

pathogens are being identified increasingly as not only common causes of CAP, but possibly as being overall more common that bacteria.[2,3] With more sensitive tests has also come confirmation that patients with CAP frequently have multiple pathogens present, particularly the combination of bacterial and viral infection.

The term "atypical pneumonia" was coined in first half of the 20th century and used to describe pneumonia owing to pathogens that were not detectable by standard Gram staining or traditional culture methods and typically associated with headache, low-grade fever, cough, and malaise. The predominant pathogens that have become associated with atypical pneumonia are *Mycoplasma pneumoniae* (first identified in human lung in 1944),[4] *Legionella pneumophila* (first identified as a significant pneumonia pathogen in 1977 after the outbreak at a convention in Philadelphia in 1976)[5] and *Chlamydophila pneumoniae* (first identified in the respiratory tract

Disclosure Statement: The author has nothing to disclose.
[a] Univeristy of Western Australia, Level 4 MRF Building, Royal Perth Hospital, Wellington Street, Perth 6000, Australia; [b] Northwestern University, 420 East Superior Street, Chicago, IL 60611, USA
* Univeristy of Western Australia, Level 4 MRF Building, Royal Perth Hospital, Wellington Street, Perth 6000, Australia.
E-mail address: grant.waterer@uwa.edu.au

in 1984).[6] A variety of different species of these genera are now recognized as pneumonia pathogens.

This review covers the main approaches to the diagnosis of atypical and viral infections in the setting of pneumonia. The most common approach has been the use of pathogen-specific assays for use in urine, blood, or sputum. Although serologic tests based on detecting antibodies to specific pathogens were the predominant technique for decades, they all have limitations in early disease before an adaptive immune response being constituted as well as issues of cross-reactivity reducing specificity. Polymerase chain reaction (PCR)–based techniques are now the primary modality for the detection of atypical pathogens in most settings. More recently, there has been the development of multipathogen detection platforms that have become used increasingly in the setting of pneumonia.

CLINICAL DIAGNOSIS

Before moving to laboratory tests, it is worth briefly looking at the evidence of whether there are any specific clinical or radiological features in CAP that help to deduce reliably the pathogen. There are definitely clinical features that are seen more commonly in some of the atypical pathogens than with disease owing to *Streptococcus pneumoniae*. Examples include erythema multiforme with *M pneumoniae*, diarrhea with *L pneumophila*, and rhinorrhea with influenza. However, there is ample evidence that no set of clinical symptoms or signs has sufficient predictive ability to rule in or out any atypical or viral pathogens, especially *M pneumoniae*[7] and *Legionella*.[8–10]

A number of nonmicrobiological tests have also been proposed as being able to discriminate between "atypical" and "typical" pathogens, including the peripheral white cell count and procalcitonin. Although peripheral white cell counts do tend to be lower in viral infections compared with bacterial infections, this is not particularly discriminating at an individual patient level and certainly not accurate enough to use to determine empiric therapy.[11] Procalcitonin seems to be more accurate than white cell count,[11] but does not discriminate between atypical bacterial infection and viral infection[12] and may be misleading, particularly in critically ill patients or in patients with bacterial and viral coinfection.[13] A definitive diagnosis based on detecting the infection pathogen(s), therefore, remains critical if we are to improve the accuracy of empiric therapy.

PATHOGEN-SPECIFIC APPROACHES
Legionella

Very little has changed in the diagnosis of *Legionella* infection since we reviewed this topic comprehensively 15 years ago.[14] In most settings, *Legionella* is underdiagnosed and therefore underrecognized owing to routine testing not being performed.[15] *Legionella* infections seem to be increasing in the United States,[16,17] possibly owing to recent climate change, including a number of severe outbreaks with multiple fatalities,[18] which has led to increased interest in its diagnosis.

Because *Legionellae* will not grow on standard culture media, the diagnosis has traditionally rested on either positive serology or a positive urinary antigen test. Both of these tests have significant limitations. In the case of serology, 20% or more of patients with culture-proven *Legionella* infection do not ever seroconvert,[19,20] and seroconversion may take months, requiring testing out to at least 2 months if not longer.[21] Urinary antigen testing is quite specific, but will only reliably detection *L pneumophila* serogroup 1, and usually serogroup 6, but in many areas other species (particularly *Legionella longbeachae* and *Legionella micdadei*) are more predominant. Despite these limitations, urinary antigen testing for *Legionella* is recommended in all patients with severe CAP (ie, admitted to the intensive care unit) for both diagnostic and public health reasons.[22]

The mainstay of diagnosis of *Legionella* infection has been from one or more of direct antigen detection or nucleic acid detection in respiratory secretions. Direct fluorescent antigen detection was developed in the pre-PCR era but have now largely been replaced by PCR because the latter is more sensitive, less technician dependent, and easier to automate. PCR tests for *Legionella* are a mix of "home-grown" assays and commercially available products, with reported sensitivity and specificity (using all other tests as the gold standard) in the range of 91% to 99% and 94% to 99%, respectively.[23] Because PCR tests for *Legionella* are generally able to detect all species,[24] not surprisingly they have a greater degree of sensitivity than urinary antigen testing.[23,25] There is, however, a reasonable argument for performing both urinary antigen testing and PCR on respiratory secretions because there is an increased diagnostic yield from this approach.[26] It is worth noting that both nasopharyngeal aspirates[27–29] and throat swabs[15] have substantially lower yields for the detection of *Legionella* by PCR, but may be of use in patients in whom it is not possible to get spontaneous or induced sputum samples.

Mycoplasma

Traditionally, *Mycoplasma* infections have most often been diagnosed on the basis of serology; however, as with serologic tests for many pathogens, this has significant limitations early in disease when false-negative results are common. Difficulties in making the diagnosis as well as the marked season to season variation in its prevalence probably explain the enormous variation in the estimated proportion of cases of CAP owing to *M pneumoniae*, which range from less than 1% to greater than 50%.

PCR does overcome some of the limitations of serology for the diagnosis of *Mycoplasma* infection and the nuances of assay development and relative performance characteristics has been reviewed comprehensively elsewhere.[30] The performance characteristics for PCR assays for *M pneumoniae* seem to be at least as good as those for *Legionella* infections and possibly better.[31,32] As with other pathogens, the detection rate of *M pneumoniae* using PCR on nasopharyngeal aspirates is lower than in sputum samples.[28] Recently, there has been interest in antigen detection assays for the diagnosis of *M pneumoniae* because these offer the potential for point-of-care testing, but so far these have yet to enter the clinical mainstream.[33,34]

Chlamydophila

The nomenclature for the *Chlamydia* has changed recently with *Chlamydia* and *Chlamydophila* being combined back into a single genus.[35] Both *Chlamydia psittaci* and *C pneumoniae* are well-accepted as causes of CAP, although almost always being identified as much less common than either *Mycoplasma* or *Legionella* infections. A number of other *Chlamydophila*-like pathogens such as *Parachlamydia acanthamoebae* and *Simkania negevensis*) also been suggested as potential causes of the 50% or more of cases of CAP where no pathogen is identified.[36,37]

The specificity of positive serology for *C pneumoniae* has also been questioned, because studies using PCR-based diagnosis typically find much lower rates of infection than earlier serology-based studies and a large variety of assays with different performance characteristics have been used.[38] As with *Mycoplasma*, in early disease *Chlamydophila* serology is often negative making PCR a superior diagnostic test.[39]

Unlike *Legionella* and *Mycoplasma*, *Chlamydophila* cannot be detected by 16S-based PCR assays. Because culture of *Chlamydophila* is difficult and has a low yield, it is rarely done[40]; therefore, PCR assays that have been developed are

generally compared with serologic tests, with their known limitations as discussed. The true sensitivity of PCR for *Chlamydophila* species is, therefore, unknown. However the reported specificity of most assays is well over 95%[41] and, therefore, a positive result in the right clinical context should be acted on.

Influenza

All major etiologic studies of CAP have identified influenza as a significant cause of CAP, particularly in hospitalized patients. Since the recent H1N1 09 influenza pandemic, there is evidence that the use of empiric antiinfluenza therapy in the setting of CAP has increased significantly, with an unclear impact on outcome.[42] A fast and reliable diagnostic test for influenza is, therefore, attractive not only to prescribe antivirals appropriately (for treatment and prophylaxis), but also to aid in the allocation of respiratory isolation beds, which are often in limited supply, especially in influenza season. For this reason, the diagnostic tools available for influenza have significantly outpaced those for the other causes of atypical pneumonia.

In the United States, there are more than a dozen approved rapid influenza tests primarily based on the detection of influenza antigens in respiratory samples. Most available assays have been compared with a gold standard of real-time reverse transcription PCR in the same sample. The sensitivity of these assays varies between 10% and 75% depending on age, quality of the sample, and duration of symptoms. Complicating the assessment of the usefulness of these assays is that the performance seems to vary between influenza strains and, unfortunately, during the H1N1 09 pandemic they were less than optimal.[43–47] A recent metaanalysis of 159 published studies of rapid influenza tests found the pooled sensitivity, sensitivity, specificity, and positive and negative predictive values to be 62%, 98%, 34%, and 38%, respectively.[47]

Not surprisingly, given these data, there is little evidence that rapid influenza tests are currently used by clinicians to alter patient management.[48] However, this is a rapidly changing field and more recent publications suggest that there are incremental improvements with a range of sensitivity from 68% to 79% and specificity of 99% to 100%.[49–51] This is clearly an area where we can expect to see significant advances over the next few years.

In the absence of rapid diagnostic tests, existing commercial PCR assays for influenza have well-documented good performance characteristics for influenza A and B, and these data are well-reviewed elsewhere.[52] What is interesting from etiologic studies is the high degree of copathogen involvement with influenza, particularly the codetection of bacterial infection with S pneumoniae.[2,3] Whether this is genuine coinfection or sequential infection is a current controversy and major area of research interest. Unlike bacterial pathogens, the constant genomic shifts in influenza A do affect the performance of assays and they need to be revalidated constantly as new strains appear.[53]

A variety of point-of-care platforms have been developed for detecting influenza, of which the GeneXpert system (Cepheid, Sunnyvale, CA) is perhaps so far the best studied.[54] GeneXpert is an "all-in-one" platform requiring minimal technical expertise, and is a potential point-of-care platform for diagnosing influenza. A sputum sample is placed in a cartridge that plugs into the platform without the need for further processing or expert microbiological assistance. With a turnaround time of less than 2 hours, results can be available fast enough to impact on empiric therapy. This system has been evaluated extensively for the diagnosis of tuberculosis, including multidrug-resistant tuberculosis, where it has been proven to have excellent sensitivity and specificity.[55] The influenza A and B GeneXpert assay has been evaluated in comparison to a number of commercially available rapid antigen tests and PCR tests and found to have excellent sensitivity (97% −100%) and specificity (99%–100%).[56–60] The potential clinical usefulness has been studied in the emergency department setting, again with good performance and efficiency.[61,62] Point-of-care testing for influenza is a highly competitive area with potential new products regularly entering the market offering greater speed, lower cost, and/or greater accuracy (for example[63–66]).

Other Viruses

A large number of other viruses are well-known to cause pneumonia, with the most common being adenovirus, respiratory syncytial virus, metapneumonvirus, parainfluenza, and coronaviruses. In the absence of specific treatments for any of these viruses, discussion of specific diagnostic tests is relatively superfluous; however, many of the multipathogen approaches are discussed herein and include 1 or more of these viruses in their "panels."

MULTIPATHOGEN APPROACHES

With an ever-expanding list of pneumonia-causing pathogens, it is both time consuming and expensive to test for each organism individually. The ability to detect multiple pathogens in a single test is, therefore, highly appealing and has been the subject of significant research, development, and validation in the setting of respiratory tract infection. Starting with "home-grown" multiplex PCR assays, a variety of new platforms have been developed to speed up pathogen identification, and in some cases combining this with antibiotic sensitivity testing. Because the focus of multipathogen detection tools is to find the cause of the pneumonia, they all combine assays for "typical" pathogens such as S pneumoniae with the "atypical" pathogens.

Multipathogen detection systems can in general these can be categorized into those specifically designed to speed up pathogen recognition from positive blood cultures (eg, including systems such as The Verigene GramPositive Blood Culture Nucleic Acid Test; Nanosphere, Northbrook, IL), Prove-it Sepsis StripArray technology (Mobidiag, Espoo, Finland), and FilmArray (BioFire Diagnostics, Salt Lake City, UT), and those designed for clinical samples such as sputum, blood, or urine (eg, GeneXpert, SeptiFast [Roche Diagnostics, Manheim, Germany], SepsiTest [Molzym, Bremen, Germany], Curetis Unyvero [Curetis AG, Holzgerlingen, Germany], and VYOO [SIRS Lab, Jena, Germany]). The systems designed to speed up blood culture results are not particularly relevant to a discussion of atypical pathogens. Systems designed to work on clinical samples are, however, of interest, especially those with point-of-care applications. Unfortunately data in the specific setting of CAP are relatively limited at present, so only those with relevant published studies on viral and atypical pathogens are discussed briefly herein.

GeneXpert

The GeneXpert system has already been discussed, but it is worth noting that the range of pathogen assays is steadily increasing and now includes respiratory syncytial virus and methicillin-resistant Staphylococcus aureus, which are clearly relevant to pneumonia.

FilmArray

FilmArray is another novel "all-in-one" multiplex PCR platform with minimal technical expertise required and a turnaround time of approximately 1 hour. Manual handling is very limited, as with GeneXpert, and a variety of panels are available. The commercially available respiratory panel detects 17 viral and 3 bacterial pathogens. The performance of the respiratory panel has been compared with "in-house" PCR tests with favorable results[67,68] and the system seems to be robust enough to be useful in routine clinical practice.[69,70]

Curetis Unyvero

The Curetis Unyvero P50 pneumonia cartridge can detect 17 bacterial and fungal pathogens and 22 antibiotic resistance markers from respiratory samples in a single run in approximately 4 hours.[71] The panel includes *L pneumophila* and *M pneumoniae*, but specific performance data on these pathogens from clinical studies has not been reported. A preliminary study in critically ill patients found the performance of the Curetis Unyvero to be questionable, but noted the system was still under development.[72]

Mass Spectrometry

Mass spectrometry has been available for decades, but improvements in size, speed, and cost have brought this technology to a point where it can be used for both broadrange and target-specific identification of pathogens. PCR-electrospray ionization mass spectrometry holds particular promise given that it can identify minute quantities and mixtures of nucleic acids from microbial isolates or directly from clinical specimens. The performance of PCR-electrospray ionization mass spectrometry for detecting influenza in clinical samples seems at least as good as conventional PCR assays.[73] A single study from Taiwan indicates that PCR-electrospray ionization mass spectrometry has promise for the detection of multiple viruses in the setting of respiratory tract infection but this was done retrospectively rather than in real time.[74]

A different use of mass spectrometry, matrix-assisted laser desorption/ionization time of flight mass spectrometry (MALDI-TOF-MS) is also a protein/peptide diagnostic tool that has been shown to have usefulness in identifying microorganisms at a species level. MALDI-TOF-MS has been assessed predominantly as a means of rapidly identifying the identity of both bacteria and their bacterial products from positive blood cultures, up to 24 hours faster than conventional methods. A comparison of the diagnostic accuracy of MALDI-TOF-MS with liquid chromatography MS for influenza A, metapneumovirus, and respiratory syncytial virus suggested the latter may be superior.[75] A potential and significant limitation of current MALDI-TOF-MS is that when a large mixture of bacteria are present, as occurs more commonly in hospital-acquired pneumonia and ventilator-acquired pneumonia, the sensitivity and specificity become suboptimal.[76]

Next-Generation Sequencing

Next-generation sequencing, also known as high-throughput sequencing, is a generic term used to describe a group of different modern sequencing technologies including Illumina (Solexa, San Diego, CA) sequencing, Roche 454 sequencing, Ion torrent: Proton/PGM Sequencing (Thermo-Fisher Scientific, Waltham, MA), and SOLiD sequencing (ThermoFisher Scientific, Waltham, MA). These recent technologies allow sequencing of DNA and RNA much more quickly and cheaply than the previously used Sanger sequencing (ThermoFisher Scientific, Waltham, MA). To date, there are few data on the applicability of next-generation sequencing to immediate clinical care, but it has been particularly useful in diagnosing new and/or novel pathogens for which there are no available assays.

SUMMARY

As technology has improved, we have moved from relying on serologic tests to diagnose atypical and viral pathogens to direct detection of these pathogens in clinical specimens. Starting from a base of homegrown PCR assays, an increasing array of commercial assays have appeared, first as single pathogen assays, and increasingly as multiplexed tests. Increasing focus on point-of-care testing, or at least rapid enough turnaround time to influence initial clinical management, has driven development of a host of new platforms and technologies that are likely to change the way we manage pneumonia over the coming decade.

REFERENCES

1. Shope RE. The etiology of swine influenza. Science 1931;73(1886):214–5.
2. Jain S, Self WH, Wunderink RG, et al. Community-acquired pneumonia requiring hospitalization among U.S. adults. N Engl J Med 2015;373(5): 415–27.
3. Holter JC, Muller F, Bjorang O, et al. Etiology of community-acquired pneumonia and diagnostic yields of microbiological methods: a 3-year prospective study in Norway. BMC Infect Dis 2015; 15:64.
4. Eaton M, Meiklejohn G, va Herick W. Studies on the etiology of primary atypical pneumonia: a filterable agent transmissible to cotton rats, hamsters and chick embryos. J Exp Med 1944;79(6):649–68.
5. McDade JE, Shepard CC, Fraser DW, et al. Legionnaires' disease: isolation of a bacterium and demonstration of its role in other respiratory disease. N Engl J Med 1977;297(22):1197–203.

6. Grayston JT, Kuo CC, Wang SP, et al. A new Chlamydia psittaci strain, TWAR, isolated in acute respiratory tract infections. N Engl J Med 1986;315(3):161–8.

7. Wang K, Gill P, Perera R, et al. Clinical symptoms and signs for the diagnosis of Mycoplasma pneumoniae in children and adolescents with community-acquired pneumonia. Cochrane Database Syst Rev 2012;(10):CD009175.

8. Wingfield T, Rowell S, Peel A, et al. Legionella pneumonia cases over a five-year period: a descriptive, retrospective study of outcomes in a UK district hospital. Clin Med (Lond) 2013;13(2):152–9.

9. Viasus D, Di Yacovo S, Garcia-Vidal C, et al. Community-acquired Legionella pneumophila pneumonia: a single-center experience with 214 hospitalized sporadic cases over 15 years. Medicine 2013; 92(1):51–60.

10. Sopena N, Sabria-Leal M, Pedro-Botet ML, et al. Comparative study of the clinical presentation of Legionella pneumonia and other community-acquired pneumonias. Chest 1998;113(5):1195–200.

11. Jereb M, Kotar T. Usefulness of procalcitonin to differentiate typical from atypical community-acquired pneumonia. Wien Klin Wochenschr 2006; 118(5–6):170–4.

12. Kruger S, Ewig S, Marre R, et al. Procalcitonin predicts patients at low risk of death from community-acquired pneumonia across all CRB-65 classes. Eur Respir J 2008;31(2):349–55.

13. Wu MH, Lin CC, Huang SL, et al. Can procalcitonin tests aid in identifying bacterial infections associated with influenza pneumonia? A systematic review and meta-analysis. Influenza Other Respir Viruses 2013;7(3):349–55.

14. Waterer GW, Baselski VS, Wunderink RG. Legionella and community-acquired pneumonia: a review of current diagnostic tests from a clinician's viewpoint. Am J Med 2001;110(1):41–8.

15. Maze MJ, Slow S, Cumins AM, et al. Enhanced detection of Legionnaires' disease by PCR testing of induced sputum and throat swabs. Eur Respir J 2014;43(2):644–6.

16. Centers for Disease Control and Prevention (CDC). Legionellosis — United States, 2000-2009. MMWR Morb Mortal Wkly Rep 2011;60(32):1083–6.

17. Adams D, Fullerton K, Jajosky R, et al. Summary of notifiable infectious diseases and conditions - United States, 2013. MMWR Morb Mortal Wkly Rep 2015;62(53):1–122.

18. Garrison LE, Kunz JM, Cooley LA, et al. Vital signs: deficiencies in environmental control identified in outbreaks of legionnaires' disease - North America, 2000-2014. MMWR Morb Mortal Wkly Rep 2016; 65(22):576–84.

19. Edelstein PH, Meyer RD, Finegold SM. Laboratory diagnosis of Legionnaires' disease. Am Rev Respir Dis 1980;121(2):317–27.

20. Zuravleff JJ, Yu VL, Shonnard JW, et al. Diagnosis of Legionnaires' disease. An update of laboratory methods with new emphasis on isolation by culture. JAMA 1983;250(15):1981–5.

21. Monforte R, Estruch R, Vidal J, et al. Delayed seroconversion in Legionnaire's disease. Lancet 1988; 2(8609):513.

22. Mandell LA, Wunderink RG, Anzueto A, et al. Infectious Diseases Society of America/American Thoracic Society consensus guidelines on the management of community-acquired pneumonia in adults. Clin Infect Dis 2007;44(Suppl 2):S27–72.

23. Avni T, Bieber A, Green H, et al. Diagnostic accuracy of PCR alone and compared to urinary antigen testing for detection of Legionella spp.: a systematic review. J Clin Microbiol 2016;54(2):401–11.

24. Benitez AJ, Winchell JM. Rapid detection and typing of pathogenic nonpneumophila Legionella spp. isolates using a multiplex real-time PCR assay. Diagn Microbiol Infect Dis 2016;84(4):298–303.

25. Botelho-Nevers E, Grattard F, Viallon A, et al. Prospective evaluation of RT-PCR on sputum versus culture, urinary antigens and serology for Legionnaire's disease diagnosis. J Infect 2016;73(2): 123–8.

26. Gadsby NJ, Russell CD, McHugh MP, et al. Comprehensive molecular testing for respiratory pathogens in community-acquired pneumonia. Clin Infect Dis 2016;62(7):817–23.

27. Blaschke AJ, Allison MA, Meyers L, et al. Non-invasive sample collection for respiratory virus testing by multiplex PCR. J Clin Virol 2011;52(3):210–4.

28. Herrera M, Aguilar YA, Rueda ZV, et al. Comparison of serological methods with PCR-based methods for the diagnosis of community-acquired pneumonia caused by atypical bacteria. J Negat Results Biomed 2016;15:3.

29. Cho MC, Kim H, An D, et al. Comparison of sputum and nasopharyngeal swab specimens for molecular diagnosis of Mycoplasma pneumoniae, Chlamydophila pneumoniae, and Legionella pneumophila. Ann Lab Med 2012;32(2):133–8.

30. Parrott GL, Kinjo T, Fujita J. A compendium for Mycoplasma pneumoniae. Front Microbiol 2016;7:513.

31. Loens K, Beck T, Ursi D, et al. Evaluation of different nucleic acid amplification techniques for the detection of M. pneumoniae, C. pneumoniae and Legionella spp. in respiratory specimens from patients with community-acquired pneumonia. J Microbiol Methods 2008;73(3):257–62.

32. Chou RC, Zheng X. A comparison of molecular assays for Mycoplasma pneumoniae in pediatric patients. Diagn Microbiol Infect Dis 2016;85(1):6–8.

33. Li W, Liu Y, Zhao Y, et al. Rapid diagnosis of Mycoplasma pneumoniae in children with pneumonia by an immuno-chromatographic antigen assay. Sci Rep 2015;5:15539.

34. Miyashita N, Kawai Y, Kato T, et al. Rapid diagnostic method for the identification of Mycoplasma pneumoniae respiratory tract infection. J Infect Chemother 2016;22(5):327–30.

35. Pannekoek Y, Qin QL, Zhang YZ, et al. Genus delineation of Chlamydiales by analysis of the percentage of conserved proteins (POCP) justifies the reunifying of the genera Chlamydia and Chlamydophila into one single genus Chlamydia. Pathog Dis 2016;74 [pii:ftw071].

36. Friedman MG, Dvoskin B, Kahane S. Infections with the chlamydia-like microorganism Simkania negevensis, a possible emerging pathogen. Microbes Infect 2003;5(11):1013–21.

37. Greub G. Parachlamydia acanthamoebae, an emerging agent of pneumonia. Clin Microbiol Infect 2009;15(1):18–28.

38. Villegas E, Sorlozano A, Gutierrez J. Serological diagnosis of Chlamydia pneumoniae infection: limitations and perspectives. J Med Microbiol 2010;59(Pt 11):1267–74.

39. Benitez AJ, Thurman KA, Diaz MH, et al. Comparison of real-time PCR and a microimmunofluorescence serological assay for detection of chlamydophila pneumoniae infection in an outbreak investigation. J Clin Microbiol 2012;50(1):151–3.

40. She RC, Thurber A, Hymas WC, et al. Limited utility of culture for Mycoplasma pneumoniae and Chlamydophila pneumoniae for diagnosis of respiratory tract infections. J Clin Microbiol 2010;48(9): 3380–2.

41. Rodriguez-Dominguez M, Sanbonmatsu S, Salinas J, et al. Microbiological diagnosis of infections due to Chlamydia spp. and related species. Enferm Infecc Microbiol Clin 2014;32(6):380–5 [in Spanish].

42. Aziz M, Vasoo S, Aziz Z, et al. Oseltamivir overuse at a Chicago hospital during the 2009 influenza pandemic and the poor predictive value of influenza-like illness criteria. Scand J Infect Dis 2012;44(4):306–11.

43. Gao F, Loring C, Laviolette M, et al. Detection of 2009 pandemic influenza A(H1N1) virus Infection in different age groups by using rapid influenza diagnostic tests. Influenza Other Respir Viruses 2012;6(3):e30–4.

44. Nutter S, Cheung M, Adler-Shohet FC, et al. Evaluation of indirect fluorescent antibody assays compared to rapid influenza diagnostic tests for the detection of pandemic influenza A (H1N1) pdm09. PLoS One 2012;7(3):e33097.

45. Ciblak MA, Kanturvardar M, Asar S, et al. Sensitivity of rapid influenza antigen tests in the diagnosis of pandemic (H1N1)2009 compared with the standard rRT-PCR technique during the 2009 pandemic in Turkey. Scand J Infect Dis 2010;42(11–12): 902–5.

46. Ganzenmueller T, Kluba J, Hilfrich B, et al. Comparison of the performance of direct fluorescent antibody staining, a point-of-care rapid antigen test and virus isolation with that of RT-PCR for the detection of novel 2009 influenza A (H1N1) virus in respiratory specimens. J Med Microbiol 2010;59(Pt 6):713–7.

47. Chartrand C, Leeflang MM, Minion J, et al. Accuracy of rapid influenza diagnostic tests: a meta-analysis. Ann Intern Med 2012;156(7):500–11.

48. Nicholson KG, Abrams KR, Batham S, et al. Randomised controlled trial and health economic evaluation of the impact of diagnostic testing for influenza, respiratory syncytial virus and Streptococcus pneumoniae infection on the management of acute admissions in the elderly and high-risk 18- to 64-year-olds. Health Technol Assess 2014; 18(36):1–274, vii–viii.

49. Peci A, Winter AL, King EC, et al. Performance of rapid influenza diagnostic testing in outbreak settings. J Clin Microbiol 2014;52(12):4309–17.

50. Busson L, Hallin M, Thomas I, et al. Evaluation of 3 rapid influenza diagnostic tests during the 2012-2013 epidemic: influences of subtype and viral load. Diagn Microbiol Infect Dis 2014;80(4): 287–91.

51. Ryu SW, Lee JH, Kim J, et al. Comparison of two new generation influenza rapid diagnostic tests with instrument-based digital readout systems for influenza virus detection. Br J Biomed Sci 2016;73:1–6.

52. Vemula SV, Zhao J, Liu J, et al. Current approaches for diagnosis of influenza virus infections in humans. Viruses 2016;8(4):96.

53. Huzly D, Korn K, Bierbaum S, et al. Influenza A virus drift variants reduced the detection sensitivity of a commercial multiplex nucleic acid amplification assay in the season 2014/15. Arch Virol 2016; 161(9):2417–23.

54. Salez N, Nougairede A, Ninove L, et al. Xpert Flu for point-of-care diagnosis of human influenza in industrialized countries. Expert Rev Mol Diagn 2014; 14(4):411–8.

55. Steingart KR, Schiller I, Horne DJ, et al. Xpert(R) MTB/RIF assay for pulmonary tuberculosis and rifampicin resistance in adults. Cochrane Database Syst Rev 2014;(1):CD009593.

56. Miller S, Moayeri M, Wright C, et al. Comparison of GeneXpert FluA PCR to direct fluorescent antibody and respiratory viral panel PCR assays for detection of 2009 novel H1N1 influenza virus. J Clin Microbiol 2010;48(12):4684–5.

57. Wahrenbrock MG, Matushek S, Boonlayangoor S, et al. Comparison of cepheid xpert Flu/RSV XC and BioFire FilmArray for detection of influenza A, influenza B, and respiratory syncytial virus. J Clin Microbiol 2016;54(7):1902–3.

58. Popowitch EB, Miller MB. Performance characteristics of xpert Flu/RSV XC assay. J Clin Microbiol 2015;53(8):2720–1.

59. Salez N, Nougairede A, Ninove L, et al. Prospective and retrospective evaluation of the Cepheid Xpert(R) Flu/RSV XC assay for rapid detection of influenza A, influenza B, and respiratory syncytial virus. Diagn Microbiol Infect Dis 2015;81(4):256–8.

60. DiMaio MA, Sahoo MK, Waggoner J, et al. Comparison of Xpert Flu rapid nucleic acid testing with rapid antigen testing for the diagnosis of influenza A and B. J Virol Methods 2012;186(1–2):137–40.

61. Dugas AF, Valsamakis A, Gaydos CA, et al. Evaluation of the Xpert Flu rapid PCR assay in high-risk emergency department patients. J Clin Microbiol 2014;52(12):4353–5.

62. Soto M, Sampietro-Colom L, Vilella A, et al. Economic impact of a new rapid PCR assay for detecting influenza virus in an emergency department and hospitalized patients. PLoS One 2016;11(1): e0146620.

63. Jokela P, Vuorinen T, Waris M, et al. Performance of the Alere i influenza A&B assay and mariPOC test for the rapid detection of influenza A and B viruses. J Clin Virol 2015;70:72–6.

64. Wang CH, Chang CP, Lee GB. Integrated microfluidic device using a single universal aptamer to detect multiple types of influenza viruses. Biosens Bioelectron 2016;86:247–54.

65. Liu J, Zhao J, Petrochenko P, et al. Sensitive detection of influenza viruses with Europium nanoparticles on an epoxy silica sol-gel functionalized polycarbonate-polydimethylsiloxane hybrid microchip. Biosens Bioelectron 2016;86:150–5.

66. Hirama T, Minezaki S, Yamaguchi T, et al. HIRA-TAN: a real-time PCR-based system for the rapid identification of causative agents in pneumonia. Respir Med 2014;108(2):395–404.

67. Pierce VM, Elkan M, Leet M, et al. Comparison of the Idaho Technology FilmArray system to real-time PCR for detection of respiratory pathogens in children. J Clin Microbiol 2012;50(2):364–71.

68. Andersson ME, Olofsson S, Lindh M. Comparison of the FilmArray assay and in-house real-time PCR for detection of respiratory infection. Scand J Infect Dis 2014;46(12):897–901.

69. Rappo U, Schuetz AN, Jenkins SG, et al. Impact of early detection of respiratory viruses by multiplex PCR assay on clinical outcomes in adult patients. J Clin Microbiol 2016;54(8):2096–103.

70. Gilbert D, Gelfer G, Wang L, et al. The potential of molecular diagnostics and serum procalcitonin levels to change the antibiotic management of community-acquired pneumonia. Diagn Microbiol Infect Dis 2016;86(1):102–7.

71. Jamal W, Al Roomi E, AbdulAziz LR, et al. Evaluation of Curetis Unyvero, a multiplex PCR-based testing system, for rapid detection of bacteria and antibiotic resistance and impact of the assay on management of severe nosocomial pneumonia. J Clin Microbiol 2014;52(7):2487–92.

72. Kunze N, Moerer O, Steinmetz N, et al. Point-of-care multiplex PCR promises short turnaround times for microbial testing in hospital-acquired pneumonia–an observational pilot study in critical ill patients. Ann Clin Microbiol Antimicrob 2015;14:33.

73. Mengelle C, Mansuy JM, Da Silva I, et al. Evaluation of a polymerase chain reaction-electrospray ionization time-of-flight mass spectrometry for the detection and subtyping of influenza viruses in respiratory specimens. J Clin Virol 2013;57(3): 222–6.

74. Shih HI, Wang HC, Su IJ, et al. Viral respiratory tract infections in adult patients attending outpatient and emergency departments, Taiwan, 2012-2013: a PCR/electrospray ionization mass spectrometry study. Medicine 2015;94(38):e1545.

75. Majchrzykiewicz-Koehorst JA, Heikens E, Trip H, et al. Rapid and generic identification of influenza A and other respiratory viruses with mass spectrometry. J Virol Methods 2015;213:75–83.

76. La Scola B, Raoult D. Direct identification of bacteria in positive blood culture bottles by matrix-assisted laser desorption ionisation time-of-flight mass spectrometry. PLoS One 2009;4(11):e8041.

Respiratory Syncytial Virus Infection
An Illness for All Ages

Edward E. Walsh, MD

KEYWORDS

- Respiratory syncytial virus • Bronchiolitis • Chronic obstructive pulmonary disease • Antivirals
- Asthma • Vaccines • Adults

KEY POINTS

- Respiratory syncytial virus (RSV) is an important respiratory pathogen at both ends of the age spectrum, with approximately 100,000 hospitalizations in infants and approximately 177,000 in adults. However, general awareness of RSV in adults among internists and general practitioners is lacking.
- The interaction of RSV with pathogenic bacteria, specifically *Streptococcus pneumoniae* and *Hemophilus influenzae*, seem to influence disease severity and contribute to morbidity, especially in the developing world.
- Prophylaxis with Palivizumab provides effective prevention in specific high-risk infants but there are currently no effective specific therapies or vaccines for most susceptible infants and adults.

Respiratory syncytial virus (RSV) was first identified in 1956 by Robert Chanock and is currently recognized as the most important cause of severe respiratory illness in infants and young children, clinically manifesting most often as bronchiolitis.[1] The virus has also more recently been identified as a significant contributor to morbidity and mortality in older adults and severely immunocompromised persons.[2]

VIRUS STRUCTURE AND GENOME

RSV is an enveloped negative-sense, single-strand RNA virus classified in the family *Pneumoviridae* along with human metapneumovirus, another cause of respiratory infections. The RSV genome contains 10 distinct genes that encode 11 individual proteins, each with distinct roles in viral infection and immune evasion (**Fig. 1**).[3] Surface glycoproteins protruding from the envelope include the viral attachment protein (G) and the fusion protein (F) that mediate entry of the viral

genome into cells while transitioning from a thermolabile prefusion F to a stable postfusion F. G may play a role in modulation of the immune and inflammatory response to infection through its CX3C chemokine homologue that binds the CX3C receptor on immune cells and primary ciliated respiratory epithelial cells.[4,5] Two nonstructural RSV proteins (NS1 and NS2) inhibit cellular antiviral innate type I interferons, providing defense against the host immune response.

There are 2 major viral groups, designated A and B, each with numerous subgroups, best identified by G gene sequence variation.[6] However, a causal relationship between antigenic variation in G and reinfections has not been firmly established. Antibody to F and the G proteins is considered a primary determinant of immunity.

EPIDEMIOLOGY

In the temperate climates, annual epidemics occur during the winters. In the United States, epidemics

Infectious Diseases Division, Department of Medicine, Rochester General Hospital, University of Rochester School of Medicine, 1425 Portland Avenue, Rochester, NY 14621, USA
E-mail address: Edward.walsh@rochesterregional.org

Clin Chest Med 38 (2017) 29–36
http://dx.doi.org/10.1016/j.ccm.2016.11.010
0272-5231/17/© 2016 Elsevier Inc. All rights reserved.

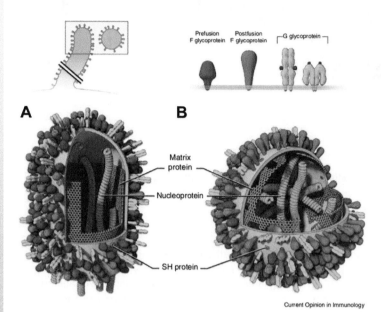

Fig. 1. The filamentous and spherical forms of RSV, indicating the (*A*) prefusion and (*B*) postfusion forms of F and the G glycoprotein. (*From* Graham BS, Modjarrad K, McLellan JS. Novel antigens for RSV vaccines. Curr Opin Immunol 2015;35:30–8; with permission.)

generally begin in the southeast in late summer and spread north and westward reaching a peak in January and February in the northeast and Pacific Northwest.[7] RSV circulation generally persists for 16 to 22 weeks in a community, and overlaps with the more sharply defined 6 to 8 week influenza epidemics. In the tropics, RSV circulation is more variable, frequently being more common during the rainy season and circulating throughout the year.[8] Group A and B RSV viruses cocirculate, with group A viruses tending to be more frequent.

Older children commonly introduce the virus into the family with spread to infants and parents.[9] RSV is most effectively transmitted by large fomites (nasal secretions) whereas aerosol is less important. The virus is stable for several hours on hard surfaces and hands, allowing transmission by direct contact with contaminated objects. The introduction of strict infection control policies in hospital settings (isolation and hand washing) and personal protective equipment (gowns, gloves, and possibly goggles) reduces nosocomial transmission.[10]

PEDIATRIC RESPIRATORY SYNCYTIAL VIRUS INFECTION

The importance of RSV on the health of infants and young children cannot be underestimated. It causes acute illness and, importantly, may be causally related to the development of subsequent wheezing in childhood and asthma later in life. Fifty percent to 70% of newborn infants become infected during their first winter, and virtually all become infected by age 2 years. Reinfections with RSV continue throughout childhood, although their severity diminishes. In the United States, approximately 1% to 2% of infants in their first year of life are hospitalized with RSV infection, whereas another 20% will be seen in pediatric offices or emergency rooms for acute respiratory symptoms.[11] Pediatric mortality from RSV in developed countries is low (~50–100 annually in the United States); however, in the developing world, RSV is estimated to result in 66,000 to 199,000 deaths and more than 3 million hospitalizations in children younger than age 5 years.[12,13]

The course of RSV illness and its manifestations follow a similar pattern in most infants, although disease severity is highly variable. Following an incubation period of 4 to 6 days, nasal congestion with mucus discharge and fever are followed by cough, tachypnea, and respiratory distress with chest retractions and wheezing, the hallmark of bronchiolitis. In young preterm infants, apnea will occasionally be an early manifestation of RSV. The clinical picture of RSV in young infants can change during observation, with hypoxia and physical findings fluctuating even in a matter of several minutes. Radiographs reveal air trapping and infiltrates related to obstructive atelectasis or viral pneumonia. This variability in the clinical appearance of an infant with RSV can make decisions about further observation or whether to hospitalize difficult.

Bacterial coinfection with *Streptococcus pneumoniae* or *Hemophilus influenzae*, either as otitis media or pneumonia, can complicate RSV infection, although the precise relationship of the interaction, incidence, and significance of bacteria in respiratory secretions is not firmly established. A review of 2396 infants and children admitted with RSV bronchiolitis noted bacterial infection was uncommon (1.6%).[14] However, in a United Kingdom study, 42% of lower airway secretions had pathogenic bacteria in mechanically ventilated infants and 21.8% were considered to have bacterial coinfection.[15] A recent study of the nasal microbiome of RSV-infected infants found that abundance of *Streptococcus pneumoniae* and *H influenzae* but not *Staphylococcus aureus* was associated with changes in the host immune response as measured by gene expression of peripheral blood mononuclear cells.[16] Finally, studies from the United States and South Africa reported 18% and 32% reductions, respectively, in RSV-confirmed hospitalization following introduction of conjugate pneumococcal vaccine.[17–19]

Many risk factors associated with severe disease, most importantly including gestational age less than 29 weeks, chronic lung disease, and cyanotic heart disease.[1] The incidence of hospitalization among preterm infants with chronic lung disease was 12.8% in 1 study.[20] Nevertheless, approximately 70% of hospitalized infants are full-term, previously healthy infants. Although lack of breast feeding, exposure to environmental tobacco smoke, crowding, day care attendance, and lower socioeconomic status have been associated with risk of severe disease, a recent population-based surveillance study of 2539 hospitalizations among 32,000 infants found only young chronologic age associated with increased hospitalization rates in full-term infants, with the peak rate in 0 to 5-month-old infants.[11,21]

Laboratory diagnosis is often sought in hospitalized infants because several other respiratory viruses, especially human metapneumovirus, can also manifest as classic bronchiolitis. A specific diagnosis allows proper institution of appropriate infection prevention measures. Nucleic acid detection tests using reverse transcriptase-polymerase chain reaction (RT-PCR) are considered the gold standard, whereas rapid antigen tests have a sensitivity of approximately 70% compared with RT-PCR.[22] Viral titers are highest on admission and peak at day 3 of illness, with shedding typically lasting 11 days.[23–25]

Treatment is primarily supportive, mostly oxygen for oxygen saturation less than 90%. Despite numerous large multicenter randomized trials, no specific therapy has been found to consistently lessen severity or shorten the natural course of the illness.[1] Inhaled ribavirin is licensed for treatment of RSV infection in infants based on early studies demonstrating modest benefit but is not recommended for most hospitalized infants.

Prophylaxis with palivizumab (Synagis), a humanized murine monoclonal antibody directed at a neutralizing epitope on the postfusion F protein, is licensed for specific groups of infants.[20] Current recommendations by the American Academy of Pediatrics advise giving up to 5 monthly injections to premature infants less than 29 weeks gestation during their first winter, to infants less than 32 weeks gestation with chronic lung disease of prematurity who required supplemental oxygen, and to children with acyanotic congenital heart disease. Treatment of established infection with monoclonal antibody has not been associated with clinical benefit despite a reduction in viral load in severely ill intubated infants.[26]

Long-term sequelae of RSV infection are a topic of great interest and controversy, specifically with regard to the development of asthma.[27] Following RSV infection, many infants will develop wheezing with other viral infections, a situation that tends to abate by age 7 years. However, children with severe RSV bronchiolitis early in life have been shown to have a higher risk of developing childhood asthma, a greater incidence of asthma in young adulthood, and greater deficits in peak airway flow if they are smokers.[28] It has been postulated that severe RSV in infancy may also predispose to the development of chronic obstructive pulmonary disease (COPD) later in life.[29] However, it is still unclear if these sequelae are causally related to RSV infection or are simply reflections of a genetic predisposition to airway obstruction during any viral infection of antigenic stimulation.[1,27]

ADULT RESPIRATORY SYNCYTIAL VIRUS INFECTION

Although RSV in adults was described shortly after its identification in 1956, the impact and burden of RSV in this population was not appreciated until recently. As previously noted, immunity to RSV is incomplete and thus reinfection is common despite relatively high levels of serum neutralizing antibodies in adults. Nevertheless, reinfection with RSV and disease severity has been associated with lower levels of serum neutralizing antibody and nasal immunoglobulin A.[30] RSV infects adults at any age, although severe illness occurs primarily in elderly persons, especially those with underlying cardiopulmonary disease or those who are frail. It is postulated that waning cell-mediated immunity plays a role in susceptibility in this age group.[31] Importantly, immunocompromised adults, especially hematopoietic stem cell transplant (HSCT) recipients, those undergoing intensive chemotherapy, and lung transplant patients are at serious risk of severe RSV infection.[32]

The burden of RSV in adults has been determined in a combination of population-based prospective surveillance studies, analysis of acute illness presenting for medical care, and modeling of large medical databases. In prospective surveillance studies in healthy elderly adults and high-risk adults with underlying cardiopulmonary disease, the annual wintertime RSV attack rate ranged from 3% to 7% and 2% to 10%, respectively.[2,33] In a 3-year study of acute respiratory illnesses seen by general practitioners in the United Kingdom, 19% of 45 to 64 year olds and 15% of those 65 years or older were diagnosed with RSV.[34] In a recent retrospective analysis of respiratory samples from 2225 subjects with medically attended acute respiratory illness (MAARI) in Marshfield, Wisconsin, RSV was identified in 8.2% of those 50 to 64 years old, 10.2% of those 65 to 79 years old, and 10.5% of those 80 years or older.[35]

The incidence of RSV among hospitalized adults during the winter season ranges from 6% to 10% in various studies.[2,35–37] Statistical modeling studies from several countries using large clinical databases coupled with laboratory viral diagnostic data calculated the morbidity and mortality of RSV in adults to be 12% to 80% (average 43%) of the concurrently measured impact of influenza (**Tables 1** and **2**).[12,38–44]

Clinical findings in adults are variable and depend on age but, more significantly, on the presence of underlying medical conditions. Infection often begins with typical upper respiratory symptoms but fever is often absent or low-grade, and significantly less than in influenza.[2,35] Illness progresses more slowly than influenza and patients present for medical care between 4 to 7 days after symptom onset. As in infants, wheezing is often noted.[45] Constitutional symptoms are less frequent than with influenza, with fever occurring in only 28%. In a study of adults older than age 50 years with RSV-associated MAARI, 61% had fever and 67% wheezed.[35] In 3 large studies of hospitalized adults with RSV, approximately 80% had a high-risk medical condition, with underlying COPD present in 58% to 68%.[2,36,37] In these studies, mortality rates were

Table 1
Summary of epidemiologic modeling studies comparing mortality and hospitalization rates for respiratory syncytial virus and influenza in adults age 65 years and older

Author (Reference)	Location	Dates (Years)	Outcome Measure	Results
Thompson et al,[39] 2003	USA	1990–1999[9]	Respiratory & circulatory deaths per 100,000	RSV 26.5 Flu A + B 98.5
Mullooly et al,[38] 2007	Portland, OR	1996–2000[4]	Annual pneumonia & influenza[a] hospitalization per 10,000	RSV 23.4 Flu 55.6
Zhou et al,[12] 2012	USA	1993–2008[15]	Annual hospitalizations per 100,000	RSV 86.1 Flu 309
van Asten et al,[40] 2012	Netherlands	1999–2007[8]	Total deaths	RSV 13902 Flu A + B 21635
Matias et al,[42] 2014	USA	1997–2009[12]	Annual deaths from respiratory illness	RSV 9673 Flu 16505
Fleming et al,[41] 2015	UK	1995–2009[14]	Annual hospitalizations (ratio of RSV/flu)	RSV 14039 (0.8)
Chan et al,[43] 2015	Hong Kong	1998–2012[15]	Annual hospitalizations per 10,000	RSV 5.2 (M) 6.1 (F) Flu A 19.5 (M) 17.3 (F)
Goldstein et al,[44] 2015	New York City, NY	2003–2011[9]	Annual hospitalizations per 100,000	RSV 15.3 Flu 125.8

Abbreviations: F, female; Flu, influenza, M, male.
[a] Influenza, unvaccinated high-risk individuals.

Table 2
Symptoms in outpatients with laboratory-confirmed respiratory syncytial virus versus influenza A over 4 seasons, 1999 to 2003, in Rochester, NY

Symptom	Healthy, Age ≥65 y		High-Risk[a], Age ≥21 y[b]	
	RSV (%) n = 48	Influenza A (%) n = 18	RSV (%) n = 54	Influenza A (%) n = 16
Nasal congestion	83	83	65	79
Cough	79	83	78	87
Sputum production	64	61	66	80
Dyspnea	9	28	58	71
Wheeze	23	17	50	50
Constitutional	53	72	59	71
Fever	18	44	31	47

[a] High-risk defined as having physician-diagnosed congestive-heart failure or chronic pulmonary disease.
[b] 10% age less than 54 years, 17% age 55 to 64 years, 73% age ≥65 years.
   Data from Falsey AR, Hennessey PA, Formica MA, et al. Respiratory syncytial virus infection in elderly and high-risk adults. N Engl J Med 2005;352(17):1749–59.

6.5% to 10%. In a prospective surveillance study of a high-risk cohort, of whom 65% had COPD, RSV infection resulted in office visits in 60% and 20% were hospitalized.[2] Radiographic abnormalities are common in adults hospitalized with RSV, with consolidation or ground glass infiltrates in 31% to 49%.[2,37]

Immunocompromised individuals have the highest morbidity and mortality from RSV.[32,46] Upper respiratory symptoms give way to lower respiratory involvement in 30% to 40% of infected persons around day 7 of illness. High-dose total body irradiation and total lymphocyte count less than 100/mm but not serum-neutralizing antibody levels or corticosteroid use were associated with progression from upper-tract to lower-tract disease.[47]

Because the attack rate in adults during the RSV season is relatively low and the clinical syndrome nonspecific, laboratory confirmation of RSV is critical to accurate diagnosis. RT-PCR is most sensitive (~80%) whereas virus culture (33%) and rapid enzyme linked antigen detection tests (10%) have poor sensitivity, even in HSCT patients.[2,48,49] Sputum RT-PCR testing can also increase yield by 22%.[50] The mean duration of RSV shedding in adults is approximately 10 days, with mean nasal secretion titers of 2.0 to 2.8 $\log_{10}$ per milliliter, with higher titers and longer shedding noted in older patients and in those with more severe illness.[51–53]

Management of adults with RSV infection is supportive. The use of antibiotics is common among both outpatients and inpatients with RSV, even when the chest radiograph is clear.[2,37] The precise incidence of bacterial coinfection during RSV-associated hospitalization has not been extensively studied but is reported to be 12% to 15%.[2,37] In a comprehensive analysis of hospitalized adults with viral infections, 31% of RSV-infected persons had evidence of invasive bacterial infection based on either standard tests or a high serum procalcitonin.[54] Use of ribavirin (aerosolized, oral, or intravenously) is not recommended in adults, with the exception of severely immunocompromised persons in whom early ribavirin treatment, often coupled with immune globulin, was the most significant factor in reducing mortality.[46]

FUTURE VACCINE AND ANTIVIRAL PROSPECTS FOR RESPIRATORY SYNCYTIAL VIRUS

Currently, there are no licensed vaccines for prevention in any age group. As of September 2016, there are over 40 vaccines in preclinical development and more than 15 in various clinical phases of study. Vaccine approaches include live, attenuated vaccines; vectored vaccines expressing protective RSV antigens; inactivated subunit vaccines, primarily prefusion or postfusion forms of F, with and without novel adjuvants; DNA-based vaccines; and newer monoclonal antibodies with a prolonged half-life (see www.path. org). Live attenuated vaccines developed using reverse genetics are currently in clinical trials in young infants.[55] Subunit vaccines are being developed for use in adults, including maternal immunization during late pregnancy to protect infants from RSV infection early in life by increasing placental transport of neutralizing antibody to the newborn. These studies are currently in phase 2 studies. A new development in the evolution of subunit and vectored vaccines is the recognition that the prefusion form of F protein carries potent neutralizing epitopes not found in the postfusion F that has been studied in several prior vaccine trials.[3]

Several new small molecule antivirals have also entered early phase 1 and 2 clinical trials in pediatric and adult age groups, including immunocompromised persons. They include a fusion inhibitor with a half-life that allows a single dose and a nucleoside analogue that inhibits the RSV polymerase.[56,57] Both of these drugs can be administered orally, and have been demonstrated to have good safety profiles and antiviral and clinical efficacy in a human challenge model of RSV infection. Finally, as previously noted, there are 2 new long half-life monoclonal antibodies currently being evaluated for prophylaxis in high-risk infants.[58]

REFERENCES

1. Meissner HC. Viral Bronchiolitis in Children. N Engl J Med 2016;374(1):62–72.
2. Falsey AR, Hennessey PA, Formica MA, et al. Respiratory syncytial virus infection in elderly and high-risk adults. N Engl J Med 2005;352(17):1749–59.
3. Graham BS, Modjarrad K, McLellan JS. Novel antigens for RSV vaccines. Curr Opin Immunol 2015; 35:30–8.
4. Johnson SM, McNally BA, Ioannidis I, et al. Respiratory syncytial virus uses CX3CR1 as a receptor on primary human airway epithelial cultures. PLoS Pathog 2015;11(12):e1005318.
5. Chirkova T, Boyoglu-Barnum S, Gaston KA, et al. Respiratory syncytial virus G protein CX3C motif impairs human airway epithelial and immune cell responses. J Virol 2013;87(24):13466–79.
6. Bose ME, He J, Shrivastava S, et al. Sequencing and analysis of globally obtained human respiratory syncytial virus A and B genomes. PLoS One 2015; 10(3):e0120098.
7. Panozzo CA, Fowlkes AL, Anderson LJ. Variation in timing of respiratory syncytial virus outbreaks: lessons from national surveillance. Pediatr Infect Dis J 2007;26(11 Suppl):S41–5.
8. Bloom-Feshbach K, Alonso WJ, Charu V, et al. Latitudinal variations in seasonal activity of influenza and respiratory syncytial virus (RSV): a global comparative review. PLoS One 2013;8(2):e54445.
9. Hall CB, Geiman JM, Biggar R, et al. Respiratory syncytial virus infections within families. N Engl J Med 1976;294(8):414–9.
10. French CE, McKenzie BC, Coope C, et al. Risk of nosocomial respiratory syncytial virus infection and effectiveness of control measures to prevent transmission events: a systematic review. Influenza Other Respir Viruses 2016;10(4):268–90.
11. Hall CB, Weinberg GA, Iwane MK, et al. The burden of respiratory syncytial virus infection in young children. N Engl J Med 2009;360(6):588–98.
12. Zhou H, Thompson WW, Viboud CG, et al. Hospitalizations associated with influenza and respiratory syncytial virus in the United States, 1993-2008. Clin Infect Dis 2012;54(10):1427–36.
13. Nair H, Nokes DJ, Gessner BD, et al. Global burden of acute lower respiratory infections due to respiratory syncytial virus in young children: a systematic review and meta-analysis. Lancet 2010;375(9725): 1545–55.
14. Purcell K, Fergie J. Concurrent serious bacterial infections in 2396 infants and children hospitalized with respiratory syncytial virus lower respiratory tract infections. Arch Pediatr Adolesc Med 2002;156(4): 322–4.
15. Thorburn K, Harigopal S, Reddy V, et al. High incidence of pulmonary bacterial co-infection in children with severe respiratory syncytial virus (RSV) bronchiolitis. Thorax 2006;61(7):611–5.
16. de Steenhuijsen Piters WA, Heinonen S, Hasrat R, et al. Nasopharyngeal microbiota, host transcriptome and disease severity in children with respiratory syncytial virus infection. Am J Respir Crit Care Med 2016;194(9):1104–15.
17. Weinberger DM, Klugman KP, Steiner CA, et al. Association between respiratory syncytial virus activity and pneumococcal disease in infants: a time series analysis of US hospitalization data. PLoS Med 2015; 12(1):e1001776.
18. Madhi SA, Klugman KP, Vaccine Trialist Group. A role for *Streptococcus pneumoniae* in virus-associated pneumonia. Nat Med 2004;10(8):811–3.
19. Madhi SA, Kuwanda L, Cutland C, et al. Five-year cohort study of hospitalization for respiratory syncytial virus associated lower respiratory tract infection in African children. J Clin Virol 2006 Jul;36(3): 215–21.
20. American Academy of Pediatrics Committee on Infectious Diseases, American Academy of Pediatrics Bronchiolitis Guidelines Committee. Updated guidance for palivizumab prophylaxis among infants and young children at increased risk of hospitalization for respiratory syncytial virus infection. Pediatrics 2014;134(2):e620–38.
21. Hall CB, Weinberg GA, Blumkin AK, et al. Respiratory syncytial virus-associated hospitalizations among children less than 24 months of age. Pediatrics 2013;132(2):e341–8.
22. Chartrand C, Tremblay N, Renaud C, et al. Diagnostic accuracy of rapid antigen detection tests for

respiratory syncytial virus infection: systematic review and meta-analysis. J Clin Microbiol 2015; 53(12):3738–49.

23. DeVincenzo JP, El Saleeby CM, Bush AJ. Respiratory syncytial virus load predicts disease severity in previously healthy infants. J Infect Dis 2005; 191(11):1861–8.

24. El Saleeby CM, Bush AJ, Harrison LM, et al. Respiratory syncytial virus load, viral dynamics, and disease severity in previously healthy naturally infected children. J Infect Dis 2011;204(7):996–1002.

25. Munywoki PK, Koech DC, Agoti CN, et al. Influence of age, severity of infection, and co-infection on the duration of respiratory syncytial virus (RSV) shedding. Epidemiol Infect 2015;143(4):804–12.

26. Malley R, DeVincenzo J, Ramilo O, et al. Reduction of respiratory syncytial virus (RSV) in tracheal aspirates in intubated infants by use of humanized monoclonal antibody to RSV F protein. J Infect Dis 1998;178(6):1555–61.

27. Feldman AS, He Y, Moore ML, et al. Toward primary prevention of asthma. Reviewing the evidence for early-life respiratory viral infections as modifiable risk factors to prevent childhood asthma. Am J Respir Crit Care Med 2015;191(1):34–44.

28. Voraphani N, Stern DA, Wright AL, et al. Risk of current asthma among adult smokers with respiratory syncytial virus illnesses in early life. Am J Respir Crit Care Med 2014;190(4):392–8.

29. Martinez FD. Early-life origins of chronic obstructive pulmonary disease. N Engl J Med 2016;375(9):871–8.

30. Walsh EE, Falsey AR. Humoral and mucosal immunity in protection from natural respiratory syncytial virus infection in adults. J Infect Dis 2004;190(2): 373–8.

31. Malloy AM, Falsey AR, Ruckwardt TJ. Consequences of immature and senescent immune responses for infection with respiratory syncytial virus. Curr Top Microbiol Immunol 2013;372:211–31.

32. Chemaly RF, Shah DP, Boeckh MJ. Management of respiratory viral infections in hematopoietic cell transplant recipients and patients with hematologic malignancies. Clin Infect Dis 2014;59(Suppl 5): S344–51.

33. Falsey AR, Walsh EE, Capellan J, et al. Comparison of the safety and immunogenicity of 2 respiratory syncytial virus (RSV) vaccines–nonadjuvanted vaccine or vaccine adjuvanted with alum–given concomitantly with influenza vaccine to high-risk elderly individuals. J Infect Dis 2008;198(9): 1317–26.

34. Zambon MC, Stockton JD, Clewley JP, et al. Contribution of influenza and respiratory syncytial virus to community cases of influenza-like illness: an observational study. Lancet 2001;358:1410–6.

35. Sundaram ME, Meece JK, Sifakis F, et al. Medically attended respiratory syncytial virus infections in

adults aged >/= 50 years: clinical characteristics and outcomes. Clin Infect Dis 2014;58(3):342–9.

36. Widmer K, Griffin MR, Zhu Y, et al. Respiratory syncytial virus- and human metapneumovirus-associated emergency department and hospital burden in adults. Influenza Other Respir Viruses 2014;8(3):347–52.

37. Lee N, Lui GC, Wong KT, et al. High morbidity and mortality in adults hospitalized for respiratory syncytial virus infections. Clin Infect Dis 2013;57(8): 1069–77.

38. Mullooly JP, Bridges CB, Thompson WW, et al. Influenza- and RSV-associated hospitalizations among adults. Vaccine 2007;25(5):846–55.

39. Thompson WW, Shay DK, Weintraub E, et al. Mortality associated with influenza and respiratory syncytial virus in the United States. JAMA 2003;289(2): 179–86.

40. van Asten L, van den Wijngaard C, van Pelt W, et al. Mortality attributable to 9 common infections: significant effect of influenza A, respiratory syncytial virus, influenza B, norovirus, and parainfluenza in elderly persons. J Infect Dis 2012;206(5):628–39.

41. Fleming DM, Taylor RJ, Lustig RL, et al. Modelling estimates of the burden of Respiratory Syncytial virus infection in adults and the elderly in the United Kingdom. BMC Infect Dis 2015;15:443.

42. Matias G, Taylor R, Haguinet F, et al. Estimates of mortality attributable to influenza and RSV in the United States during 1997-2009 by influenza type or subtype, age, cause of death, and risk status. Influenza Other Respir Viruses 2014;8(5):507–15.

43. Chan PK, Tam WW, Lee TC, et al. Hospitalization incidence, mortality, and seasonality of common respiratory viruses over a period of 15 years in a developed subtropical city. Medicine (Baltimore) 2015; 94(46):e2024.

44. Goldstein E, Greene SK, Olson DR, et al. Estimating the hospitalization burden associated with influenza and respiratory syncytial virus in New York City, 2003-2011. Influenza Other Respir Viruses 2015; 9(5):225–33.

45. Hall CB, Long CE, Schnabel KC. Respiratory syncytial virus infections in previously healthy working adults. Clin Infect Dis 2001;33(6):792–6.

46. Shah DP, Ghantoji SS, Shah JN, et al. Impact of aerosolized ribavirin on mortality in 280 allogeneic haematopoietic stem cell transplant recipients with respiratory syncytial virus infections. J Antimicrob Chemother 2013;68(8):1872–80.

47. Kim YJ, Guthrie KA, Waghmare A, et al. Respiratory syncytial virus in hematopoietic cell transplant recipients: factors determining progression to lower respiratory tract disease. J Infect Dis 2014;209(8): 1195–204.

48. Casiano-Colon AE, Hulbert BB, Mayer TK, et al. Lack of sensitivity of rapid antigen tests for the

diagnosis of respiratory syncytial virus infection in adults. J Clin Virol 2003;28(2):169–74.

49. Englund JA, Piedra P, Jewell A, et al. Rapid diagnosis of respiratory syncytial virus infections in immunocompromised adults. J Clin Microbiol 1996; 34(7):1649–53.

50. Branche AR, Walsh EE, Formica MA, et al. Detection of respiratory viruses in sputum from adults by use of automated multiplex PCR. J Clin Microbiol 2014; 52(10):3590–6.

51. Walsh EE, Peterson DR, Kalkanoglu AE, et al. Viral shedding and immune responses to respiratory syncytial virus infection in older adults. J Infect Dis 2013;207(9):1424–32.

52. Duncan CB, Walsh EE, Peterson DR, et al. Risk factors for respiratory failure associated with respiratory syncytial virus infection in adults. J Infect Dis 2009; 200(8):1242–6.

53. Lee N, Chan MC, Lui GC, et al. High viral load and respiratory failure in adults hospitalized for respiratory syncytial virus infections. J Infect Dis 2015;212(8):1237–40.

54. Falsey AR, Becker KL, Swinburne AJ, et al. Bacterial complications of respiratory tract viral illness: a comprehensive evaluation. J Infect Dis 2013; 208(3):432–41.

55. Karron RA, Buchholz UJ, Collins PL. Live-attenuated respiratory syncytial virus vaccines. Curr Top Microbiol Immunol 2013;372:259–84.

56. DeVincenzo JP, McClure MW, Symons JA, et al. Activity of oral ALS-008176 in a respiratory syncytial virus challenge study. N Engl J Med 2015;373(21):2048–58.

57. DeVincenzo JP, Whitley RJ, Mackman RL, et al. Oral GS-5806 activity in a respiratory syncytial virus challenge study. N Engl J Med 2014;371(8):711–22.

58. Mejias A, Garcia-Maurino C, Rodriguez-Fernandez R, et al. Development and clinical applications of novel antibodies for prevention and treatment of respiratory syncytial virus infection. Vaccine 2016. [Epub ahead of print].

Other Community Respiratory Viruses

Richard G. Wunderink, MD

KEYWORDS

- Respiratory viral panel • Pneumonia • Acute respiratory distress syndrome • Ribavirin • Cidofovir
- Adenovirus • Coronavirus • Human metapneumovirus

KEY POINTS

- Polymerase chain reaction–based diagnosis has become the standard for viral pneumonia and other respiratory tract infections.
- Expanded respiratory viral panels (RVPs) lead to diagnosis of viral respiratory infections for which no specific treatment exists outside of influenza and, possibly, respiratory syncytial virus.
- Careful clinical evaluation, including source of sample, pattern of respiratory tract involvement and tempo of progression, degree of immunocompromise, and extrapulmonary involvement, of the patient with a positive RVP is critical, given the limited repertoire of treatments.
- Generic treatments with intravenous immunoglobulin, ribavirin, and interferons may benefit select severe viral pneumonia patients, whereas cidofovir has activity for severe adenoviral pneumonia.

INTRODUCTION

The advent of clinical use of polymerase chain reaction (PCR) technology has revolutionized the diagnosis of viral respiratory infections. Early studies demonstrated much greater sensitivity than viral culture with a clinically actionable time to results. PCR has, therefore, essentially replaced viral culture for acute clinical diagnosis. PCR has an unclear relationship to acute and convalescent serology, a prior diagnostic standard that was not clinically useful except for retrospective diagnosis. PCR detects presence of viral genomic material at the time of specimen acquisition. This usually represents acute infection, although prolonged shedding of viral genomic material after an acute infection can occur, especially in immunocompromised patients.

Multiplex platforms that perform a respiratory viral panel (RVP) have become the norm for many hospitals. The initial driving force for multiplex panels was the 2007 to 2008 seasonal influenza outbreak. During that year, 2 strains of influenza A were circulating: an H1 strain that was resistant to oseltamivir and an H3 strain that remained sensitive.[1] At that time, differentiation between influenza A and B, and between the 2 strains of influenza A, became critical in order to discontinue dual antiviral therapy. In the subsequent year, the pandemic strain of influenza A(H1N1) virus added an additional target for multiplex RVP assays.

To completely replace respiratory viral cultures, the RVPs included other clinically important viral assays used for epidemiologic purposes, such as respiratory syncytial virus (RSV) and adenovirus. Panels became progressively more extensive, including addition of newly discovered human respiratory viral pathogens such as the coronaviruses responsible for severe acute respiratory syndrome (SARS) and human metapneumovirus (HMPV). Initially perceived as simply a positive alternative when more significant pathogens were not detected, the frequent association of rhinovirus with respiratory tract disease[2] led to its

Disclosure: Dr R.G. Wunderink has consulted for GenMark Diagnostics and bioMerieux.
Department of Medicine, Pulmonary and Critical Care, Northwestern University Feinberg School of Medicine, 676 North Saint Clair Street, Arkes 14-015, Chicago, IL 60611, USA
E-mail address: r-wunderink@northwestern.edu

Clin Chest Med 38 (2017) 37–43
http://dx.doi.org/10.1016/j.ccm.2016.11.003

routine inclusion in RVP panels. Increasingly, sub-species of viruses other than influenza A were added. This was made dramatically clear with the recent epidemic of enterovirus (EV)-D68[3] which was detected as human rhinovirus in some multiplex assays and not in others. The EV species seem to have distinct trophism with C and D, mainly causing respiratory tract disease. Finally, PCR for bacterial species difficult to grow, such as *Mycoplasma* spp and *Chlamydophila* spp, and in the differential of respiratory tract infections, such as *Bordetella pertussis*, were added for con-venience and increased diagnostic yield. A spec-trum of causes covered by most multiplex RVPs is listed in **Box 1**.

Unfortunately, current multiplex RVP panels now provide laboratory diagnoses of viral respira-tory tract diseases that have few, if any, clinical treatment options. This disconnect between diag-nosis and specific treatment raises difficult man-agement issues and a tendency to ignore the results. For a positive assay on an RVP panel, influenza and atypical bacterial pathogens (if included) are clearly actionable and covered in other articles in this issue. In this article, evaluation

and management of the other respiratory viruses commonly detected with multiplex RVPs are reviewed.

PCR is also the standard for diagnosis of many other viral infections that are either rare (eg, hanta-virus syndrome or Middle East respiratory syn-drome [MERS]) or which rarely involve the lung. Because high clinical suspicion for these infections is required before ordering a PCR assay, they will not be specifically discussed in this article.

GENERAL APPROACH

Given the limited repertoire of treatment options for viral respiratory tract infections, careful assess-ment of the clinical significance of a positive PCR for any virus other than influenza is needed. In gen-eral, the indication for treatment of a positive RVP (other than influenza) is presence of or high risk of subsequently developing lower respiratory tract (LRT) infection (LRTI). **Box 2** gives a general approach to evaluating a positive RVP.

Colonization Versus Active Infection

One of the major questions is whether a positive RVP represents disease or is simply colonization or prolonged shedding from a prior unrelated infection. Many viral syndromes may have minimal symptoms, yet lead to positive screening tests. Several viruses have also been demonstrated to have prolonged shedding after symptomatic illness. Prolonged shedding is a particular problem in the immunocompromised, the exact population in which viral pneumonia is most likely to require treatment.

A perspective on the frequency of colonization or prolonged asymptomatic shedding can be gained from studies of healthy patients presenting for noninfectious clinic visits. Colonization is clearly more common in asymptomatic children than in adults.[4] A pediatric case control study of community-acquired pneumonia (CAP) compared with normal healthy controls demonstrated that

---

Box 1
Pathogens included in usual respiratory viral panels

Influenza A

- H1 lineage
- H3 lineage
- pdm2009 H1 lineage

Influenza B

Adenovirus

HMPV

Rhinovirus or EV

RSV

Parainfluenza

- Types 1 to 4

Coronavirus

- OC43, NL63, 229E, HKU1

Bocavirus

Atypical bacterial pathogens occasionally included

Mycoplasma pneumoniae

Chlamydophila pneumoniae

Bordetella pertussis

Box 2
Clinical evaluation of a positive respiratory viral panel

Colonization versus active infection

Upper respiratory tract versus LRT

Temporal pattern of symptoms

Immune status

Pattern of LRTI involvement

Extrarespiratory tract involvement

he odds ratio was greater than 10 for influenza, RSV, and HMPV, and at least greater than 1 for adenovirus.[5] For bocavirus, coronaviruses, EV, parainfluenza, and rhinovirus, the frequency of positive nasopharynx (NP) PCR tests was actually greater in asymptomatic controls than cases of pneumonia. In contrast, detection of any common respiratory virus in asymptomatic adults was only 2.1%.[4] In adults, even rhinovirus is highly associated with pneumonia with an odds ratio of greater than 13. The most common virus detected in asymptomatic adults was coronaviruses, although detection was still associated with an odds ratio for pneumonia of greater than 3.

Upper Versus Lower Respiratory Tract Disease

The second critical issue is the site of sampling. A positive sample from the LRT carries more significance than a positive sample from the NP or oropharynx (OP). Most positive viral samples are from NP or OP swabs because of the ease of obtaining the specimen. The lower in the respiratory tract that the sample is obtained, the greater the significance; that is, a positive bronchoalveolar lavage sample is much more likely to indicate viral pneumonia than an NP or OP swab. Expectorated sputum and endotracheal aspirates can represent viral tracheobronchitis or an intermediate risk of viral pneumonia.

Probably the most concerning aspect of site of sampling is the finding that patients with positive LRTI can occasionally have negative NP or OP swabs. This may result from poor sampling technique with the NP or OP swab or may actually represent a transition from upper respiratory tract (URT) to LRT disease. Of major concern is that this has been seen in patients with influenza A-induced acute respiratory distress syndrome (ARDS). Preliminary data suggest that high quality sputum samples in patients with radiographic pneumonia may be positive more often than NP or OP swabs, even for common viruses such as influenza. Obtaining an LRT sample from patient with CAP-induced respiratory failure is prudent even if the NP or OP swab is negative for influenza.

The risks for progression from viral URT infection to pneumonia or ARDS are generally unclear or nonspecific. Presence of peripheral monocytosis has been demonstrated to be associated with pneumonia in adenoviral infection.[6] For stem cell transplants, smoking, steroids, total body irradiation, and lymphopenia are associated with progression to LRTI.[7] Other investigators have suggested that detection of multiple respiratory viruses portends poor prognosis and may be a marker for occult immuncompromise.[8]

Temporal pattern of symptoms

Assessing the tempo of disease progression is also key to understanding the significance of a positive RVP. A long duration or interval since onset of URT symptoms followed by new or changed symptoms consistent with LRT or systemic infection suggests a pulmonary infiltrate in a patient with a positive NP or OP swab is more likely bacterial superinfection than primary viral pneumonia. In this case, the positive NP or OP RVP likely represents persistent shedding after an antecedent viral URI. Conversely, a negative RVP in this situation may result in seroconversion, leading to the discordant results between serology and RVPs seen in epidemiologic studies. Persistent or worsening URI symptoms suggest that a positive NP or OP RVP may be the cause of tracheobronchitis or pneumonia.

Immune status

By far the most important factor on the decision to treat a positive RVP is the immune status of the patient. Up to 50% of patients with viral pneumonia may be immunocompromised.[8] Disseminated disease, including viremia, is much more likely in the severely immunocompromised.

The type of immunocompromise associated with progression to viral pneumonia is poorly studied. Probably the greatest risk is to recent human stem cell and bone marrow transplant patients.[8] Recovery of T- and B-lymphocytes is delayed more than neutrophils and recent hematologic transplant patients may have low immunoglobulin levels. Lung transplant patients are also particularly prone to serious viral pneumonia. Use of B-cell suppressive therapy, for example, rituximab, may also predispose to progressive LRT viral infections when used for both malignancies and other immunoglobulin-mediated disease. Conversely, acute leukemia or chemotherapy-induced neutropenia may not have as important a role in severe viral infections as they do bacterial and fungal infections.

Despite the increased risk in hematologic and lung transplant recipients, most patients with viral pneumonia or viral-induced ARDS are not overtly immunocompromised. Given the frequency of infection with common respiratory viruses in both adults and children, the proportion developing LRTI is very small. Specific genetic defects in the normal host response to viral URT infection are likely in patients with these extreme manifestations.

Pattern of lower respiratory tract involvement

Four general patterns of LRTI with viruses are commonly seen: acute bronchitis or bronchiolitis in adults and children without prior lung disease, acute exacerbation of obstructive lung diseases (asthma and chronic obstructive lung disease [COPD]), pneumonia, and ARDS. The potential benefit of nonspecific therapies increases with the latter 2, whereas supportive therapy alone is usually adequate for airway-only involvement.

Acute bronchiolitis in children and exacerbation of asthma or COPD are by far the most common reasons for hospitalization with an acute viral illness. Whether specific antiviral therapy improves outcome in these entities is still under investigation. The data on influenza antivirals in exacerbations of asthma or COPD are very mixed. Data on response to the various novel agents for RSV are pending. However, RSV is a major cause of pediatric hospitalizations and justification for treatment of airway disease alone should be available from the ongoing trials.

Extrarespiratory involvement

Involvement of extrapulmonary sites with a respiratory viral infection clearly increases the propensity to treat. Sites that may be involved with respiratory viruses are listed in **Table 1**.

Viremia occurs frequently in some viral LRTIs although it has not been reported in others. However, the technology for assessing viremia in the past has been poor and incompletely studied. Experience with human immunodeficiency virus (HIV) and hepatitis viruses, in which assessing serum viral load is commonplace, may lead to greater use of whole blood viral load for assessing indication and response to therapy of respiratory viruses. A serum assay for adenovirus is commercially available.

Neurologic complications are classic for EV, including the prototypical EV D68 strain,[3] with flaccid paralysis, encephalitis, and aseptic meningitis being the most prominent features. Central nervous system involvement in influenza includes encephalitis; transverse myelitis; aseptic meningitis; and, rarely, Guillain-Barré syndrome. Up to 10% of cases of viral encephalitis may be influenza, in both adults and children.[9] Encephalitis has been associated with HMPV in case reports.

Pericarditis and myocarditis are classic for the EV strain previously called coxsackievirus. Coxsackievirus is not routinely detected with the current commercially available RVPs. Myocarditis and pericarditis were reported in the 1918 influenza pandemic but have been infrequently reported since. However, during the Asian epidemic in 1957, signs of focal or diffuse myocarditis were found in a third of autopsies.

Hepatitis can clearly complicate several viral respiratory tract infections with the classic being adenovirus. EV is also a significant risk because the group includes hepatitis A, and EV A and B groups are also associated with hepatitis.

Rhabdomyolysis has been reported with viral pneumonia, particularly from the 2009 pandemic influenza A strain. A multicenter report of patients admitted to the intensive care units found that creatinine kinase was elevated in 24%, with greater risk of renal replacement therapy and prolonged ventilation.[10] In vitro studies suggest that muscle cells also express the $\alpha 2,3$ and $\alpha 2,6$-linked sialic acid receptors, identical to the receptors influenza use to bind respiratory epithelial cells.[11] Rhabdomyolysis, therefore, seems to likely be a manifestation of viremia. Case reports have associated rhabdomyolysis with other respiratory viruses as well.

Clinical Decisions

The clinical response to a positive RVP can take a variety of forms. In many ways, the most straightforward responses occur when specific treatments are available, such as for influenza and, potentially, RSV. Management of infection with other viruses in an RVP panel requires a much more nuanced approach. The primary clinical question is "Does providing a viral diagnosis lead to differential treatment?"

Antibiotic discontinuation

A major clinical question is whether a positive viral diagnosis in patients with LRTI allows safe avoidance or discontinuation of antibiotics. No randomized controlled trial has specifically addressed this issue. The most pertinent publications are before-and-after studies of introduction of a multiplex PCR into a specific institution. One large study suggested that a positive RVP did not decrease antibiotic utilization but did have a significant impact on increased antiviral use

Table 1
Extrapulmonary site of infection with respiratory viruses

Manifestation	Viruses Involved
Viremia	? all: influenza, adenovirus, rhinovirus, EV
Encephalitis or cerebritis	Adenovirus, EV, influenza, RSV
Hepatitis	Adenovirus, influenza, RSV
Pericarditis	Influenza
Myocarditis	Adenovirus, influenza, EV, RSV
Rhabdomyolysis	Influenza

(purely oseltamivir) and a 6% decrease in chest computed tomography (CT) scans.[12]

The most pertinent study was a pilot randomized controlled trial of the combination of serum procalcitonin and multiplex RVP in subjects with nonpneumonic LRTI.[13] In this study, subjects with a positive RVP had significantly less discharge antibiotics and a trend toward shorter duration of antibiotic therapy, especially with high protocol adherence. The combination of a low procalcitonin and positive RVP is also demonstrated to be too few antibiotics in an observational study of pneumonia.[14]

Until true randomized control trials are available, the current data suggest that a positive RVP alone is insufficient evidence to discontinue antibiotics. However, a positive RVP seems to have a synergistic effect with procalcitonin, a biomarker that has independently been associated with decreased antibiotic therapy, to decrease the duration of antibiotic therapy. Avoiding all antibiotic therapy in patients with pneumonia seems to be an unlikely use of RVP. In addition, a positive RVP may give enough clinical assurance to avoid additional diagnostic procedures, such as chest CT scans or bronchoscopy for patients who are failing empirical antibiotic therapy. In contrast, avoidance of antibiotics in other LRTIs, including acute exacerbations of COPD and acute simple bronchitis based on a positive RVP and low procalcitonin may be clinically safe.

GENERIC TREATMENT

In addition to decisions regarding antibiotics, several other clinically relevant generic treatments may be affected by a positive RVP.

Anticholinergics for Bronchospasm

The initial resurgence use of anticholinergic bronchodilators was the recognition that postviral cough and bronchospasm seemed to respond better to anticholinergics than the then standard β-agonist bronchodilators. For COPD exacerbations, anticholinergics are now standard therapies, although significantly less so for asthma. Therefore, a positive RVP may suggest the need to add anticholinergics that the patient was not previously taking. More importantly, a positive RVP may generate less concern about prolonged exacerbation because certain viruses are associated with prolonged bronchospasm, including rhinovirus, influenza, parainfluenza, and RSV. In this situation, avoidance of escalation in corticosteroid dose or duration may result from knowledge of the viral trigger. No prospective randomized trial has addressed this issue.

Extracorporeal Membrane Oxygenation

Documentation of viral pneumonia causing ARDS is increasingly being recognized as an indication for venovenous (VV) extracorporeal membrane oxygenation (ECMO). Improvements in technical aspects of ECMO, including simplification of the membrane oxygenator, VV circuits, and use of a single catheter, have taken this from a rare intervention to becoming part of the standard armamentarium in tertiary referral centers.

In recent years, pneumonia secondary to the pandemic A(H1N1) strain has become the leading nontransplant indication for VV-ECMO. The LRT trophism of this influenza strain and the predilection for previously healthy young patients may be the main reasons. However, other respiratory viruses are associated with severe ARDS and need for rescue therapies. Viral-induced ARDS is less likely to respond to other rescue therapies such as prone positioning or high PEEP. In addition, lack of a reliable treatment of the underlying disease, as seen with bacterial pneumonia, may have pushed clinical care more toward this type of support.

GENERIC ANTIVIRAL THERAPIES

Lack of specific antiviral therapies has led to use of several more generic forms. Generally, these are reserved for patients with pneumonia or ARDS, or for patients with severe immunocompromise. In addition, they are often used in combination, making dissecting out to individual benefits very difficult.

A positive RVP may be a contraindication to other generic antiviral therapies. Patients infected with both SARS coronavirus and severe pandemic A(H1N1) virus seem to be worsened with the use of systemic corticosteroids.[15,16] Therefore, a positive RVP may be an indication to avoid steroids in patients with ARDS.

In patients with organ transplant, a positive RVP may be a consideration for decreasing the degree of immunosuppression. Although this may be possible in renal transplant and some other solid organ transplants, the combination of organ rejection or graft versus host disease and a positive RVP is often a lethal combination, mainly because high-dose immunosuppression cannot be decreased.

Intravenous Immunoglobulin

The rationale for use of intravenous immunoglobulin (IVIG) is the probability of virus-specific antibodies present in the pooled immunoglobulin extracted from multiple people. Because of the pooled specimens and variable exposure and titers of virus-specific antibodies, the benefit may be inconsistent. Plasma from patients who have recently recovered from serious viral infections may have much more effectiveness but limited availability. Data from RSV antibody work suggest that the benefit of IVIG may be greatest when viremia is still occurring but may not stop direct cell-to-adjacent-cell spread of viruses.

Ribavirin

Ribavirin, a guanosine analog, seems to have activity against a broad spectrum of both RNA and DNA viruses and has been used for a variety of viral respiratory tract infections.[17] Greatest use has been in the immunocompromised population, often in combination with IVIG. Ribavirin treatment has been attempted in severe pneumonia from almost all the viruses in the usual RVP. Unfortunately, most of the studies are uncontrolled and nonblinded, making estimation of the true benefit of ribavirin difficult to determine. Also, most gave other immunomodulators, including IVIG and corticosteroids, further obscuring the potential benefit.

Aerosolized ribavirin has generally fallen into disfavor secondary to the significant teratogenic effects and difficulty in venting the drug from the patient's room without potentially affecting caregivers or visitors. Oral or intravenous ribavirin has been associated with hemolytic anemia and severe hypomagnesemia, requiring drug discontinuation in as many as 15% of cases.

Interferon

Recently, the availability of different interferon formulations has been explored in the treatment of severe viral respiratory infections. These pharmaceutical interferon medications have been developed principally for the treatment of chronic hepatitis. Interferon is a critical part of the normal host response to respiratory viral infections as well. Although it is tempting to suspect that immunocompetent patients who develop severe viral pneumonia or ARDS may have alterations in their interferon response, only limited data support this concept.[18]

The greatest support for interferon combination therapy in respiratory viral infections comes from a historical-control cohort series of treatment of the coronavirus-induced MERS.[19] Pegylated interferon alfa-2a weekly for 2 weeks and daily ribavirin were used to treat 20 subjects with documented MERS. Early survival at 14 days was significantly higher (70%) than a historical control at the same

site (29%). However, sustained survival was not demonstrated. The combination of interferon and ribavirin also seems to be synergistic for SARS coronavirus.[20]

Interferon-β-1a has been used to treat patients with ARDS,[21] many of which had pneumonia although the frequency of viral pneumonia was unknown. In a small pilot study, 28 day mortality was significantly improved compared with control. Interferon-β has also been used as an aerosol to treat viral-induced exacerbations of asthma with equivocal results.[22] The combination of interferon α2a and ribavirin has also been used to treat refractory serious rhinovirus respiratory tract infections in patients with hypogammaglobulinemia with good results.[23]

SPECIFIC ANTIVIRALS

The only specific antiviral treatment of pathogens, other than influenza and RSV, is cidofovir for serious adenoviral pneumonia. Released for treatment of cytomegalovirus retinitis in HIV patients, intravenous cidofovir has been used in both immunocompromised and immunocompetent patients. Treatment is clearly more effective in immunocompetent[24] than immunocompromised patients.[25,26] Cidofovir has significant nephrotoxicity. Adenoviral serum titer measurement is commercially available and can assist in determining the duration of therapy, although 1 or 2 doses weekly is usually sufficient for those patients likely to respond.

Pleconaril has been studied in neonatal EV sepsis with successful results.[27] Possible use in serious enteroviral or rhinoviral respiratory tract infections has not been studied and the drug is not clinically available yet. Side effects seem to be very tolerable.

SUMMARY

PCR-based diagnosis has become the standard for viral pneumonia and other respiratory tract infections. Expansion of RVPs outside of influenza, and possibly RSV, has led to the ability to diagnose viral infections for which no approved specific antiviral treatment exists. Careful clinical evaluation of the patient with a positive RVP is, therefore, critical given the limited repertoire of treatments. Generic treatments with IVIG, ribavirin, and interferons may benefit select severe viral pneumonia patients, whereas cidofovir has activity for severe adenoviral pneumonia. Development of new treatments will add significant value to the ability to detect viral respiratory pathogens.

REFERENCES

1. Dharan NJ, Gubareva LV, Meyer JJ, et al. Infections with oseltamivir-resistant influenza A(H1N1) virus in the United States. JAMA 2009;301(10):1034–41.

2. Royston L, Tapparel C. Rhinoviruses and respiratory enteroviruses: not as simple as ABC. Viruses 2016;8(1):E16.

3. Holm-Hansen CC, Midgley SE, Fischer TK. Global emergence of enterovirus D68: a systematic review. Lancet Infect Dis 2016;16(5):e64–75.

4. Self WH, Williams DJ, Zhu Y, et al. Respiratory viral detection in children and adults: comparing asymptomatic controls and patients with community-acquired pneumonia. J Infect Dis 2016;213(4):584–91.

5. Rhedin S, Lindstrand A, Hjelmgren A, et al. Respiratory viruses associated with community-acquired pneumonia in children: matched case-control study. Thorax 2015;70(9):847–53.

6. Yoon H, Jhun BW, Kim SJ, et al. Clinical characteristics and factors predicting respiratory failure in adenovirus pneumonia. Respirology 2016;21(7): 1243–50.

7. Kim YJ, Guthrie KA, Waghmare A, et al. Respiratory syncytial virus in hematopoietic cell transplant recipients: factors determining progression to lower respiratory tract disease. J Infect Dis 2014;209(8): 1195–204.

8. Crotty MP, Meyers S, Hampton N, et al. Epidemiology, co-infections, and outcomes of viral pneumonia in adults: an observational cohort study. Medicine (Baltimore) 2015;94(50):e2332.

9. Kolski H, Ford-Jones EL, Richardson S, et al. Etiology of acute childhood encephalitis at the hospital for sick children, Toronto, 1994-1995. Clin Infect Dis 1998;26(2):398–409.

10. Borgatta B, Perez M, Rello J, et al. Elevation of creatine kinase is associated with worse outcomes in 2009 pH1N1 influenza A infection. Intensive Care Med 2012;38(7):1152–61.

11. Desdouits M, Munier S, Prevost MC, et al. Productive infection of human skeletal muscle cells by pandemic and seasonal influenza A(H1N1) viruses. PLoS One 2013;8(11):e79628.

12. Mulpuru S, Aaron SD, Ronksley PE, et al. Hospital resource utilization and patient outcomes associated with respiratory viral testing in hospitalized patients. Emerg Infect Dis 2015;21(8):1366–71.

13. Branche AR, Walsh EE, Vargas R, et al. Serum procalcitonin measurement and viral testing to guide antibiotic use for respiratory infections in hospitalized adults: a randomized controlled trial. J Infect Dis 2015;212(11):1692–700.

14. Gelfer G, Leggett J, Myers J, et al. The clinical impact of the detection of potential etiologic pathogens of community-acquired pneumonia. Diagn Microbiol Infect Dis 2015;83(4):400–6.

15. Brun-Buisson C, Richard JC, Mercat A, et al. Early corticosteroids in severe influenza A/H1N1 pneumonia and acute respiratory distress syndrome. Am J Respir Crit Care Med 2011;183(9): 1200–6.

16. Diaz E, Martin-Loeches I, Canadell L, et al. Corticosteroid therapy in patients with primary viral pneumonia due to pandemic (H1N1) 2009 influenza. J Infect 2012;64(3):311–8.

17. Gross AE, Bryson ML. Oral ribavirin for the treatment of noninfluenza respiratory viral infections: a systematic review. Ann Pharmacother 2015;49(10): 1125–35.

18. Everitt AR, Clare S, Pertel T, et al. IFITM3 restricts the morbidity and mortality associated with influenza. Nature 2012;484(7395):519–23.

19. Omrani AS, Saad MM, Baig K, et al. Ribavirin and interferon alfa-2a for severe Middle East respiratory syndrome coronavirus infection: a retrospective cohort study. Lancet Infect Dis 2014;14(11): 1090–5.

20. Chen F, Chan KH, Jiang Y, et al. In vitro susceptibility of 10 clinical isolates of SARS coronavirus to selected antiviral compounds. J Clin Virol 2004; 31(1):69–75.

21. Bellingan G, Maksimow M, Howell DC, et al. The effect of intravenous interferon-beta-1a (FP-1201) on lung CD73 expression and on acute respiratory distress syndrome mortality: an open-label study. Lancet Respir Med 2014;2(2):98–107.

22. Djukanovic R, Harrison T, Johnston SL, et al. The effect of inhaled IFN-beta on worsening of asthma symptoms caused by viral infections. A randomized trial. Am J Respir Crit Care Med 2014;190(2): 145–54.

23. Ruuskanen O, Waris M, Kainulainen L. Treatment of persistent rhinovirus infection with pegylated interferon alpha2a and ribavirin in patients with hypogammaglobulinemia. Clin Infect Dis 2014;58(12): 1784–6.

24. Kim SJ, Kim K, Park SB, et al. Outcomes of early administration of cidofovir in non-immunocompromised patients with severe adenovirus pneumonia. PLoS One 2015;10(4):e0122642.

25. Symeonidis N, Jakubowski A, Pierre-Louis S, et al. Invasive adenoviral infections in T-cell-depleted allogeneic hematopoietic stem cell transplantation: high mortality in the era of cidofovir. Transpl Infect Dis 2007;9(2):108–13.

26. Lion T. Adenovirus infections in immunocompetent and immunocompromised patients. Clin Microbiol Rev 2014;27(3):441–62.

27. Abzug MJ, Michaels MG, Wald E, et al. A randomized, double-blind, placebo-controlled trial of pleconaril for the treatment of neonates with enterovirus sepsis. J Pediatric Infect Dis Soc 2016; 5(1):53–62.

Atypical Pneumonia
Updates on *Legionella*, *Chlamydophila*, and *Mycoplasma* Pneumonia

Lokesh Sharma, PhD[a,1], Ashley Losier, MD[b,1],
Thomas Tolbert, MD[c,1], Charles S. Dela Cruz, MD, PhD[a],
Chad R. Marion, DO, PhD[a],*

KEYWORDS

- Community-acquired pneumonia (CAP) • Walking pneumonia • *Legionella* • Legionnaires' disease
- Pontiac fever • *Chlamydophila* • *Mycoplasma*

KEY POINTS

- The clinical diagnosis of atypical pneumonia remains elusive but recent advances in rapid diagnostic platforms show promise of earlier identification of the infectious organism.
- Macrolides and respiratory fluoroquinolones remain the antibiotics of choice for atypical pneumonia but there are several new antibiotics currently under development or clinical trials.
- Both *Chlamydophila* and *Mycoplasma* have been associated with chronic diseases, but *Legionella* seems to occur sporadically and is not associated with chronic diseases.

INTRODUCTION

Pneumonia is a common cause of hospital admission and mortality and is categorized based on the clinical context in which a patient develops symptoms of infection. These categories include community-acquired pneumonia (CAP), CAP with risk factors of resistant organisms, hospital-acquired pneumonia, and ventilator-associated events. CAP is defined as contracting pneumonia with minimal or no recent contact with the healthcare system CAP is one of the most common infectious diseases and is caused by various infectious pathogens, including viruses, typical bacteria, and atypical pathogens. This article reviews the clinical considerations of atypical causes of CAP that include *Legionella*, *Mycoplasma*, and *Chlamydophila* and discusses current controversies surrounding the diagnosis and treatment of atypical CAP.

LEGIONELLA PNEUMOPHILA
Clinical Presentation

Legionella infections are manifested mainly in 2 forms:

1. Legionnaires' disease, which is a severe form of pneumonia due to infection with *Legionella*. Legionnaires' disease can manifest as a multisystem disease most commonly involving the lungs and gastrointestinal tract and is associated with significant mortality.[1]

2. Pontiac fever, which is a mild and self-resolving flu-like disease. The characteristics of Pontiac fever are mild fever, chills, myalgia, and

[a] Section of Pulmonary, Critical Care and Sleep Medicine, Yale University School of Medicine, 300 Cedar Street, TAC S440, New Haven, CT 06510, USA; [b] Department of Internal Medicine, Norwalk Hospital, 34 Maple Street, Norwalk, CT 06856, USA; [c] Department of Internal Medicine, Yale University School of Medicine, 330 Cedar Street, New Haven, CT 06510, USA
[1] Contributed equally to this article.
* Corresponding author.
E-mail address: chad.marion@yale.edu

Clin Chest Med 38 (2017) 45–58
http://dx.doi.org/10.1016/j.ccm.2016.11.011

headache that lasts 2 to 5 days and often resolves itself without significant mortality.[2]

Legionella mostly affects people above 50 years of age but cases have been reported in infants and neonates.[3] Legionnaires' disease is hard to distinguish from pneumonia caused by other pathogens because it presents similar clinical symptoms; however, presence of diarrhea and elevated creatinine kinase levels can be indicators of infection by *Legionella*.[4] Pneumonia due to *Legionella* is usually found in clusters that are not associated with person-to-person transmissions but is related to exposure to the same source of infection. Most of the *Legionella* infections are acquired by contaminated water or soil. Rainfall, high humidity, and work in gardens with compost are risk factors for acquiring *Legionella* disease.[5–7] Most of the cases of legionnaires' disease are associated with *Legionella pneumophila*, but many other bacterial species have been found to cause *Legionella* lung infections.[7,8]

Diagnostic Considerations

Because many manifestations of *Legionella* are similar to other typical and atypical pneumonias, clinical symptoms or radiologic evidences are of little value for diagnostic purposes. The Centers for Disease Control and Prevention defines confirmation of infection if *Legionella* can be cultured from sputum or bronchoalveolar lavage, a positive urine antigen test, or a 4-fold increase in antibodies specific to *Legionella*.[9,10] Details about these tests are summarized in **Table 1**. Polymerase chain reaction (PCR)-based diagnostic tests are being tested and some of them show specificity and sensitivity, although these tests are yet to be approved by Food and Drug Administration

(FDA). Other tools, such as direct immunostaining, are used to detect the presence of bacterium but frequently require invasive procedures to collect tissue for testing.[11]

Prognosis

Legionnaires' disease has significant mortality rates if untreated or if there is delay in administrating appropriate antibiotic therapy. The risk factors associated with mortality are acquiring the infection in nosocomial settings, diabetes, immunosuppression, and malignancies.[12,13] Complete recovery from the infection in these susceptible populations might be prolonged and signs of stress and trauma might persist for years.[14]

Treatment

Antibiotics are the first-line therapy for *Legionella* pneumonia. Failure to administer appropriate antimicrobial therapies at early stage of infection is associated with high mortality rates.[15,16] The correct choice of antibiotic depends not only on its in vitro bactericidal or bacteriostatic activity but also on its ability to penetrate the cell membrane of host tissues because *Legionella* resides within host tissue cells. Fluoroquinolones and macrolides are the 2 most commonly used and highly effective antibiotics to treat patients with legionnaires' disease. Including these agents in initial treatment regimen is prudent if *Legionella* infection is suspected based on an ongoing outbreak in the area, travel history, or extrapulmonary symptoms.[17]

It was found during the first reported outbreak of legionnaires' disease that tetracycline and erythromycin are more effective than other antibiotics, such as β-lactam antibiotics, whereas the use of steroids has been associated with unfavorable outcome.[1] Erythromycin has been the antibiotic

Table 1
Diagnostic tests for *Legionella* species

Test	Sensitivity (%)	Advantages	Limitations
Culture	20–80	Detects all the *Legionella* species	Takes technical expertise, longer duration >5 d
Urinary antigen	70–100	Quick, same-day results, not affected by antibiotic treatment	Kits available are limited mostly to *Legionella pneumophila*; other species may go undetected
Serology	80–90	Little effect of antibiotic treatment	Paired samples are required
Direct fluorescence assay	25–75	Performed on pathologic tissue	Technically difficult

of choice for the treatment of legionnaires' disease that is highly effective but has been associated with significant side effects, especially when used intravenously.[16,18–20] Azithromycin, another macrolide, has been shown highly effective in treating patients with *Legionella* infection, with minor side effects.[21] Azithromycin has been successfully used to treat *Legionella* infection not responding to erythromycin and is frequently chosen to treat patients infected with *Legionella*.[22] Other antibiotics that are effective against *Legionella* are clarithromycin, rifampin, ciprofloxacin, and doxycycline, and these are used either alone or with erythromycin.[18] In a prospective study, it has been shown that fluoroquinolones are at least as effective as erythromycin in treating patients with legionnaires' disease.[23] Levofloxacin, either 500 mg for 10 days or 750 mg for 5 days, can cure most of the patients (>95%) and is becoming the antibiotic of choice for legionnaires' disease.[24] Use of levofloxacin is increasing to treat *Legionella* infection and is associated with early clinical response and shorter hospital stay.[25] A meta-analysis by Burdet and colleagues[26] revealed quinolones may be superior to macrolides in treating the *Legionella* infection.

The usual duration of therapy for most of the antibiotics is 5 to 10 days and is often sufficient to completely treat patients with *Legionella* infection, but duration of therapy up to 3 weeks may be considered in immunocompromised patients.[17] The route of administration used for the antibiotics depends on the severity of the infection, with parenteral therapy preferred for severe infections. If intravenous therapy is initiated early in infection, then therapy can be transitioned to oral route to complete therapy once a desirable response is observed. Treatment options are outlined in Table 2.

Acquired antibiotic resistance among *Legionella* species can be seen in vitro but is rarely reported in vivo, although a recent report has shown the presence of fluoroquinolone resistance in *Legionella* in patients who are treated with these antibiotics.[27,28] These reports warrant special attention toward ineffectiveness or relapse of disease during ongoing antibiotic therapy.

Conflicts and Controversies

Most cases of legionnaires' disease reported are due to *Legionella* pneumophila serotype 1 (80%).[29] This might reflect a diagnosis bias because most of the commercial kits available detect *Legionella* serotype-1 antigen in urine samples but not for other species. Efforts are under way to develop rapid diagnostic test for *Legionella* species, such

as multiplex PCR assays, and may be more efficacious than detection of *Legionella* pneumophila serotype-1 antigen in patients' urine.[11,30]

To date, there are few reported cases of *Legionella* species that are resistant to conventional antibiotics resistance and there is little evidence that combination therapy is superior to monotherapy.[31,32] *Legionella* resistant to ciprofloxacin has been reported. It was unclear if the strain of *Legionella* was resistant at the presentation of disease or developed resistance during treatment because the patient was treated with ciprofloxacin and clinically improved from severe infection.[27] Regardless, several new antibiotics are under development that target intracellular organisms, such as *Legionella*, either by favoring a low pH enthronement or by inhibiting bacterial protein synthesis.[33–35] Currently, these therapies are not available for clinical use.

Person-to-person transfer is usually not considered a route of transmission for *Legionella*; however, reports are emerging showing person-to-person transfer.[36,37] Despite these reports, person-to-person contact seems to be the exception. The best means of preventing disease is by thwarting the contamination of water supplies. Water temperature, pipe age, and pipe configuration have been

Table 2
Antibiotic therapy for *Legionella*, *Chlamydophila*, and *Mycoplasma* community-acquired pneumonia

Medication	Dose
Azithromycin	1.5 g over 5 d (500 mg on day 1 followed by 250 mg for 4 d)
Clarithromycin	500 mg PO bid for 10 d
Doxycycline	100 mg bid for 7–21 d
Tetracycline	250 mg qid for 7–21 d
Levofloxacin	750 mg PO/IV for 5–10 d or 500 mg PO/IV daily for 7–14 d
Moxifloxacin	400 mg daily for 10 d
Nemonoxacin[a]	500 mg daily for 7 d or 750 mg daily for 7 d
Slorithromycin[a]	800 mg on day 1 followed by 400 mg daily for 4 d

[a] Nemonoxacin and slorithromycin remain in the trial phase and are not yet FDA approved. Nemonoxacin treatment was associated with clinical in all patients with *C pneumoniae* identified as etiologic pathogen between 22 phase II clinical trials (n = 9). Slorithromycin shows in vitro activity against *C pneumoniae* but has not been specifically tested in vivo.

Data from Refs.[60,62,66]

shown to play a role in the contamination of water supplies with Legionella.[38,39] Current recommendations to prevent Legionella contamination include maintaining water temperature outside the optimal temperature for Legionella growth, preventing stagnation, superheat-and-flush or point-of-use filters, UV irradiation, and chemical disinfection.[40] Currently there are no clear recommendations as to optimal combination of preventative measures; therefore, despite the method of prevention utilized, the World Health Organization recommends quarterly water testing.[41]

CHLAMYDOPHILA PNEUMONIAE
Clinical Presentation

Chlamydophila pneumoniae has been implicated in upper respiratory infections, acute bronchitis, and pneumonia.[42] The common symptoms of C pneumoniae pneumonia and their frequencies are presented in **Table 3**. Classically, pneumonia due to C pneumoniae presents as a mild illness predominated by fever and cough, often preceded by upper respiratory symptoms of rhinitis and sore throat. In a 2013 study of an outbreak by Conklin

and colleagues,[43] duration of cough ranged from 1 to 64 days with a mean of 21 days. Although the classic presentation is associated with nonproductive cough, approximately 70% of patients presented with sputum production in outbreaks of C pneumoniae infection in 2006 and 2013. The presentation is especially difficult to distinguish from pneumonia due to Mycoplasma pneumoniae or respiratory viruses. Despite previous suggestions that hoarseness and laryngitis are more common in infection from C pneumoniae than from M pneumoniae, comparison of clinical features of both causes have shown the opposite.[44,45] Punji and colleagues[45] demonstrated that cough, rhinitis, and hoarseness were significantly more common in M pneumoniae infection than in C Pneumoniae infection. In the same study, C-reactive protein and aspartate aminotransferase elevations were significantly greater in C pneumoniae infection than in M pneumoniae infection. Other clinical symptoms and laboratory findings due to the 2 pathogens were not significantly different. C-reactive protein and white blood cell values have been previously shown significantly lower in both C pneumoniae and M pneumoniae pneumonia than in pneumonia due to Streptococcus pneumoniae.[44] No single symptom, laboratory finding, or collection of findings can reliably distinguish pneumonia due to C pneumoniae from pneumonia due to other respiratory pathogens. Additionally, C pneumoniae infection may occur concomitantly with other pathogens, which may influence clinical presentation.[44]

Imaging

A list of roentgenographic manifestations of C pneumoniae is presented in **Table 4**. On initial chest radiograph, a unilateral pattern of alveolar infiltrates or bronchopneumonia predominates. Findings are usually confined to a single lobe with lower lobe involvement more frequent than middle or upper lobe involvement.[46–48] A pattern of interstitial pneumonia is comparatively rare. Up to a quarter of patients may demonstrate a small to moderate-size pleural effusion. Hilar or mediastinal lymphadenopathy is an uncommon finding on chest radiograph. Findings may depend on the timing of imaging in the course of the illness, the method of diagnosis, and whether concomitant infection with another respiratory pathogen is excluded. In 1 review of 17 patients classified as having primary infection, admission chest radiographs showed predominantly unilateral findings with repeat chest radiographs taken an average of 3.8 days later showing predominantly bilateral findings.[46]

Table 3
Major symptoms encountered in Chlamydophila pneumoniae community-acquired pneumonia

	Frequency (%)
Constitutional	
Fever	68.1–97.8
Myalgias/arthralgias	37.5–40.5
Confusion	7.5
Upper respiratory/ear, nose and throat	
Headache	25–60
Rhinorrhea	6.7–72.9
Sinus pain	43.2
Sore throat	9–72.9
Hoarseness	15.7
Lower respiratory	
Cough	82–98
Sputum production	67.5–68.8
Dyspnea	25–58.3
Wheezing	58.7
Chest pain	9–17.5
Hemoptysis	7.5
Gastrointestinal	
Nausea ± vomiting	5–19.1
Diarrhea	5–12.5

Data from Refs.[43–45]

Table 4
Major imaging findings in *Chlamydophila pneumoniae* community-acquired pneumonia

Imaging Type	Chest Radiograph (%)	CT Scan (%)
Distribution		
Unilateral	42–75	50
Bilateral	24–25	50
Involvement of only 1 lobe	62–86	33
Lower lobe	88	71
Middle lobe	25	46
Upper lobe	21	67
Chest radiograph patterns		
Bronchopneumonia	88	—
Alveolar infiltrates	29–86	—
Interstitial infiltrates	0–4	—
Air bronchogram	57	—
CT parenchymal findings		
Consolidation	—	83
Bronchovascular bundle thickening	—	71
Reticular or linear opacity	—	62
Ground-glass opacities	—	54
Pulmonary emphysema	—	46
Airway dilatation	—	38
Lymphadenopathy	0–17	33
Pleural effusion	14–38	25

Data from [Chest radiograph] Kauppinen MT, Lahde S, Syrjala H. Roentgenographic findings of pneumonia caused by Chlamydia pneumoniae. A comparison with streptococcus pneumonia. Arch Intern Med 1996;156(16):1851–6; Boersma WG, Daniels JM, Löwenberg A, et al. Reliability of radiographic findings and the relation to etiologic agents in community-acquired pneumonia. Respir Med 2006;100(5):926–32; and *[CT scan]* Nambu A, Saito A, Araki T, et al. Chlamydia pneumoniae: comparison with findings of Mycoplasma pneumoniae and Streptococcus pneumoniae at thin-section CT. Radiology 2006;238(1):330–8.

In a retrospective review of thin-section CT scans of 24 patients serologically diagnosed with *C pneumonia* CAP, Nambu and colleagues[49] found a significant increase in airway dilatation compared with patients with pneumonia due to *S pneumoniae* or *M pneumoniae* as well as an increased rate of pulmonary emphysema compared with *M pneumoniae* but not *S pneumoniae*. The study speculated that the increased rate of airway dilatation and pulmonary emphysema may reflect obstructive lung disease as a predisposing risk factor for *C pneumoniae* pneumonia and may not be caused by the infection itself. Despite the statistically significant increase in airway dilatation and/or pulmonary emphysema, neither these findings nor any other on CT was able to reliably distinguish pneumonia from *C pneumoniae* from pneumonia due to other pathogens. Overall, findings in *C pneumoniae* on CT scan were widely variable. Involvement of more than 1 lobe, usually upper and/or lower lobe involvement, with consolidation and bronchovascular bundle thickening were the predominant findings. Bilateral lung involvement was seen in half of patients. Ultimately, the imaging findings on either radiograph or CT scan are nonspecific for *C pneumoniae* and cannot be reliably used to identify the pathogen in the etiology of pneumonia.[46–48]

Diagnostic Considerations

Accepted techniques for identifying *Chlamydophila* infection include serologic studies and culture or PCR of respiratory tract samples. Historically, diagnosis of *Chlamydophila* infection has relied on serologic studies, requiring a 4-fold rise in IgG or IgA levels between acute and convalescent serum samples. Serologic methods in general are cumbersome because patients must return 4 to 6 weeks after initial presentation to retrospectively confirm the diagnosis. Moreover, the retrospective nature of diagnosis means serologic results have little effect on treatment decisions. Alternative serologic criteria allowing diagnosis on initial presentation, such as a serum IgM antibody titer of 1:16 or greater, rely on the timing of sample collection, because a rise in titers may not be observed early in the course of acute infection or reinfection.[50,51] Relying solely on initial serologic samples for diagnosis (that is, forgoing retrospective confirmation with convalescent serum samples) risks missing 25% to 33% of infections.[52] Additionally, initial serologic testing may take days to result, further limiting their use in initial management decisions. Serologic techniques are limited in specificity by potential cross-reactivity between C pneumoniae antigens and antigens of other Chlamydia species.

Microimmunofluorescence is considered the reference standard for serologic diagnosis.[42,51] ELISA is also available and may be less technically demanding and more objectively interpretable than microimmunofluorescence.[51] Complement fixation is not a recommended diagnostic technique owing to a limited sensitivity and specificity.[42,52]

Although considered specific due to a low rate of asymptomatic carriage, the sensitivity of culture is markedly limited by the fastidious and slow growth of Chlamydophila, which may require weeks.[42,50,53] Previous studies have shown a very low frequency of growth in culture, even from specimens where infection is identified by serology and/or PCR.[52] In a 2010 study, She and colleagues[50] recommended against the routine use of culture for diagnosis after failing to identify any positive culture results from 6981 specimens from patients with respiratory symptoms despite a rate of Chlamydophila as the cause of CAP and other respiratory infections of 5% to 22%.

Given the limitations of serology and culture, PCR of respiratory tract specimens has emerged as the favored method of diagnosis. Specimens may be assessed with multiplex PCR, allowing for the detection of multiple potential respiratory pathogens without significant diminishment in sensitivity compared with singleplex PCR testing.[54] In 2012, the FDA approved the FilmArray Respiratory Panel (BioMérieux, France), which uses multiplex PCR for the detection of C pneumoniae in addition to M pneumoniae, Bordetella pertussis, and 17 respiratory viruses on nasopharyngeal swab (NPS) specimens.[55] PCR remains limited in specificity, however, by asymptomatic carriage, which approaches 5% in healthy adults.[53] Specificity is further limited by a pattern of persistence of Chlamydophila identified on respiratory swabs well after resolution of clinical symptoms in some patients. In a recent outbreak, approximately 80% of patients who were positive for Chlamydophila infection by PCR of respiratory samples remained positive for up to 8 weeks after resolution of symptoms.[43] Patients may continue to harbor the pathogen in the absence of symptoms for up to 11 months, even after appropriate antibiotic therapy.[56] Positive PCR results in patients with a history of C pneumoniae infection may, therefore, be challenging to attribute definitively to reinfection, persistent infection or ongoing asymptomatic carriage with other potential pathogens causing new symptoms.[57] Furthermore, the identification of Chlamydophila in respiratory samples does not rule out coinfection with other pathogens, which has been noted to occur in multiple studies and may affect clinical presentation.[44,46,47,52,53]

Alternative methods of detection include identification of circulating Chlamydophila lipopolysaccharide in serum, C pneumoniae presence in circulating phagocytes or atheromas, and seroresponse to C pneumoniae antigens. These methods are technically demanding, however, and currently used only in research settings.[51]

Prognosis

Compared with infection with typical bacterial respiratory pathogens, such as Streptococcus, Klebsiella, and Pseudomonas species, the course and outcomes for pneumonia due to C pneumoniae are thought to be benign. Outcomes are typically reported for patients with atypical pneumonias as a group, however, and there are few data available on outcomes specific to C pneumoniae.

A 2012 study of etiologic agents in CAP and their effect on outcomes by Capelastegui and colleagues[58] identified 151 patients with pneumonia due to atypical pathogens, 37 of whom (or 24%) had C pneumoniae.[49] Atypical pneumonia had a hospitalization rate of 25.8%, an ICU admission rate of 0.7%, and a mechanical ventilation rate of 0.7%. With the exception of mechanical ventilation, these rates were significantly lower for atypical pneumonias than for pneumonia due to typical bacteria; 30-day mortality was 1.3% compared with 4.3% for pneumonia due to typical bacteria, although this difference was not statistically significant. Outcomes more specific to C pneumoniae were not reported. The mortality rate of C pneumoniae pneumonia is likely low, with 30-day mortality rates for atypical pneumonias in general ranging from 0% to 2.2%.[59] In the 2013 outbreak studied by Conklin and colleagues[43] no deaths were reported among 52 patients. However, 22 of these patients had persistently positive oropharyngeal swabs (OPSs) or *C pneumoniae* up to 8 weeks after the outbreak, and many of these patients experienced cough symptoms for several weeks after completion of antibiotic treatment. Patients should be advised that cough could persist even after completion of an appropriate antibiotic course.

Treatment

Recommendations for antibiotic treatment of *C pneumoniae* are limited by an absence of standardized diagnostic criteria and the use of serology alone for diagnosis in most previous studies. Infectious Diseases Society of America (IDSA) guidelines from 2007 note a lack of strong evidence to recommend specific antibiotic therapy for the pathogen.[17] Treatment recommendations continue to rely on expert opinion. Given a pattern of reappearance of symptoms after a standard course of therapy, longer courses of antibiotics have been recommended when *Chlamydophila* is identified.[42] A list of antibiotics, their doses, and treatment courses as recommended by expert opinion is given in **Table 2**.[60]

Because *C pneumoniae* is an obligate intracellular microbe, antibiotics must achieve intracellular penetration to achieve efficacy. Antibiotics that interfere with DNA and protein synthesis, including macrolides, tetracyclines, and fluoroquinolones, demonstrate in vitro activity against the pathogen and are the recommended drug classes for clinical treatment. Ciprofloxacin, however, demonstrates a higher minimum inhibitory concentration than other fluoroquinolones and may, therefore, be less efficacious. *C pneumoniae* is resistant to trimethoprim, sulfonamides, aminoglycosides, and glycopeptides. Penicillin and amoxicillin have demonstrated in vitro activity against *Chlamydia* species but are not recommended as part of routine therapy against *C pneumoniae*.

Resistance to the recommended therapies is considered rare and does not seem to play a role in either treatment failure or in the persistence of *C pneumoniae* identified on respiratory samples after completion of therapy because isolates obtained from patients after appropriate therapy demonstrate in vitro sensitivity.

Three novel antibiotics, nemonoxacin, slorithromycin, and AZD0914, have all demonstrated in vitro activity against *Chlamydophila* but are currently in trial stages and have not yet received FDA approval for treatment.[61–63] Nemonoxacin is a novel fluoroquinolone with in vitro activity comparable to azithromycin, doxycycline, and levofloxacin.[62] In 2 phase II clinical trials of 256 and 192 patients with mild to moderately severe CAP, nemonoxacin led to clinical treatment success in all patients identified as having *C pneumoniae*, although this totaled only 9 patients between the 2 trails.[64,65] Slorithromycin is a novel fourth-generation macrolide with in vitro activity against *Chlamydophila* that demonstrated noninferiority to moxifloxacin for the treatment of CAP in a recent phase III clinical trial.[66] No patients with *Chlamydophila* were specifically identified in the study. AZD0914 is a bacterial DNA gyrase/topoisomerase inhibitor that demonstrates high activity against *Chlamydophila* and other respiratory pathogens in vitro but is not yet under clinical investigation for treatment of respiratory infections.[63]

Conflicts and Controversies

C pneumoniae infection has been identified as a possible contributing factor in a multitude of chronic conditions. A 2013 meta-analysis by Orrskog and colleagues[67] identified *C pneumoniae* infection as potentially linked with 26 chronic conditions, most strongly with conditions of the circulatory system. Research interest into a causal link between *Chlamydophila* infection and atherosclerosis has been intense since 1988, when Saikku and colleagues[68] identified a higher rate of serologic evidence of infection in patients with a history of coronary heart disease. Subsequently, *C pneumoniae* was identified by culture, PCR, and immunohistochemical methods in macrophages, endothelial cells, and smooth muscle cells in atherosclerotic vessel walls. Each of these techniques has been criticized, however, given that isolation in culture is rare and inconsistent, PCR identification is widely variable and potentially prone to contamination, and immunohistochemical staining is plagued by cross-reactivity with human proteins.[69] Furthermore, identification of *C pneumoniae* in atherosclerotic lesions has not correlated well with seropositivity. It has been suggested that the initially identified serologic markers, such as elevations in IgG, may be more reflective of atherosclerotic processes other than persistent *C pneumoniae* infection, such as smoking and inflammation.[70] In recent meta-analyses, elevated titers of IgG or IgA to *C pneumoniae* have been associated with increased stroke risk and increased inflammatory markers.[71,72]

The connection between *C pneumoniae* infection and atherosclerosis has been most strongly shaken by disappointing results in studies of antibiotic therapy. A 2005 meta-analysis of 11 randomized controlled trials, including 19,217 patients with established coronary artery disease, showed that antibiotic therapy had no effect on rates of myocardial infarction or all-cause mortality.[73] The CLARICOR trial, which demonstrated an unexpected increase in long-term mortality after short-term treatment with clarithromycin in patients with stable coronary heart disease, further contributed to doubt in the association.[70] The failure of antibiotic therapies to influence cardiovascular outcomes may reflect a lack of an association but could also result from the limited efficacy of antibiotics to penetrate atherosclerotic plaques or eradicate infection. Alternatively, the initiation of atherosclerosis may depend on transient *C pneumoniae* infection rather than chronic infection. Ultimately, the hypothesized association remains to be definitively demonstrated.[74]

Definitively implicating persistent *C pneumoniae* infection in the pathogenesis of chronic diseases will first require a method of reliably identifying persistent infection. No standardized method yet exists, but potential methods have been investigated.[51] In a 2008 study by Bunk and colleagues[75] using proteomics, 12 *C pneumoniae* antigens were identified that produce a serologic IgG antibody response in patients shown to have persistent infection by PCR of either circulating phagocytes or atheromas. Two antigens, Cpaf-c and RpoA, produced the strongest response and could potentially be used in the future as evidence of chronic infection. The possibility that *C pneumoniae* infection, however, may play an initiating role in the pathogenesis of chronic conditions that does not require chronic infection remains.

MYCOPLASMA PNEUMONIAE
Clinical Manifestations

Pneumonia due to *M pneumoniae* can often have a misleading clinical picture with its mild and indistinct symptoms, such as myalgias, cervical adenopathy, nonproductive cough, and fatigue, making it difficult to distinguish from other upper respiratory infections caused by viruses and other atypical bacterium.[76–78] The age group most often affected by *M pneumoniae* include school-aged children and young adults with outbreaks typically occurring during the autumn season.[76–79] Outbreaks occur among close contacts and members within the same household or confined spaces.[80] Apart from its atypical symptoms, *M pneumoniae* presentations can vary dramatically ranging from the mild upper respiratory symptoms to pneumonia and other extrapulmonary manifestations in absence of pneumonia,[6] including dermatologic, cardiovascular, and central nervous system findings.[81] The extrapulmonary manifestations of *M pneumoniae* are outlined in **Table 5**.

Imaging characteristics of *M pneumoniae* infections also follow along with its indistinct nature. The chest radiograph often shows diffuse

Table 5
Extrapulmonary manifestations of *Mycoplasma pneumoniae*

Skin	Erythema Nodosum, Cutaneous Leukocytoclastic Vasculitis, Stevens-Johnson Syndrome
Gastrointestinal	Acute hepatitis
Central nervous system	Encephalitis, aseptic meningitis
Cardiovascular	Cardiac thrombi, Kawasaki disease

interstitial patterns sometimes out of proportion to a patient's physical findings. On CT of the chest, the interstitial changes seen in the chest radiograph show up as tree-in-bud formation.[82] In 2016, Gong and colleagues[82] completed a prospective study that looked at a population of 1280 pediatric cases with *M pneumoniae* pneumonia between the years 2010 to 2014 and found that there were a high proportion of the patients with extensive patchy infiltrates both unilaterally and bilaterally indicating that the diagnosis of pneumonia could not be made on imaging characteristics alone and should occur with clinical findings. Other findings found on CT chest imaging include bronchial wall thickening and ground-glass consolidation.

Diagnostic Considerations

The diagnosis of pneumonia has long been considered a clinical diagnosis as encouraged by the IDSA where a patient should have suggestive symptoms and associated imaging findings correlating with pneumonia and other associated diagnostic techniques have remained controversial due to frequent low yield results.[17] For an overview of diagnostic techniques, see **Table 6**.

Confirmatory diagnostic testing plays an important role in delineating epidemiology of infection and antibiotic resistance patterns. Traditionally diagnosis of *M pneumoniae* has come from cultures and serology where isolation via culture was considered the gold standard. Given the fastidious nature of *M pneumoniae* it is not routinely cultured anymore because it is slow growing and culture results are often inconsistent and provide poor clinical utility given the length of time the organism takes to grow.[77,79]

Alternative methods of diagnosing *M pneumoniae* include serologic studies using ELISA to quantify expression of antibodies to the bacteria,

Table 6
Diagnosis of *Mycoplasma pneumoniae*

Diagnostic Test	Sample Type	Advantages/Disadvantages of Test
Culture	Sputum	Advantages • If positive, 100% specific and considered the gold standard Disadvantages • Long growth period that provides limited clinical utility
Serology	Serum	Advantages • Test has ability to quantify expression amount Disadvantages • Poor sensitivity and specificity • Requires paired sera (acute and convalescent phases) leading to retrospective results High false-positive rate likely due to carrier state
Molecular	Sputum, NPA, NPS, OPS	Advantages • Readily available with fast results; high specificity Disadvantages • Expensive commercial kits • Improved standardization among kits required to determine optimal sample specimen

microparticle agglutination studies and complement fixation assays. For a definitive diagnosis in the serologic studies paired sera were needed to demonstrate a significant 4-fold elevation of IgG or a subsequent seroconversion of IgG in the sera collected 3 to 4 weeks later.[83–86] Due to the delay in antibody production during initial infection and the time needed to allow for seroconversion, the serologic tests also have poor utility in diagnosing acute *M pneumoniae* infections in clinical practice and functioned more as a retrospective confirmation for epidemiologic studies.[79,83–85] With the many disadvantages of culture and serology in diagnosing *M pneumoniae* infections, diagnostics are evolving toward more rapid molecular techniques including nucleic acid amplification techniques.

Molecular diagnostic techniques allow for a timely diagnosis of *M pneumoniae* infections and are quickly becoming the mainstay for diagnosis in clinical practice with the development of a vast repertoire of laboratory techniques including nucleic acid amplification techniques, multilocus variable number tandem-repeat analysis, multilocus sequence typing, among many others.[79] These tests have quickly become preferential with their ability to produce fast results with high specificity and sensitivity.[79,83] Many of the new tests undergo real-time PCR to look at specific gene regions of *M pneumoniae* as the regions encoding 16S ribosomal RNA, P1 gene, ATPase operon, and the community-acquired respiratory distress syndrome (CARDS) toxin.[79,83–86] This technology allowed for the development of multiplex PCR, which often allow for the detection of several atypical pathogens, including *C pneumoniae*, *C psittaci*, and *Legionella* species, among other respiratory viruses.[54,79] There still remains some debate over which sample type has the best sensitivity and specificity while performing these assays, with current studies showing that sputum samples yield more positive results than both nasopharyngeal aspirates (NPAs) and NPSs as well as OPSs.[85,87]

Prognosis

The clinical course of *M pneumoniae* infections is usually mild and self-limiting in nature and resolves within 2 to 4 weeks regardless of treatment.[77,78,83,84] There have been cases of severe infections, however, resulting in acute respiratory distress syndrome and severe neurologic complications that are associated with increased morbidity and mortality.[88]

Treatment

Infection from *M pneumoniae* is often underdiagnosed, where patients tend to not seek treatment given the subacute nature of their symptoms.[76–79] The bacterium has a long incubation of approximately 3 weeks with prolonged bacterial shedding where symptoms can last up to 4 months; however, most cases resolve naturally within 2 to 4 weeks without treatment.[77,79,83]

When patients present for clinical care, treatment is often guided by the IDSA guidelines for CAP based on a patient's symptoms and imaging results.[17] M pneumoniae, as a small, self-replicating bacteria that lacks a cell wall, is inherently resistant to the family of β-lactam type of antimicrobials but is routinely covered in the empiric treatment of CAP treatment with macrolide therapy, usually without a formal laboratory diagnosis. Treatment with such antimicrobials can shorten the course of the illness by using a 5-day to 2-week course of antibiotic therapy dependent on the choice of antibiotic in infected individuals.[89,90] Because M pneumoniae often affects children and young adults, macrolides have become the treatment of choice because both tetracyclines and fluoroquinolones have unfavorable side-effect profiles that can occur in the younger patient population, such as discoloration of dentition with tetracyclines and tendinitis with fluoroquinolones.[90]

The treatment of extrapulmonary symptoms or complicated M pneumoniae pneumonia remains unclear apart from the administration of antibiotics. In patients with extrapulmonary conditions associated with M pneumoniae, it is important to understand the inflammatory nature of the bacteria where, through pathways associated with Toll-like receptor 2, the bacteria are able to induce proinflammatory cytokines and inflammasome activity.[91] This partially helps explain why the symptoms are present more often in young adults who express a more robust immune response rather than infants or geriatric patients who are unable to mount the same level of response.[92] In patients with central nervous system syndromes from M pneumoniae, such as encephalitis and stroke, case reports have suggested the use of steroids and immunoglobulin therapy may be of benefit, although this has not been validated in clinical trials.[5,93] Similar reports have been made for patients with severe M pneumoniae pneumonia resulting in acute respiratory distress syndrome, suggesting possible benefit from extracorporeal membrane oxygenation and steroids.[5,84,88] Antimicrobial options are summarized in **Table 2**.

Conflicts and Controversies

Infections with M pneumoniae are usually mild, which can make it a difficult diagnosis; however, complications can occur with severe infections that sometimes correlate with macrolide-resistant strains and reiterate the importance of therapy guidelines.

With its mild clinical presentation, M pneumoniae can be a challenging clinical diagnosis as one that often mimics mild respiratory viruses; or, patients fail to present for evaluation due to their low-grade symptoms, making it an underdiagnosed infection. With the development of many novel molecular diagnostic techniques, it is becoming faster and easier for clinicians to make a formal diagnosis; however, with the many new techniques, there is still no standardized test recommended by IDSA guidelines. Several barriers that may arise in the primary care settings are that many of these molecular tests are expensive and many of these techniques require specialized laboratory equipment. There have been several assays developed that allow for the convenience of testing for multiple pathogens, with current tests approved for clinical use, including the Bioscience USA illumigene assay (Meridian Bioscience, USA) approved by the FDA in the United States and the FilmArray Respiratory Panel (BioMérieux, France) approved in parts of Europe.[83,87] These multiplex assays can often detect a positive result, which may not always correlate with the presence of disease because many patients may be a carrier, have a coinfection, or have overcome the clinical infection but still are undergoing a prolonged period of bacterial shedding.[87,94] It remains unclear whether the asymptomatic carriage of M pneumoniae or colonization can be differentiated from active infection with the new diagnostic techniques. Such results can cause confusion, make interpretation of results difficult, and may lead to unnecessary treatment with antibiotics and increased health care resources based on initiation of respiratory precautions in hospitalized patients.

Macrolide resistance in M pneumoniae has been a rapidly emerging phenomenon with reports of increasing resistance in Asia, Europe, and the United States.[79,95–97] Countries in Asia have shown a large amount of macrolide resistance; in Beijing it has been reported that as many as 98% of certain populations infected with M pneumoniae between 2008 and 2012 are resistant to macrolide therapy.[95] The emerging resistance patterns have also been found in the United States, where up to 13% to 27% of M pneumoniae infections have been resistant to macrolide therapy.[96,98] Resistance to macrolides can come by various mechanisms, including the most common, a single-nucleotide polymorphism at one of the residues around the binding site of the peptidyl transferase loop of the 23s ribosomal RNA subunit preventing binding, which ultimately can inhibit protein synthesis.[99] It remains unclear as to how the emerging resistance patterns are going to affect clinical prescribing patterns in the near future in the United States; however, at this time, there are no formal recommendations for macrolide prophylaxis in close contacts of infected individuals. The mainstay of preventing infection spread remains handwashing and respiratory droplet isolation to limit transmission of the bacteria.

There have also been studies linking *M pneumoniae* to asthma, supporting that the presence of the bacteria can precede the onset of asthma and also cause acute exacerbations in those with preexisting asthma. Biscardi and colleagues[100] showed that 20% of pediatric patients requiring hospitalizations due to acute exacerbations of asthma were positive for *M pneumoniae* and 50% of those patients were having their initial exacerbation. A similar study in adult patients showed that 18% of the patients hospitalized for acute asthma exacerbations were positive for *M pneumoniae*.[101] Chronic stable asthmatics have been found to have *M pneumoniae* present in their airways significantly more than control patients and this may help explain some of the chronic inflammation that asthmatics experience and decreased forced expiratory volume in the first second of expiration (FEV_1) due to the IgE-mediated hypersensitivity effect that *M pneumoniae* has on the airways.[102] Treatment with macrolides, such as clarithromycin, can improve FEV_1, it is suspected that either the antimicrobial aspect of macrolides on *M pneumoniae* or their ability to modulate inflammation may be responsible for this improvement.[103]

SUMMARY

CAP due to *Legionella*, *Chlamydophyla*, or *Mycoplasma* continues to be a diagnostic challenge due to the nonspecific clinical and radiographic presentations. The vague clinical presentations of atypical CAP contribute to its underdiagnosis and under-reporting. Advancements in diagnostic techniques bring hope to rapid and accurate diagnosis of atypical CAP. Macrolides and respiratory fluoroquinolones are currently the antibiotics of choice, but this may change in the near future as more antibiotics resistance patterns emerge for atypical CAP. Several controversies still exist in atypical CAP, underscoring the need for continued investigation of preventing atypical CAP and determine its association with chronic lung diseases.

REFERENCES

1. Fraser DW, Tsai TR, Orenstein W, et al. Legionnaires' disease: description of an epidemic of pneumonia. N Engl J Med 1977;297(22):1189–97.
2. Glick TH, Gregg MB, Berman B, et al. Pontiac fever. An epidemic of unknown etiology in a health department: I. Clinical and epidemiologic aspects. Am J Epidemiol 1978;107(2):149–60.
3. Levy I, Rubin LG. Legionella pneumonia in neonates: a literature review. J Perinatol 1998;18(4):287–90.
4. Sopena N, Sabrià-Leal M, Pedro-Botet ML, et al. Comparative study of the clinical presentation of Legionella pneumonia and other community-acquired pneumonias. Chest 1998;113(5):1195–200.
5. Garcia AV, Fingeret AL, Thirumoorthi AS, et al. Severe Mycoplasma pneumoniae infection requiring extracorporeal membrane oxygenation with concomitant ischemic stroke in a child. Pediatr Pulmonol 2013;48(1):98–101.
6. Fisman DN, Lim S, Wellenius GA, et al. It's not the heat, it's the humidity: wet weather increases legionellosis risk in the greater Philadelphia metropolitan area. J Infect Dis 2005;192(12):2066–73.
7. Graham FF, White PS, Harte DJ, et al. Changing epidemiological trends of legionellosis in New Zealand, 1979-2009. Epidemiol Infect 2012;140(8):1481–96.
8. Stout JE, Yu VL. Legionellosis. N Engl J Med 1997;337(10):682–7.
9. Prevention, C.D.C. Legionella (Legionnaires' Disease and Pontiac Fever). Available at: http://www.cdc.gov/legionella/clinicians/diagnostic-testing.html. Accessed July 7, 2016.
10. Phin N, Parry-Ford F, Harrison T, et al. Epidemiology and clinical management of Legionnaires' disease. Lancet Infect Dis 2014;14(10):1011–21.
11. Avni T, Bieber A, Green H, et al. Diagnostic accuracy of PCR alone and compared to urinary antigen testing for detection of legionella spp.: a systematic review. J Clin Microbiol 2016;54(2):401–11.
12. Marston BJ, Lipman HB, Breiman RF. Surveillance for Legionnaires' disease. Risk factors for morbidity and mortality. Arch Intern Med 1994;154(21):2417–22.
13. Farnham A, Alleyne L, Cimini D, et al. Legionnaires' disease incidence and risk factors, New York, New York, USA, 2002-2011. Emerg Infect Dis 2014;20(11):1795–802.
14. Lettinga KD, Verbon A, Nieuwkerk PT, et al. Health-related quality of life and posttraumatic stress disorder among survivors of an outbreak of Legionnaires disease. Clin Infect Dis 2002;35(1):11–7.
15. Gacouin A, Le Tulzo Y, Lavoue S, et al. Severe pneumonia due to Legionella pneumophila: prognostic factors, impact of delayed appropriate antimicrobial therapy. Intensive Care Med 2002;28(6):686–91.
16. Heath CH, Grove DI, Looke DF. Delay in appropriate therapy of Legionella pneumonia associated with increased mortality. Eur J Clin Microbiol Infect Dis 1996;15(4):286–90.
17. Mandell LA, Wunderink RG, Anzueto A, et al. Infectious Diseases Society of America/American Thoracic Society consensus guidelines on the management of community-acquired pneumonia in adults. Clin Infect Dis 2007;44(Suppl 2):S27–72.
18. Edelstein PH. Legionnaires' disease. Clin Infect Dis 1993;16(6):741–7.

19. Swanson DJ, Sung RJ, Fine MJ, et al. Erythromycin ototoxicity: prospective assessment with serum concentrations and audiograms in a study of patients with pneumonia. Am J Med 1992; 92(1):61–8.

20. Howden BP, Stuart RL, Tallis G, et al. Treatment and outcome of 104 hospitalized patients with legionnaires' disease. Intern Med J 2003;33(11):484–8.

21. Plouffe JF, Breiman RF, Fields BS, et al. Azithromycin in the treatment of Legionella pneumonia requiring hospitalization. Clin Infect Dis 2003; 37(11):1475–80.

22. Dorrell L, Fulton B, Ong EL. Intravenous azithromycin as salvage therapy in a patient with Legionnaire's disease. Thorax 1994;49(6):620–1.

23. Sabria M, Pedro-Botet ML, Gómez J, et al. Fluoroquinolones vs macrolides in the treatment of Legionnaires disease. Chest 2005;128(3):1401–5.

24. Dunbar LM, Khashab MM, Kahn JB, et al. Efficacy of 750-mg, 5-day levofloxacin in the treatment of community-acquired pneumonia caused by atypical pathogens. Curr Med Res Opin 2004;20(4): 555–63.

25. Viasus D, Di Yacovo S, Garcia-Vidal C, et al. Community-acquired Legionella pneumophila pneumonia: a single-center experience with 214 hospitalized sporadic cases over 15 years. Medicine (Baltimore) 2013;92(1):51–60.

26. Burdet C, Lepeule R, Duval X, et al. Quinolones versus macrolides in the treatment of legionellosis: a systematic review and meta-analysis. J Antimicrob Chemother 2014;69(9):2354–60.

27. Bruin JP, Koshkolda T, IJzerman EP, et al. Isolation of ciprofloxacin-resistant Legionella pneumophila in a patient with severe pneumonia. J Antimicrob Chemother 2014;69(10):2869–71.

28. Shadoud L, Almahmoud I, Jarraud S, et al. Hidden selection of bacterial resistance to fluoroquinolones in vivo: the case of legionella pneumophila and humans. EBioMedicine 2015;2(9):1179–85.

29. Fields BS, Benson RF, Besser RE. Legionella and Legionnaires' disease: 25 years of investigation. Clin Microbiol Rev 2002;15(3):506–26.

30. Benitez AJ, Winchell JM. Clinical application of a multiplex real-time PCR assay for simultaneous detection of Legionella species, Legionella pneumophila, and Legionella pneumophila serogroup 1. J Clin Microbiol 2013;51(1):348–51.

31. Varner TR, Bookstaver PB, Rudisill CN, et al. Role of rifampin-based combination therapy for severe community-acquired Legionella pneumophila pneumonia. Ann Pharmacother 2011;45(7–8): 967–76.

32. Rello J, Gattarello S, Souto J, et al. Community-acquired Legionella Pneumonia in the intensive care unit: impact on survival of combined antibiotic therapy. Med Intensiva 2013;37(5):320–6.

33. Draper MP, Weir S, Macone A, et al. Mechanism of action of the novel aminomethylcycline antibiotic omadacycline. Antimicrob Agents Chemother 2014;58(3):1279–83.

34. Sader HS, Paukner S, Ivezic-Schoenfeld Z, et al. Antimicrobial activity of the novel pleuromutilin antibiotic BC-3781 against organisms responsible for community-acquired respiratory tract infections (CARTIs). J Antimicrob Chemother 2012;67(5): 1170–5.

35. Lemaire S, Van Bambeke F, Tulkens PM. Activity of finafloxacin, a novel fluoroquinolone with increased activity at acid pH, towards extracellular and intracellular Staphylococcus aureus, Listeria monocytogenes and Legionella pneumophila. Int J Antimicrob Agents 2011;38(1):52–9.

36. Correia AM, Ferreira JS, Borges V, et al. Probable person-to-person transmission of legionnaires' disease. N Engl J Med 2016;374(5):497–8.

37. Borges V, Nunes A, Sampaio DA, et al. Legionella pneumophila strain associated with the first evidence of person-to-person transmission of Legionnaires' disease: a unique mosaic genetic backbone. Sci Rep 2016;6:26261.

38. Bargellini A, Marchesi I, Righi E, et al. Parameters predictive of Legionella contamination in hot water systems: association with trace elements and heterotrophic plate counts. Water Res 2011;45(6): 2315–21.

39. Borella P, Montagna MT, Romano-Spica V, et al. Legionella infection risk from domestic hot water. Emerg Infect Dis 2004;10(3):457–64.

40. Borella P, Bargellini A, Marchegiano P, et al. Hospital-acquired Legionella infections: an update on the procedures for controlling environmental contamination. Ann Ig 2016;28(2):98–108.

41. WHO. W.H.O. Legionella and the prevention of legionellosis. 2007. Available at: http://www.who.int/water_sanitation_health/emerging/legionella.pdf.

42. Burillo A, Bouza E. Chlamydophila pneumoniae. Infect Dis Clin North Am 2010;24(1):61–71.

43. Conklin L, Adjemian J, Loo J, et al. Investigation of a Chlamydia pneumoniae outbreak in a Federal correctional facility in Texas. Clin Infect Dis 2013; 57(5):639–47.

44. Miyashita N, Fukano H, Okimoto N, et al. Clinical presentation of community-acquired Chlamydia pneumoniae pneumonia in adults. Chest 2002; 121(6):1776–81.

45. Puljiz I, Kuzman I, Dakovic-Rode O, et al. Chlamydia pneumoniae and Mycoplasma pneumoniae pneumonia: comparison of clinical, epidemiological characteristics and laboratory profiles. Epidemiol Infect 2006;134(3):548–55.

46. McConnell CT Jr, Plouffe JF, File TM, et al. Radiographic appearance of Chlamydia pneumoniae (TWAR strain) respiratory infections. CBPIS Study

Group. Community-based pneumonia incidence study. Radiology 1994;192(3):819–24.

47. Kauppinen MT, Lahde S, Syrjala H. Roentgeno-graphic findings of pneumonia caused by Chlamydia pneumoniae. A comparison with streptococcus pneumonia. Arch Intern Med 1996;156(16):1851–6.

48. Boersma WG, Daniels JM, Löwenberg A, et al. Reliability of radiographic findings and the relation to etiologic agents in community-acquired pneumonia. Respir Med 2006;100(5):926–32.

49. Nambu A, Saito A, Araki T, et al. Chlamydia pneumoniae: comparison with findings of Mycoplasma pneumoniae and Streptococcus pneumoniae at thin-section CT. Radiology 2006;238(1):330–8.

50. She RC, Thurber A, Hymas WC, et al. Limited utility of culture for Mycoplasma pneumoniae and Chlamydophila pneumoniae for diagnosis of respiratory tract infections. J Clin Microbiol 2010;48(9):3380–2.

51. Puolakkainen M. Laboratory diagnosis of persistent human chlamydial infection. Front Cell Infect Microbiol 2013;3:99.

52. Verkooyen RP, Willemse D, Hiep-van Casteren SC, et al. Evaluation of PCR, culture, and serology for diagnosis of Chlamydia pneumoniae respiratory infections. J Clin Microbiol 1998;36(8):2301–7.

53. Hyman CL, Roblin PM, Gaydos CA, et al. Prevalence of asymptomatic nasopharyngeal carriage of Chlamydia pneumoniae in subjectively healthy adults: assessment by polymerase chain reaction-enzyme immunoassay and culture. Clin Infect Dis 1995;20(5):1174–8.

54. Thurman KA, Warner AK, Cowart KC, et al. Detection of Mycoplasma pneumoniae, Chlamydia pneumoniae, and Legionella spp. in clinical specimens using a single-tube multiplex real-time PCR assay. Diagn Microbiol Infect Dis 2011;70(1):1–9.

55. FDA news release: FDA expands use for FilmArray Respiratory Panel. U.S. Food and Drug Administration website. 2012. http://www.fda.gov/NewsEvents/Newsroom/PressAnnouncements/ucm304177.htm. Accessed February 22, 2016.

56. Hammerschlag MR, Chirgwin K, Roblin PM, et al. Persistent infection with Chlamydia pneumoniae following acute respiratory illness. Clin Infect Dis 1992;14(1):178–82.

57. Jain S, Self WH, Wunderink RG. Community-acquired pneumonia requiring hospitalization. N Engl J Med 2015;373(24):2382.

58. Capelastegui A, España PP, Bilbao A, et al. Etiology of community-acquired pneumonia in a population-based study: link between etiology and patients characteristics, process-of-care, clinical evolution and outcomes. BMC Infect Dis 2012;12:134.

59. Lee YT, Chen SC, Chan KC, et al. Impact of infectious etiology on the outcome of Taiwanese patients hospitalized with community acquired pneumonia. J Infect Dev Ctries 2013;7(2):116–24.

60. Kohlhoff SA, Hammerschlag MR. Treatment of Chlamydial infections: 2014 update. Expert Opin Pharmacother 2015;16(2):205–12.

61. Roblin PM, Kohlhoff SA, Parker C, et al. In vitro activity of CEM-101, a new fluoroketolide antibiotic, against Chlamydia trachomatis and Chlamydia (Chlamydophila) pneumoniae. Antimicrob Agents Chemother 2010;54(3):1358–9.

62. Chotikanatis K, Kohlhoff SA, Hammerschlag MR. In vitro activity of nemonoxacin, a novel nonfluorinated quinolone antibiotic, against Chlamydia trachomatis and Chlamydia pneumoniae. Antimicrob Agents Chemother 2014;58(3):1800–1.

63. Biedenbach DJ, Huband MD, Hackel M, et al. In vitro activity of AZD0914, a novel bacterial DNA gyrase/topoisomerase IV inhibitor, against clinically relevant gram-positive and fastidious gram-negative pathogens. Antimicrob Agents Chemother 2015;59(10):6053–63.

64. van Rensburg DJ, Perng RP, Mitha IH, et al. Efficacy and safety of nemonoxacin versus levofloxacin for community-acquired pneumonia. Antimicrob Agents Chemother 2010;54(10):4098–106.

65. Liu Y, Zhang Y, Wu J, et al. A randomized, double-blind, multicenter Phase II study comparing the efficacy and safety of oral nemonoxacin with oral levofloxacin in the treatment of community-acquired pneumonia. J Microbiol Immunol Infect 2015. [Epub ahead of print].

66. Barrera CM, Mykietiuk A, Metev H, et al. Efficacy and safety of oral solithromycin versus oral moxifloxacin for treatment of community-acquired bacterial pneumonia: a global, double-blind, multicentre, randomised, active-controlled, non-inferiority trial (SOLITAIRE-ORAL). Lancet Infect Dis 2016;16(4):421–30.

67. Orrskog S, Medin E, Tsolova S, et al. Causal inference regarding infectious aetiology of chronic conditions: a systematic review. PLoS One 2013;8(7):e68861.

68. Saikku P, Leinonen M, Mattila K, et al. Serological evidence of an association of a novel Chlamydia, TWAR, with chronic coronary heart disease and acute myocardial infarction. Lancet 1988;2(8618):983–6.

69. Hoymans VY, Bosmans JM, Ieven MM, et al. Chlamydia pneumoniae-based atherosclerosis: a smoking gun. Acta Cardiol 2007;62(6):565–71.

70. Hilden J, Lind I, Kolmos HJ, et al. Chlamydia pneumoniae IgG and IgA antibody titers and prognosis in patients with coronary heart disease: results from the CLARICOR trial. Diagn Microbiol Infect Dis 2010;66(4):385–92.

71. Su X, Chen HL. Chlamydia pneumoniae infection and cerebral infarction risk: a meta-analysis. Int J Stroke 2014;9(3):356–64.

72. Filardo S, Di Pietro M, Farcomeni A, et al. Chlamydia pneumoniae-mediated inflammation in atherosclerosis: a meta-analysis. Mediators Inflamm 2015;2015:378658.

73. Andraws R, Berger JS, Brown DL. Effects of antibiotic therapy on outcomes of patients with coronary artery disease: a meta-analysis of randomized controlled trials. JAMA 2005;293(21):2641–7.

74. Joshi R, Khandelwal B, Joshi D, et al. Chlamydophila pneumoniae infection and cardiovascular disease. N Am J Med Sci 2013;5(3):169–81.

75. Bunk S, Susnea I, Rupp J, et al. Immunoproteomic identification and serological responses to novel Chlamydia pneumoniae antigens that are associated with persistent C. pneumoniae infections. J Immunol 2008;180(8):5490–8.

76. Yu Y, Fei A. Atypical pathogen infection in community-acquired pneumonia. Biosci Trends 2016;10(1):7–13.

77. Reinton N, Manley L, Tjade T, et al. Respiratory tract infections during the 2011 Mycoplasma pneumoniae epidemic. Eur J Clin Microbiol Infect Dis 2013;32(6):835–40.

78. Cilloniz C, Ewig S, Polverino E, et al. Microbial aetiology of community-acquired pneumonia and its relation to severity. Thorax 2011;66(4):340–6.

79. Diaz MH, Winchell JM. The evolution of advanced molecular diagnostics for the detection and characterization of mycoplasma pneumoniae. Front Microbiol 2016;7:232.

80. Jonas MW. Mycoplasma pneumoniae – a national public health perspective. Curr Pediatr Rev 2013; 9(4):324–33.

81. Narita M. Classification of extrapulmonary manifestations due to Mycoplasma pneumoniae infection on the basis of possible pathogenesis. Front Microbiol 2016;7:23.

82. Gong L, Zhang CL, Zhen Q. Analysis of clinical value of CT in the diagnosis of pediatric pneumonia and mycoplasma pneumonia. Exp Ther Med 2016; 11(4):1271–4.

83. Loens K, Ieven M. Mycoplasma pneumoniae: current knowledge on nucleic acid amplification techniques and serological diagnostics. Front Microbiol 2016;7:448.

84. Youn YS, Lee KY. Mycoplasma pneumoniae pneumonia in children. Korean J Pediatr 2012;55(2):42–7.

85. Loens K, Ursi D, Goossens H, et al. Molecular diagnosis of Mycoplasma pneumoniae respiratory tract infections. J Clin Microbiol 2003;41(11): 4915–23.

86. Herrera M, Aguilar YA, Rueda ZV, et al. Comparison of serological methods with PCR-based methods for the diagnosis of community-acquired pneumonia caused by atypical bacteria. J Negat Results Biomed 2016;15:3.

87. Loens K, Van Heirstraeten L, Malhotra-Kumar S, et al. Optimal sampling sites and methods for detection of pathogens possibly causing community-acquired lower respiratory tract infections. J Clin Microbiol 2009;47(1):21–31.

88. Sztrymf B, Jacobs F, Fichet J, et al. Mycoplasma-related pneumonia: a rare cause of acute respiratory distress syndrome (ARDS) and of potential antibiotic resistance. Rev Mal Respir 2013;30(1): 77–80 [in French].

89. Kashyap S, Sarkar M. Mycoplasma pneumonia: clinical features and management. Lung India 2010;27(2):75–85.

90. Cao B, Zhao CJ, Yin YD, et al. High prevalence of macrolide resistance in Mycoplasma pneumoniae isolates from adult and adolescent patients with respiratory tract infection in China. Clin Infect Dis 2010;51(2):189–94.

91. Shimizu T. Inflammation-inducing factors of Mycoplasma pneumoniae. Front Microbiol 2016;7:414.

92. Principi N, Esposito S. Emerging role of Mycoplasma pneumoniae and Chlamydia pneumoniae in paediatric respiratory-tract infections. Lancet Infect Dis 2001;1(5):334–44.

93. Sanchez-Vargas FM, Gomez-Duarte OG. Mycoplasma pneumoniae-an emerging extrapulmonary pathogen. Clin Microbiol Infect 2008; 14(2):105–17.

94. Self WH, Williams DJ, Zhu Y, et al. Respiratory viral detection in children and adults: comparing asymptomatic controls and patients with community-acquired pneumonia. J Infect Dis 2016;213(4):584–91.

95. Zhao F, Liu G, Wu J, et al. Surveillance of macrolide-resistant mycoplasma pneumoniae in Beijing, China, from 2008 to 2012. Antimicrob Agents Chemother 2013;57(3):1521–3.

96. Zheng X, Lee S, Selvarangan R, et al. Macrolide-resistant mycoplasma pneumoniae, United States. Emerg Infect Dis 2015;21(8):1470–2.

97. Steffens I. Mycoplasma pneumoniae and Legionella pneumophila. Euro Surveill 2012;17(6):27–30.

98. Wolff BJ, Thacker WL, Schwartz SB, et al. Detection of macrolide resistance in Mycoplasma pneumoniae by real-time PCR and high-resolution melt analysis. Antimicrob Agents Chemother 2008;52(10):3542–9.

99. Bebear C, Pereyre S, Peuchant O. Mycoplasma pneumoniae: susceptibility and resistance to antibiotics. Future Microbiol 2011;6(4):423–31.

100. Biscardi S, Lorrot M, Marc E, et al. Mycoplasma pneumoniae and asthma in children. Clin Infect Dis 2004;38(10):1341–6.

101. Lieberman D, Lieberman D, Printz S, et al. Atypical pathogen infection in adults with acute exacerbation of bronchial asthma. Am J Respir Crit Care Med 2003;167(3):406–10.

102. Martin RJ, Kraft M, Chu HW, et al. A link between chronic asthma and chronic infection. J Allergy Clin Immunol 2001;107(4):595–601.

103. Kraft M, Cassell GH, Pak J, et al. Mycoplasma pneumoniae and Chlamydia pneumoniae in asthma: effect of clarithromycin. Chest 2002;121(6):1782–8.

Pandemic and Avian Influenza A Viruses in Humans
Epidemiology, Virology, Clinical Characteristics, and Treatment Strategy

Hui Li, MD[a,1], Bin Cao, MD[a,b],*

KEYWORDS

- Pandemic influenza virus • Avian influenza A viruses • Epidemiology • Virology
- Clinical characteristics • Treatment

KEY POINTS

- Though great progress in the understanding of influenza has been made in the past decades, the incidence, morbidity, and mortality of influenza patients are still high.
- Clinical features of people infected with influenza A virus may range from asymptomatic, to conjunctivitis only, to influenza-like illness, to viral pneumonia complicated with acute respiratory distress syndrome, or shock.
- Severe complications of influenza A virus infection are the orchestrated results of direct viral damage and injury induced by uncontrolled immune response.
- Neuraminidase inhibitors are currently sensitive to most strains of influenza A virus and are widely used worldwide. However, strains that are resistant to clinically used antivirals drugs have emerged.
- As for adjuvant immunomodulators that have been attempted in clinical basis, controversies remain and no concrete conclusion about the efficacy of these drugs can be made based on published data so far. High-level evidence, such as that from randomized controlled trials, is urgently needed to guide clinical practice.

INTRODUCTION

Influenza has raised alarming concern for public health worldwide. From the Spanish flu in 1918 and the Asian flu in 1957 to the 2009 swine flu, millions of people died from influenza pandemics. In the 2009 H1N1 pandemic alone, it is estimated that, globally, around 201,200 patients died from respiratory diseases caused by influenza A(H1N1)pdm09, and an additional 83,300 patients died from cardiovascular disorders associated with influenza A(H1N1)pdm09 virus infection.[1]

Funding Sources: National Science Grant for Distinguished Young Scholars (grant number 81425001/H0104), National Key Technology Support Program from Ministry of Science and Technology (2015BAI12B00) (Dr B. Cao); None (Dr H. Li).
Conflict of Interest: None.
[a] Department of Respiratory Medicine, Capital Medical University, NO. 10 You-an -men-wai Xi-tou-tiao, Feng-tai District, Beijing 10069, China; [b] Lab of Clinical Microbiology and Infectious Diseases, Centre of respiratory and Critical Care Medicine, China-Japan Friendship Hospital, NO. 2 Ying-hua Dong jie, Chao yang District, Bei jing 100029, China
[1] Present address: NO. 2 Ying-hua Dong-jie, Chao-yang District, Beijing 100029, China.
* Corresponding author. NO. 2 Ying-hua Dong-jie, Chao-yang District, Beijing 100029, China.
E-mail address: caobin_ben@163.com

chestmed.theclinics.com

Normally, the influenza viruses just cause sporadic infection or seasonal epidemics among human beings. However, a pandemic might occur when a novel influenza virus with sufficient transmissibility emerges, to which most people are immune naïve. Recently, more and more novel influenza virus strains have emerged. Though most of the strains reported so far just caused sporadic infections due to the restriction of low transmissibility among human beings, the possibility that accumulative adaptive mutation would confer on a virus the ability to cause a pandemic cannot be excluded. Recent research found that some strains of influenza viruses could gain the ability to spread easily between people by specific mutations.[2]

During the past decades, great efforts have been put toward exploring new potent antiviral drugs and promoting vaccines worldwide. However, the number of influenza cases did not show any significant decrease during the past decade. Also, the efficacy of most of the current drugs is still under clinical investigation. Meantime, drug resistances have emerged to the antivirals that are commonly used. Also, though antiviral drugs are already available in most areas worldwide, there are still large numbers deaths induced by influenza each year.[3]

To step up vigilance and improve pandemic preparedness, this article elucidates the virology, epidemiology, pathogenesis, clinical characteristics, and treatment of human infections by influenza A viruses, with an emphasis on the influenza A(H1N1)pdm09, H5N1, and H7N9 subtypes.

EPIDEMIOLOGY

Since 1996, more than 14 subtypes of influenza A viruses have been reported to cause human infections (**Fig. 1**). Most of the influenza subtypes causing human infections originated from avian strains, whereas only a few strains were from swine, including influenza A(H1N1)pdm09, influenza A(H1N1)v, and influenza A(H3N2)v.[4–17] In the past 3 years, more subtypes of influenza A virus have crossed the species barrier to cause

human infections than ever before, especially in China, where live poultry markets are popular (see **Fig. 1**).

Most of the influenza A viruses only caused sporadic or small clusters of infections among human beings. Among all the influenza A viruses reported so far, influenza A(H1N1)pdm09, influenza A(H5N1) and influenza A(H7N9) were documented to have caused large-scale outbreaks in human beings and led to the highest mortality and morbidity rate. Influenza A(H1N1)pdm09, which emerged and caused a worldwide pandemic in 2009, is now established in human population and is circulating seasonally (**Fig. 2**). Human cases of influenza A(H5N1) was first detected in Hong Kong, China, in 1997 and 18 confirmed cases were reported to the World Health Organization (WHO), including 6 deaths.[18] After 6 years' absence, confirmed influenza A(H5N1) human cases re-emerged in 2003 in Southeast Asia. Since then, the influenza A(H5N1) virus has undergone evolution and generated multiple clades, and gained long-term persistence and geographic migration. As of February 2016, the influenza A(H5N1) virus has migrated to at least 16 countries and more than 846 confirmed cases, including 449 deaths, were reported to WHO.[17] The influenza A(H7N9) virus was first isolated from a human being in March 2013.[13] Since then, 4 waves of outbreaks among humans have been reported and a total of 722 confirmed cases, including 286 deaths, have been detected. Most of the influenza A(H7N9) cases were from mainland China.[17] Also, similar to the seasonal influenza, most of the influenza A(H7N9) cases emerged in the winter season, except for the first wave (see **Fig. 2**).

As for transmissibility, it has been confirmed that influenza A(H1N1)pdm09 virus can transmit from person to person efficiently, especially in enclosed environment.[19] By contrast, for most avian originated influenza viruses, including influenza A(H7N9) and influenza A(H5N1), few clustering cases are reported so far and human-to-human transmission is inefficient and nonsustainable.[20–23] However, physicians should be alerted that with the certain mutation and reassortment, some

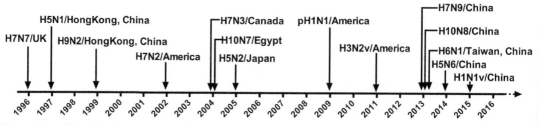

Fig. 1. Year of the first human case infected by specific subtypes of influenza A virus reported worldwide.

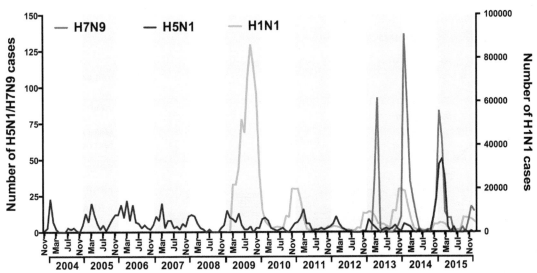

Fig. 2. Number of confirmed human cases with influenza A(H5N1), influenza A(H7N9), or influenza A(H1N1) pdm09 worldwide. (*Data from* World Health Organization. Available at: http://www.who.int/influenza/human animal interface Influenza Summary IRA HA interface. Accessed February 25, 2016; and the Global Influenza Surveillance and Response System (GISRS). Available at: http://www.who.int/influenza/gisrs laboratory/updates/summary report. Accessed February 21, 2016.)

influenza strains may obtain enhanced transmissibility among human beings.[24]

VIROLOGY AND PATHOGENESIS IN HUMANS

As a single-stranded negative-sense RNA virus, influenza A virus comprises 8 separated gene segments and a surrounding liquid envelope (**Fig. 3**). To date, 16 proteins are recognized to be encoded by the influenza genome.[25] Among them, hemagglutinin (HA) and neuraminidase (NA) protrude on the envelope, and are the basis of antigenicities. By binding to the α2,6-linked sialic acid and/orα2,3-linked sialic acid receptors on cell surface, HA initiates infection of influenza viruses. Due to the specific distribution of the 2 kinds of sialic acid receptors in different species, the binding specificity to sialic acid receptors of HA contributes to the host tropism and transmission of influenza viruses.[26,27] After entering cells by endocytosis, HA fuses under specific pH level and releases the viral genomic RNA (vRNA) from endosome, which serves as a template to synthesize complementary RNA (cRNA) with the help of polymerase, including PB1, PB2, PA, and NP. Further, progeny vRNA and messenger RNA (mRNA) are synthesized. Assembled with structural proteins synthesized in the cytoplasm, 8 unique viral RNA segments are packaged to form complete influenza virion by a selective packaging model.[28,29] Subsequently, the link between the sialic acid and HA protein is cleaved by the NA

protein and the virus particles are released (see **Fig. 3**).[30]

Humans infected with influenza usually present with asymptomatic or mild illness that is self-limited. However, a few have presented with severe pneumonia and even progressed into acute respiratory distress syndrome (ARDS). Additionally, the most prominent histopathological features observed during autopsy were epithelial necrosis, diffuse alveolar damage, edema, and intra-alveolar hemorrhage in the lung.[31–33] Except for direct cell and tissue damage induced by the virus replication previously listed,[34,35] accumulative studies have suggested that overactivated immune response also contributes to the severe complications of influenza.[36–38] In severe influenza infection, double-stranded RNA (dsRNA) or single-stranded RNA (sRNA) endocytosed or produced during viral replication are recognized by pattern-recognition receptors (PRRs), mainly Toll-like receptor (TLR)-3, TLR7/8, and RIG-I, triggering different pathways to induce production of a large amount of inflammatory cytokines.[39] Except for the direct activation of PRRs by influenza RNA, studies found that damage-associated molecular patterns (DAMPs), molecules produced from damaged cells such as S100A9, could also induce an inflammatory response during influenza A virus infection in paracrine fashion via TLR4.[40] The higher level of proinflammatory cytokines has been documented to be associated with disease severity and lung damage.[36] Besides the innate

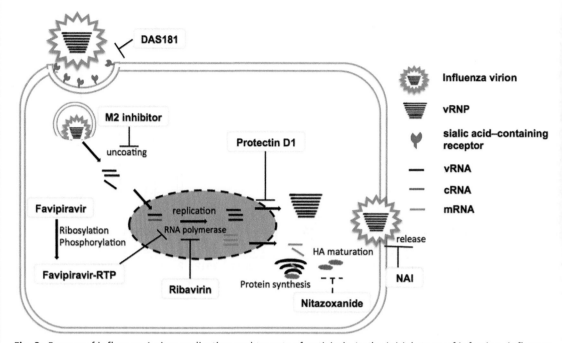

Fig. 3. Process of influenza A virus replication and targets of antivirals. In the initial stage of infection, influenza virus enters cytoplasm by endocytosis, which is mediated by hemagglutinin (HA) binding to the sialic acid receptors on the target cell. In the endosome, the virion then fuses. Viral ribonucleoprotein (vRNP) is then uncoated and travels to the nucleus. Viral genomic RNA (vRNA) is replicated into complementary RNA (cRNA), which serves as the template for vRNA and messenger RNA (mRNA) synthesis. The progeny vRNA then assembles with RNA polymerase (including PB1, PB2, and PA) and multiple copies of NP, forming the vRNP. The vRNP and mRNA are exported to the cytoplasm. Viral proteins such as HA are then synthesized. Proteins and vRNP then assemble to complete the influenza virion, which then is released from the cell. DAS181, a recombinant fusion protein with sialidase activity, prevents attachment of influenza virus by removing the sialic acid receptors on the target cell. By inhibiting the M2 ion channel, M2 inhibitors, including amantadine and rimantadine, interfere with virion uncoating. After ribosylation and phosphorylation, favipiravir evolves to its active form, favipiravir-RTP, which could interfere viral RNA replication by inhibiting the RNA polymerase. As an inhibitor of RNA polymerase, ribavirin could also inhibit the replication of influenza. The lipid mediator protectin D1 attenuates influenza replication by inhibiting nuclear export of vRNP and mRNA in animal experiments. By inhibiting HA maturation at the post-translation level, nitazoxanide could interfere with influenza virion replication. Neuraminidase inhibitors (NAIs), including Oseltamivir, Zanamivir, Peramivir, and Laninamivir, are now widely used in anti-influenza therapy via interfering with the virion release.

immune response, evidence also revealed that uncontrolled adaptive immune response was also involved in the disease pathogenesis.[41] It has been found that, in patients infected with influenza A(H1N1)pdm09, the level of circulating influenza-specific CD4$^+$T cells is positively correlated to the disease severity.[37] Though it is a consensus that uncontrolled inflammatory cytokine production is involved in severe influenza infection, currently there is no answer for how to balance the immune response to keep it at a level to effectively control virus replication with minimum immune damage. Also, the mechanism for the imparity of cytokine production phenotype during different subtypes of influenza A virus infection remains unknown.[42,43]

RISK FACTORS AND CLINICAL CHARACTERISTICS

Signs or symptoms of people infected with influenza A virus have been reported to range from asymptomatic to conjunctivitis only, to influenza-like illness, to severe respiratory illness (eg, shortness of breath, difficulty breathing, viral pneumonia) with or without ARDS, to respiratory failure and multiorgan diseases. Clinical presentation of patients infected with influenza A virus is the orchestrated result of treatment, host factors, and viral virulence. Early medical attention, especially early antiviral therapy, is essential for reducing the mortality risk and reducing the incidence of severe outcomes in patients with influenza A virus infection.[44–46] Except for medical attention, host factor plays a prominent role in the disease pathogenesis of influenza. Usually, the extremely elderly and young, as well as pregnant patients, are at higher risk to develop severe complications than otherwise healthy patients during influenza A virus infection.[47–50] The frequency of severe outcomes is also determined by the virulence of the influenza A virus itself. According to data reported to WHO, the subgroups of H5N1 and H7N9 have been responsible for the highest mortality of influenza A virus worldwide, with a case fatality rate up to 53% and 39%, respectively.[17] Though the case fatality rate reported to WHO might not be a fair reflection of the much milder cases of influenza A virus infection,[51] it at least shows the difference in virulence of different subgroups of influenza A virus.

As for laboratory findings, patients infected with different subtypes of influenza A virus share much in common. Patients usually were detected with a normal or decreased leukocyte count. Lymphopenia and thrombocytopenia occurred in more than 50% of patients hospitalized with influenza A(H1N1)pdm09, H7N9, or H5N1 infections. C-reactive protein was elevated (>10 mg/L) in more than 70% of the patients hospitalized with influenza A(H1N1)pdm09, H7N9, and H51N infections. By contrast, most patients had a normal procalcitonin (PCT) level, and no more than 37% of patients hospitalized for H7N9 were observed with a PCT level greater than 0.5 ng/mL.[47,52] Therefore, PCT was found to be a reasonably accurate marker for differentiating bacterial pneumonia during an influenza pandemic.[53,54]

Consistent with histopathological changes, in the early stage of the infection, a chest radiograph of viral pneumonia induced by influenza A virus infections is characterized by ground glass opacities, which may be accompanied by consolidation. With the deterioration of illness, partial and even areas of consolidation involved both lungs could be observed in some patients. By contrast, in the resolution phase, with the elimination of the proteinaceous exudate and inflammatory cells, the ground opacities and consolidation shadows began to resolve, and in some areas were substituted with pulmonary fibroproliferative changes, which presented as reticular shapes on the chest radiograph.[52,55,56] This abnormality most commonly presents in the peripheral region and peribronchovascular areas, with the lower zone of the lung predominant.[57]

DETECTION AND DIAGNOSIS OF INFLUENZA A VIRUS INFECTION IN HUMANS

Diagnosis of influenza virus infections in humans should be based on clinical manifestations, history of contact, and virological tests. It is difficult to diagnose influenza virus infections in humans based only on clinical characteristics. One study based on a tertiary emergency department revealed that clinical diagnosis has low sensitivity for diagnosing influenza, with sensitivity lower than 40%.[58] Therefore, laboratory tests are of great importance to help guide management in the clinical setting. To date, there are several laboratory diagnosis techniques available, including the reverse-transcription polymerase chain reaction (RT-PCR), virus isolation in cell culture or fertilized chicken eggs, immunofluorescence detection of the virus in clinical specimens or isolates, rapid antigen tests, and other molecular techniques. Among them, RT-PCR techniques are relatively rapid and have a higher sensitivity and specificity for detection and identification of influenza viruses.[59] Rapid antigen tests could detect influenza virus in a qualitative way by identifying the viral nucleoprotein antigens in respiratory specimens. Though it has advantages, such as being quick to produce results and simple to perform, the technique is limited by its common false-negative results. Moreover, quick antigen tests do not provide information on influenza A virus subtypes. Sometimes paired sera antibodies detection is also used to diagnose influenza virus infection. Due to the difficulty in obtaining convalescent serum and time constraints (1 taken during the first week of illness and another taken 3–4 weeks later), paired sera immunoglobulin-G antibody titer tests are usually performed as an epidemiologic rather than a diagnostic tool.

TREATMENT

It is a consensus that severe outcomes of influenza infection are the results of both viral replication and immune damage. The underlying mechanism hints that the treatment of severe influenza A infection should focus on controlling viral replication and overactivated immune response.

Antivirals for Influenza

Currently, a series of antivirals targeting different processes of viral replication from endocytosis (DAS181), uncoating (M2 inhibitor), RNA synthesizing (favipiravir and ribavirin), nuclear exporting (protectin D1), translation, and protein maturation (nitazoxanide), to releasing of virion (NA inhibitors [NAIs]) have been studied (see **Fig. 3**). Except for DAS181, which acts on host factors, most drugs developed to date target at the virus itself. Currently, most of the drugs including DAS181, favipiravir, and nitazoxanide are still under clinical investigation.[60] Though, the lipid mediator protectin D1 could inhibit influenza virus replication and protects against severe influenza virus infection in mice models,[61,62] its effectiveness in human beings needs further investigation. As an RNA and DNA polymerase inhibitor, ribavirin confers antiviral effectiveness for hepatitis C virus.[63] However, its efficacy in the treatment of influenza remains controversial.[64,65] As for M2 ion channel inhibitors, including amantadine and rimantadine, most of the strains of influenza A(H1N1)pdm09 virus, influenza A(H7N9) virus, and some strains of influenza A(H5N1) virus are resistant to it.[66–68] Therefore, they are not currently recommended for antiviral therapy. The most widely used in clinical practice currently are the NAIs, which target the NAs. Though NAIs remain effective against most of the currently circulating human influenza viruses, there has been rapid emergence of drug-resistant influenza A virus strains during the past few years. In 2012 to 2013, only 0.2% of human influenza virus strains submitted for surveillance by the WHO Collaborating Centers have shown highly reduced inhibition against at least 1 of the 4 NAIs (oseltamivir, zanamivir, peramivir, and laninamivir).[69] In just 1 year, the value increased to 2% in the 2013 to 2014 surveillance data. Large community clusters of drug-resistant influenza A(H1N1)pdm09 patients were also observed.[70] Therefore, in addition to monitoring the emergence of drug-resistant influenza strains, it is crucial to develop novel ways of combating influenza A viruses.

Development of Immunomodulatory Therapy

In an attempt to ameliorate immune damage induced by the excess inflammatory cytokines, physicians have prescribed some immunomodulators as adjunct therapy for patients with severe influenza. Among them, corticosteroids are the most widely used. Though the benefits of corticosteroid therapy have been observed in animal model studies of the influenza A(H1N1)pdm09 virus[71,72] and in patients with severe community-acquired pneumonia,[73,74] the use of corticosteroids in patients with severe pneumonia induced by influenza virus seems not very positive. Most of the published observational studies suggest that corticosteroid therapy could not decrease mortality and, in some cases, even increase the risk of death due to side effects, such as secondary bacterial or fungal infection, prolonged viral shedding, and hyperglycemia (**Table 1**). However, patients who received corticosteroid therapy were usually more severe at baseline than those who did not get corticosteroid treatment. With statistical methods to adjust baseline confounders, the effect of corticosteroid therapy might shift from harmful to neutral.[75] In addition, the cytokine production phenotype among different subtypes of influenza and different groups of patients with different immune conditions and disease severity are not the same.[42,43] Also, the efficacy of corticosteroids is influenced by the timing of initiation, dosing, and type of corticosteroids. However, most of the published studies did not perform any subgroup analysis based on these important factors. Therefore, it is arbitrary to conclude that corticosteroids are harmful, and more precise randomized controlled trials are needed to give more precise evidence about the effectiveness of corticosteroids on severe influenza patients.

Statins are another kind of immunomodulator that has been suggested as an adjunct treatment in influenza A virus infection, especially during pandemics. Several observational studies have shown its beneficial effects in the treatment of patients with severe influenza infection (see **Table 1**). However, Laidler and colleagues[76] found that the so-called beneficial effect might be influenced by unmeasured confounders. Macrolides, including azithromycin and clarithromycin, which exert immunomodulatory effects on the host and antibacterial effects, have also been tried to improve outcome of influenza patients. Though 1 observational study showed that clarithromycin could shorten the duration of cough in nonelderly, nonsevere patients with seasonal influenza virus A infection,[77] azithromycin could not inhibit the inflammatory cytokine production[78] and macrolide-based treatment did not decrease the risk of death among critically ill patients with influenza A(H1N1)pdm09 infection.[79] The mammalian target of rapamycin inhibitor (mTOR) inhibitor sirolimus combined with corticosteroids and oseltamivir, was found to be associated with improvement in outcomes, such as shortened ventilator days. However, no significantly beneficial effect on reducing the mortality of patient with severe influenza infection was observed.[80] Oxidative stress has been described as a characteristic of severe influenza infection and antioxidants have been speculated to be effective. However, to date, only 1 case report showed its efficacy and no large-scale clinical research confirms this speculation.[81]

Supportive Treatment Methods for Severe Influenza A Virus–Infected Cases

For severe cases of patients infected with influenza A virus, appropriate supportive care, such as timely correction of hypoxemia and appropriate rescue therapy for patients complicated with shock, is also necessary to improve the outcome.[92] Secondary or coinfections with pathogenic bacteria were found to be an important

Table 1
Summary of clinical effectiveness of immunomodulatory therapy against severe influenza A virus infection

	Study Type	Target Population	Mortality[a]		Risk of Mortality[b]
			Treatment Group	No Treatment Group	
Corticosteroids					
Linko et al,[82] 2011	Prospective, observational	Adult ICU pH1N1 subjects	8/72 (11.1)	2/60 (3.3)	OR, 3.3 (0.5–23.4)
Delaney et al,[75] 2016	Retrospective, observational	Adult ICU pH1N1 subjects	70/280 (25.0)	51/324 (15.7)	OR, 1.71 (1.05–2.78)
Lee et al,[83] 2015	Retrospective, observational	Adult hospitalized influenza subjects[c]	60/600 (10.0)	96/1689 (5.7)	HR, 1.11 (0.79–1.56)
Brun-Buisson et al,[84] 2011	Retrospective, observational	Adult ICU pH1N1 subjects with ARDS or MV	28/83 (33.8)	21/125 (16.8)	HR, 2.59 (1.42–4.73)
Kim et al,[85] 2011	Retrospective, observational	Adult and adolescent ICU pH1N1 subjects	62/107 (57.9)	37/138 (26.8)	OR, 2.20 (1.03–4.71)
Diaz et al,[86] 2012	Retrospective, observational	Adult ICU pH1N1 subjects	25/136 (18.4)	41/236 (17.4)	HR, 1.06 (0.63–1.80)
Xi et al,[87] 2010	Retrospective, observational	Adult hospitalized pH1N1 subjects	17/52 (32.7)	10/103 (9.7)	OR, 3.67 (0.99–13.64)
Cao et al,[88] 2016	Retrospective, observational	Adult hospitalized H7N9 subjects	81/204 (39.7)	11/84 (13.1)	HR, 1.81 (0.88–3.74)
Liem et al,[89] 2009	Retrospective, observational	Adult hospitalized H5N1 subjects	17/29 (58.6)	9/36 (25.0)	OR, 4.11 (1.14–14.83)
Statins					
Nelson et al,[83] 2015	Retrospective, observational	Adult hospitalized influenza subjects[c]	11/336 (3.3)	145/2313 (6.3)	HR, 0.44 (0.23–0.84)
Laidler et al,[76] 2015	Retrospective, observational	Adult hospitalized influenza subjects	—/1013	—/2030	HR, 0.41 (0.25–0.68)
			—/980	—/3458	HR, 0.77 (0.43–1.36)[d]
Vandermeer et al,[90] 2012	Retrospective, observational	Adult hospitalized influenza subjects	40/1013 (3.9)	111/2021 (5.5)[e]	OR, 0.59 (0.38–0.92)
Kwong et al,[91] 2009	Retrospective, observational	≥65 y old influenza subjects	—/1565074	—/5112211	OR, 0.84 (0.77–0.91)
Macrolides					
Martin et al,[79] 2013	Retrospective, observational	Adult ICU pH1N1 subjects	36/190 (19.2)	153/543 (28.1)[e]	OR, 0.87 (0.55–1.37)
Kakeya et al,[78] 2014	RCT	Adult influenza A subjects	0/51	0/56	No impact on cytokine production

(continued on next page)

			Mortality[a]		
	Study Type	Target Population	Treatment Group	No Treatment Group	Risk of Mortality[b]
Ishii et al,[77] 2012	Prospective, observational	Adult mild influenza subjects	0/74	0/67	No influence on the duration of disease in the total population
Sirolimus					
Wang et al,[80] 2014	RCT	Adult ICU pH1N1 subjects	3/19 (15.8)	8/19 (42.1)	OR, 0.26 (0.06–1.19)
Antioxidants					
Lai et al,[81] 2010 (NAC)	Case report	Adult hospitalized pH1N1 patient	—	—	Effective

—, Data is not available.

Abbreviations: HR, hazard ratio; ICU, intensive care unit; MV, mechanical ventilation; OR, odds ratio; RCT, randomized, placebo controlled trial.

[a] Shown as events/total (percentage).

[b] After adjusting for baseline characteristics, such as disease severity, antiviral treatments, and/or underlying diseases.

[c] Including influenza A(pH1N1, seasonal H1N1, H3N2) and influenza B subtypes.

[d] —/1013 versus —/2030, HR, 0.41 (0.25–0.68) for the 2007 to 2008 season; —/980 versus —/3458, HR, 0.77 (0.43–1.36) for the 2009 pandemic.

[e] Data are not provided, which is calculated based on the original data in the literature.

contributor in complicated outcomes in patients with influenza infection.[93,94] It was reported that the most commonly isolated bacteria complicated with severe pandemic H1N1 infection patients on admission were *Streptococcus pneumoniae*, *Staphylococcus aureus*, and *Haemophilus influenza*.[93–96] By contrast, *Acinetobacter baumannii* is the most frequently seen bacteria in hospital-acquired respiratory coinfections of patients with influenza infection.[52,97] However, the types of coinfection pathogen might be influenced by prevailing bacteria in a specific area. Therefore, the empirical antibacterial therapy for influenza patients suspected with bacterial coinfection should follow the local guidelines for community-acquired or hospital-acquired pneumonia accordingly.

SUMMARY

The intermittent outbreak of influenza pandemics and emergence of novel influenza viruses among human being have caused great concern worldwide. Though great progress in the understanding of influenza has been made in the past decades, the incidence, morbidity, and mortality and of influenza patients are still high. Antivirals that are available for clinical choice are scarce. NAIs are currently sensitive to most strains of influenza A virus and are widely used worldwide. However,

strains that are resistant to clinically used antiviral drugs have emerged. Therefore, in addition to monitoring the emergence of drug-resistant influenza strains, it is crucial to develop novel ways of combating influenza A viruses. Though consensus has been reached that uncontrolled immune response has been involved in the pathogenesis of severe influenza infection, the mechanism of the different cytokine production during different subtypes of influenza A virus remains an enigma. There is still no answer to how to balance the immune response to keep it at a level to effectively control virus replication with the less immune damage. As for adjuvant immunomodulators that have been attempted in clinical basis, controversies remain and no concrete conclusion about the efficacy of these drugs can be made based on published data to date and a high-level evidence is urgently needed to guide clinical practice.

REFERENCES

1. Dawood FS, Iuliano AD, Reed C, et al. Estimated global mortality associated with the first 12 months of 2009 pandemic influenza A H1N1 virus circulation: a modelling study. Lancet Infect Dis 2012;12: 687–95.

2. Neumann G, Kawaoka Y. Transmission of influenza A viruses. Virology 2015;479–80:234–46.

3. WHO. FluNet summary. Available at: http://www. who.int/influenza/gisrs_laboratory/updates/summary report/en/. Accessed February 21, 2016.

4. Kurtz J, Manvell RJ, Banks J. Avian influenza virus isolated from a woman with conjunctivitis. Lancet 1996;348:901–2.

5. Chan PK. Outbreak of avian influenza A(H5N1) virus infection in Hong Kong in 1997. Clin Infect Dis 2002; 34(Suppl 2):S58–64.

6. Peiris M, Yuen KY, Leung CW, et al. Human infection with influenza H9N2. Lancet 1999;354:916–7.

7. Abdelwhab EM, Veits J, Mettenleiter TC. Prevalence and control of H7 avian influenza viruses in birds and humans. Epidemiol Infect 2014;142:896–920.

8. Tweed SA, Skowronski DM, David ST, et al. Human illness from avian influenza H7N3, British Columbia. Emerg Infect Dis 2004;10:2196–9.

9. Arzey GG, Kirkland PD, Arzey KE, et al. Influenza virus A (H10N7) in chickens and poultry abattoir workers, Australia. Emerg Infect Dis 2012;18: 814–6.

10. Ogata T, Yamazaki Y, Okabe N, et al. Human H5N2 avian influenza infection in Japan and the factors associated with high H5N2-neutralizing antibody titer. J Epidemiol 2008;18:160–6.

11. Human infection with pandemic A (H1N1) 2009 influenza virus: clinical observations in hospitalized patients, Americas, July 2009-update. Wkly Epidemiol Rec 2009;84:305–8 [in English, French].

12. Centers for Disease Control and Prevention (CDC). Notes from the field: outbreak of influenza A (H3N2) virus among persons and swine at a county fair–Indiana, July 2012. MMWR Morb Mortal Wkly Rep 2012;61:561.

13. Gao R, Cao B, Hu Y, et al. Human infection with a novel avian-origin influenza A (H7N9) virus. N Engl J Med 2013;368:1888–97.

14. Chen S, Li Z, Hu M, et al. Knowledge, attitudes, and practices (KAP) relating to avian influenza (H10N8) among farmers' markets workers in Nanchang, China. PLoS One 2015;10:e0127120.

15. Shi W, Shi Y, Wu Y, et al. Origin and molecular characterization of the human-infecting H6N1 influenza virus in Taiwan. Protein Cell 2013;4:846–53.

16. Chen T, Zhang R. Symptoms seem to be mild in children infected with avian influenza A (H5N6) and other subtypes. J Infect 2015;71:702–3.

17. WHO. Influenza at the human-animal interface. Available at: http://www.who.int/influenza/human animal interface Influenza Summary IRA HA interface. Accessed February 25, 2016.

18. Yuen KY, Chan PK, Peiris M, et al. Clinical features and rapid viral diagnosis of human disease associated with avian influenza A H5N1 virus. Lancet 1998;351:467–71.

19. Casado I, Martinez-Baz I, Burgui R, et al. Household transmission of influenza A(H1N1)pdm09 in the pandemic and post-pandemic seasons. PLoS One 2014;9:e108485.

20. Qi X, Qian YH, Bao CJ, et al. Probable person to person transmission of novel avian influenza A (H7N9) virus in Eastern China, 2013: epidemiological investigation. BMJ 2013;347:f4752.

21. Li Q, Zhou L, Zhou M, et al. Epidemiology of human infections with avian influenza A(H7N9) virus in China. N Engl J Med 2014;370:520–32.

22. Wang H, Feng Z, Shu Y, et al. Probable limited person-to-person transmission of highly pathogenic avian influenza A (H5N1) virus in China. Lancet 2008;371:1427–34.

23. Ungchusak K, Auewarakul P, Dowell SF, et al. Probable person-to-person transmission of avian influenza A (H5N1). N Engl J Med 2005;352:333–40.

24. Long JS, Benfield CT, Barclay WS. One-way trip: influenza virus' adaptation to gallinaceous poultry may limit its pandemic potential. Bioessays 2015; 37:204–12.

25. Muramoto Y, Noda T, Kawakami E, et al. Identification of novel influenza A virus proteins translated from PA mRNA. J Virol 2013;87:2455–62.

26. Shinya K, Ebina M, Yamada S, et al. Avian flu: influenza virus receptors in the human airway. Nature 2006;440:435–6.

27. de Graaf M, Fouchier RA. Role of receptor binding specificity in influenza A virus transmission and pathogenesis. EMBO J 2014;33:823–41.

28. Noda T, Kawaoka Y. Packaging of influenza virus genome: robustness of selection. Proc Natl Acad Sci U S A 2012;109:8797–8.

29. Chou YY, Vafabakhsh R, Doganay S, et al. One influenza virus particle packages eight unique viral RNAs as shown by FISH analysis. Proc Natl Acad Sci U S A 2012;109:9101–6.

30. Tripathi S, Batra J, Lal SK. Interplay between influenza A virus and host factors: targets for antiviral intervention. J Virol 2015;160:1877–91.

31. Korteweg C, Gu J. Pathology, molecular biology, and pathogenesis of avian influenza A (H5N1) infection in humans. Am J Pathol 2008;172:1155–70.

32. Yu L, Wang Z, Chen Y, et al. Clinical, virological, and histopathological manifestations of fatal human infections by avian influenza A(H7N9) virus. Clin Infect Dis 2013;57:1449–57.

33. Shieh WJ, Blau DM, Denison AM, et al. 2009 pandemic influenza A (H1N1): pathology and pathogenesis of 100 fatal cases in the United States. Am J Pathol 2010;177:166–75.

34. de Jong MD, Simmons CP, Thanh TT, et al. Fatal outcome of human influenza A (H5N1) is associated with high viral load and hypercytokinemia. Nat Med 2006;12:1203–7.

35. Hu Y, Lu S, Song Z, et al. Association between adverse clinical outcome in human disease caused by novel influenza A H7N9 virus and sustained viral

shedding and emergence of antiviral resistance. Lancet 2013;381:2273–9.

36. Guo J, Huang F, Liu J, et al. The serum profile of hypercytokinemia factors identified in H7N9-infected patients can predict fatal outcomes. Sci Rep 2015; 5:10942.

37. Zhao Y, Zhang YH, Denney L, et al. High levels of virus-specific CD4+ T cells predict severe pandemic influenza A virus infection. Am J Respir Crit Care Med 2012;186:1292–7.

38. Mohn KG, Cox RJ, Tunheim G, et al. Immune responses in acute and convalescent patients with mild, moderate and severe disease during the 2009 influenza pandemic in Norway. PLoS One 2015;10:e0143281.

39. Pulendran B, Maddur MS. Innate immune sensing and response to influenza. Curr Top Microbiol Immunol 2015;386:23–71.

40. Tsai SY, Segovia JA, Chang TH, et al. DAMP molecule S100A9 acts as a molecular pattern to enhance inflammation during influenza A virus infection: role of DDX21-TRIF-TLR4-MyD88 pathway. PLoS Pathog 2014;10:e1003848.

41. Duan S, Thomas PG. Balancing immune protection and immune pathology by CD8(+) T-cell responses to influenza infection. Front Immunol 2016;7:25.

42. Meliopoulos VA, Karlsson EA, Kercher L, et al. Human H7N9 and H5N1 influenza viruses differ in induction of cytokines and tissue tropism. J Virol 2014;88:12982–91.

43. Leung YH, Nicholls JM, Ho CK, et al. Highly pathogenic avian influenza A H5N1 and pandemic H1N1 virus infections have different phenotypes in Toll-like receptor 3 knockout mice. J Gen Virol 2014;95: 1870–9.

44. Mata-Marin LA, Mata-Marin JA, Vasquez-Mota VC, et al. Risk factors associated with mortality in patients infected with influenza A/H1N1 in Mexico. BMC Res Notes 2015;8:432.

45. Ergonul O, Alan S, Ak O, et al. Predictors of fatality in pandemic influenza A (H1N1) virus infection among adults. BMC Infect Dis 2014;14:317.

46. Muthuri SG, Venkatesan S, Myles PR, et al. Effectiveness of neuraminidase inhibitors in reducing mortality in patients admitted to hospital with influenza A H1N1pdm09 virus infection: a meta-analysis of individual participant data. Lancet Respir Med 2014;2: 395–404.

47. Wang C, Yu H, Horby PW, et al. Comparison of patients hospitalized with influenza A subtypes H7N9, H5N1, and 2009 pandemic H1N1. Clin Infect Dis 2014;58:1095–103.

48. Meijer WJ, van Noortwijk AG, Bruinse HW, et al. Influenza virus infection in pregnancy: a review. Acta Obstet Gynecol Scand 2015;94:797–819.

49. Ren YY, Yin YY, Li WQ, et al. Risk factors associated with severe manifestations of 2009 pandemic influenza A (H1N1) infection in China: a case-control study. Virol J 2013;10:149.

50. Ji H, Gu Q, Chen LL, et al. Epidemiological and clinical characteristics and risk factors for death of patients with avian influenza A H7N9 virus infection from Jiangsu Province, Eastern China. PLoS One 2014;9:e89581.

51. Ip DK, Liao Q, Wu P, et al. Detection of mild to moderate influenza A/H7N9 infection by China's national sentinel surveillance system for influenza-like illness: case series. BMJ 2013;346:f3693.

52. Gao HN, Lu HZ, Cao B, et al. Clinical findings in 111 cases of influenza A (H7N9) virus infection. N Engl J Med 2013;368:2277–85.

53. Pfister R, Kochanek M, Leygeber T, et al. Procalcitonin for diagnosis of bacterial pneumonia in critically ill patients during 2009 H1N1 influenza pandemic: a prospective cohort study, systematic review and individual patient data meta-analysis. Crit Care 2014; 18:R44.

54. Rodriguez AH, Aviles-Jurado FX, Diaz E, et al. Procalcitonin (PCT) levels for ruling-out bacterial coinfection in ICU patients with influenza: A CHAID decision-tree analysis. J Infect 2016;72:143–51.

55. Qureshi NR, Hien TT, Farrar J, et al. The radiologic manifestations of H5N1 avian influenza. J Thorac Imaging 2006;21:259–64.

56. Wang Q, Zhang Z, Shi Y, et al. Emerging H7N9 influenza A (novel reassortant avian-origin) pneumonia: radiologic findings. Radiology 2013;268:882–9.

57. Bakhshayeshkaram M, Saidi B, Tabarsi P, et al. Imaging Findings in Patients With H1N1 Influenza A Infection. Iran J Radiol 2011;8:230–4.

58. Dugas AF, Valsamakis A, Atreya MR, et al. Clinical diagnosis of influenza in the ED. Am J Emerg Med 2015;33:770–5.

59. Gharabaghi F, Hawan A, Drews SJ, et al. Evaluation of multiple commercial molecular and conventional diagnostic assays for the detection of respiratory viruses in children. Clin Microbiol Infect 2011;17: 1900–6.

60. Zumla A, Memish ZA, Maeurer M, et al. Emerging novel and antimicrobial-resistant respiratory tract infections: new drug development and therapeutic options. Lancet Infect Dis 2014;14:1136–49.

61. Morita M, Kuba K, Ichikawa A, et al. The lipid mediator protectin D1 inhibits influenza virus replication and improves severe influenza. Cell 2013;153:112–25.

62. Tam VC, Quehenberger O, Oshansky CM, et al. Lipidomic profiling of influenza infection identifies mediators that induce and resolve inflammation. Cell 2013;154:213–27.

63. Paterson JC, Miller MH, Dillon JF. Update on the treatment of hepatitis C genotypes 2-6. Curr Opin Infect Dis 2014;27:540–4.

64. Kim WY, Young Suh G, Huh JW, et al. Triple-combination antiviral drug for pandemic H1N1 influenza

virus infection in critically ill patients on mechanical ventilation. Antimicrob Agents Chemother 2011;55: 5703–9.

65. Seo S, Englund JA, Nguyen JT, et al. Combination therapy with amantadine, oseltamivir and ribavirin for influenza A infection: safety and pharmacokinetics. Antivir Ther 2013;18:377–86.

66. Hurt AC. The epidemiology and spread of drug resistant human influenza viruses. Curr Opin Virol 2014;8:22–9.

67. Chen Y, Liang W, Yang S, et al. Human infections with the emerging avian influenza A H7N9 virus from wet market poultry: clinical analysis and characterisation of viral genome. Lancet 2013;381: 1916–25.

68. Govorkova EA, Baranovich T, Seiler P, et al. Antiviral resistance among highly pathogenic influenza A (H5N1) viruses isolated worldwide in 2002-2012 shows need for continued monitoring. Antiviral Res 2013;98:297–304.

69. Meijer A, Rebelo-de-Andrade H, Correia V, et al. Global update on the susceptibility of human influenza viruses to neuraminidase inhibitors, 2012-2013. Antiviral Res 2014;110:31–41.

70. Takashita E, Meijer A, Lackenby A, et al. Global update on the susceptibility of human influenza viruses to neuraminidase inhibitors, 2013-2014. Antiviral Res 2015;117:27–38.

71. Li C, Yang P, Zhang Y, et al. Corticosteroid treatment ameliorates acute lung injury induced by 2009 swine origin influenza A (H1N1) virus in mice. PloS One 2012;7:e44110.

72. Ottolini M, Blanco J, Porter D, et al. Combination anti-inflammatory and antiviral therapy of influenza in a cotton rat model. Pediatr Pulmonol 2003;36:290–4.

73. Torres A, Sibila O, Ferrer M, et al. Effect of corticosteroids on treatment failure among hospitalized patients with severe community-acquired pneumonia and high inflammatory response: a randomized clinical trial. JAMA 2015;313:677–86.

74. Blum CA, Nigro N, Briel M, et al. Adjunct prednisone therapy for patients with community-acquired pneumonia: a multicentre, double-blind, randomised, placebo-controlled trial. Lancet 2015;385:1511–8.

75. Delaney JW, Pinto R, Long J, et al. The influence of corticosteroid treatment on the outcome of influenza A(H1N1pdm09)-related critical illness. Crit Care 2016;20:75.

76. Laidler MR, Thomas A, Baumbach J, et al. Statin treatment and mortality: propensity score-matched analyses of 2007-2008 and 2009-2010 laboratory-confirmed influenza hospitalizations. Open Forum Infect Dis 2015;2:ofv028.

77. Ishii H, Komiya K, Yamagata E, et al. Clarithromycin has limited effects in non-elderly, non-severe patients with seasonal influenza virus A infection. J Infect 2012;64:343–5.

78. Kakeya H, Seki M, Izumikawa K, et al. Efficacy of combination therapy with oseltamivir phosphate and azithromycin for influenza: a multicenter, open-label, randomized study. PLoS One 2014;9: e91293.

79. Martin-Loeches I, Bermejo-Martin JF, Valles J, et al. Macrolide-based regimens in absence of bacterial co-infection in critically ill H1N1 patients with primary viral pneumonia. Intensive Care Med 2013;39: 693–702.

80. Wang CH, Chung FT, Lin SM, et al. Adjuvant treatment with a mammalian target of rapamycin inhibitor, sirolimus, and steroids improves outcomes in patients with severe H1N1 pneumonia and acute respiratory failure. Crit Care Med 2014;42:313–21.

81. Lai KY, Ng WY, Osburga Chan PK, et al. High-dose N-acetylcysteine therapy for novel H1N1 influenza pneumonia. Ann Intern Med 2010;152:687–8.

82. Linko R, Pettila V, Ruokonen E, et al. Corticosteroid therapy in intensive care unit patients with PCR-confirmed influenza A(H1N1) infection in Finland. Acta Anaesthesiol Scand 2011;55:971–9.

83. Lee N, Leo YS, Cao B, et al. Neuraminidase inhibitors, superinfection and corticosteroids affect survival of influenza patients. Eur Respir J 2015;45: 1642–52.

84. Brun-Buisson C, Richard JC, Mercat A, et al. Early corticosteroids in severe influenza A/H1N1 pneumonia and acute respiratory distress syndrome. Am J Respir Crit Care Med 2011;183:1200–6.

85. Kim SH, Hong SB, Yun SC, et al. Corticosteroid treatment in critically ill patients with pandemic influenza A/H1N1 2009 infection: analytic strategy using propensity scores. Am J Respir Crit Care Med 2011; 183:1207–14.

86. Diaz E, Martin-Loeches I, Canadell L, et al. Corticosteroid therapy in patients with primary viral pneumonia due to pandemic (H1N1) 2009 influenza. J Infect 2012;64:311–8.

87. Xi X, Xu Y, Jiang L, et al. Hospitalized adult patients with 2009 influenza A(H1N1) in Beijing, China: risk factors for hospital mortality. BMC Infect Dis 2010; 10:256.

88. Cao B, Gao H, Zhou B, et al. Adjuvant corticosteroid treatment in adults with influenza A (H7N9) viral pneumonia. Crit Care Med 2016;44(6):e318–28.

89. Liem NT, Tung CV, Hien ND, et al. Clinical features of human influenza A (H5N1) infection in Vietnam: 2004-2006. Clin Infect Dis 2009;48:1639–46.

90. Vandermeer ML, Thomas AR, Kamimoto L, et al. Association between use of statins and mortality among patients hospitalized with laboratory-confirmed influenza virus infections: a multistate study. J Infect Dis 2012;205:13–9.

91. Kwong JC, Li P, Redelmeier DA. Influenza morbidity and mortality in elderly patients receiving statins: a cohort study. PLoS One 2009;4:e8087.

92. Cao B, Hayden FG. Therapy of H7N9 pneumonia: current perspectives. Expert Rev Anti Infect Ther 2013;11:1123–6.

93. Yang M, Gao H, Chen J, et al. Bacterial coinfection is associated with severity of avian influenza A (H7N9), and procalcitonin is a useful marker for early diagnosis. Diagn Microbiol Infect Dis 2016;84:165–9.

94. Brundage JF. Interactions between influenza and bacterial respiratory pathogens: implications for pandemic preparedness. Lancet Infect Dis 2006;6: 303–12.

95. Martin-Loeches I, Sanchez-Corral A, Diaz E, et al. Community-acquired respiratory coinfection in critically ill patients with pandemic 2009 influenza A(H1N1) virus. Chest 2011;139:555–62.

96. Chertow DS, Memoli MJ. Bacterial coinfection in influenza: a grand rounds review. JAMA 2013;309: 275–82.

97. Estenssoro E, Rios FG, Apezteguia C, et al. Pandemic 2009 influenza A in Argentina: a study of 337 patients on mechanical ventilation. Am J Respir Crit Care Med 2010;182:41–8.

Epidemic and Emerging Coronaviruses (Severe Acute Respiratory Syndrome and Middle East Respiratory Syndrome)

David S. Hui, MD

KEYWORDS

- SARS-CoV • MERS-CoV • Respiratory tract infections • Clinical features • Pathogenesis
- Treatment

KEY POINTS

- Bats are the natural reservoirs of severe acute respiratory syndrome (SARS)-like coronaviruses (CoVs) and are likely the reservoir of Middle East respiratory syndrome (MERS)-CoVs.
- The clinical features of SARS-CoV infection and MERS-CoV infection are similar but patients with MERS-CoV infection progress to respiratory failure much more rapidly than those with SARS.
- Although the estimated pandemic potential of MERS-CoV is lower than that of SARS-CoV, the case fatality rate of MERS is much higher and likely related to older age and presence of comorbid illness among the sporadic cases.
- Although dromedary camels have a high seroprevalence of MERS-CoV antibody and some camels have been found to have positive nasal swabs by reverse transcription (RT)–polymerase chain reaction (PCR), the transmission route and the possibility of other intermediary animal sources remain uncertain among many sporadic primary cases.
- The more feasible clinical trial options for MERS-CoV infection at present include monotherapy and combination therapy with lopinavir/ritonavir, interferon (IFN)-β1b, passive immunotherapy with convalescent plasma, or human monoclonal or polyclonal antibody.

INTRODUCTION

CoVs (order Nidovirales, family Coronaviridae, subfamily Coronavirinae) are a group of highly diverse, single-stranded, enveloped, positive-sense, RNA viruses that may cause respiratory, hepatic, gastrointestinal, and neurologic diseases of varying severity in a wide range of animal species, including humans. There are 4 genera of CoVs: αCoV, βCoV, γCoV, and δCoV.[1] Before the SARS epidemic, the main CoVs causing respiratory tract infection in humans were human CoV-OC43 and human CoV-229E. A novel group, 2b βCoV, was discovered in March 2003 as the causative agent responsible for SARS-CoV infection.[2–4] Both SARS-CoV and MERS-CoV are βCoV and belong to lineages B and C, respectively.[1] In this article, the clinical features, laboratory aspects, pathogenesis, and potential treatment modalities of SARS-CoV infection and MERS-CoV infection are reviewed.

No conflict of interest declared.

Department of Medicine & Therapeutics, Stanley Ho Center for Emerging Infectious Diseases, Prince of Wales Hospital, The Chinese University of Hong Kong, Shatin, New Territories, Hong Kong, China
E-mail address: dschui@cuhk.edu.hk

Clin Chest Med 38 (2017) 71–86
http://dx.doi.org/10.1016/j.ccm.2016.11.007

SEVERE ACUTE RESPIRATORY INFECTION–CORONAVIRUS INFECTION

SARS-CoV first emerged in November 2002 in the Guangdong province in the southern part of China before spreading to Canada, Singapore, and Vietnam by travelers through Hong Kong (HK) in February 2003 and March 2003.[5,6] In November 2002, there was an unusual epidemic of atypical pneumonia in Foshan, Guangdong province, in China, with a high rate of nosocomial transmission to health care workers (HCWs).[7,8] A retrospective analysis of 55 patients hospitalized with atypical pneumonia in Guangzhou between January 2003 and February 2003 revealed positive SARS-CoV in their nasopharyngeal aspirates whereas 48 (87%) patients had positive serology to SARS-CoV in their convalescent sera. Genetic analysis showed that the SARS-CoV isolates from Guangzhou shared the same origin with those in other countries, with a phylogenetic pathway that matched the spread of SARS-CoV to other parts of the world.[9]

The Origin of the Virus

In March 2003, a novel CoV was confirmed as the causative agent for SARS and thus was referred to as SARS-CoV. A retrospective serologic survey suggested that cross-species transmission of SARS-CoV or its variants from animal species to humans might have occurred frequently in the wet market where a high seroprevalence of 16.7% was detected among asymptomatic animal handlers.[10] It was initially thought that masked palm civets might have contributed to transmission of SARS-CoV to humans after detection of a close variant of SARS-CoV from palm civets in Dongmen market, Shenzhen, in 2003.[11] During the small-scale SARS-CoV infection outbreaks in late 2003 and early 2004 in China, 3 of the 4 patients had direct or indirect contact with palm civets.[12,13] Viral genomic sequence analysis showed, however, that the SARS-CoV–like virus had not been present among masked civets in markets for long. CoVs highly similar to SARS-CoV were isolated in horseshoe bats in 2005.[14,15] These bat SARS-like CoVs shared 88% to 92% sequence homology with human or civet isolates and the data suggest that bats could be a natural reservoir of a close ancestor of SARS-CoV.[16]

Pathogenesis

SARS-CoV infects humans through the respiratory tract, mainly via droplet transmission. Although human intestinal cells were proved susceptible to SARS-CoV replication, the role of the intestinal tract as a portal of entry remains uncertain.[17] The surface envelope spike protein (S protein) of SARS-CoV plays an important role in establishing infection and determining the cell and tissue tropism. Entry of the virus requires receptor binding, followed by conformational change of the S protein and then cathepsin L–mediated proteolysis within the endosome.[18] The angiotensin-converting enzyme 2 (ACE2) is the host receptor mediating the entry of SARS-CoV[19] and is expressed on a wide variety of body tissues.

Several mechanisms of direct injury in infected lungs with SARS have been revealed. The ACE2 probably contributes to the diffuse alveolar damage (DAD). ACE2 is a negative regulator of the local renin-angiotensin system and data from animal study support that the DAD seen in SARS is mediated by S protein–ACE2-renin-angiotensin pathway.[20] In addition, the SARS-CoV–encoded 3a and 7a proteins were shown a strong inducer of apoptosis in cell lines derived from different organs, including lungs, kidneys, and liver.[21,22]

Activation of helper T (TH1) cell–mediated immunity and hyperinnate inflammatory response might be responsible for disease progression in SARS-CoV infection,[23,24] as shown by marked increases in the levels of the TH1 and inflammatory cytokines (IFN-γ, interleukin [IL]-1, IL-6, and IL-12) and marked increases in chemokines, such as TH1 chemokine IFN-γ–inducible protein 10 (IP-10), neutrophil chemokine IL-8, and monocyte chemoattractant protein-1 (MCP-1) in patients with SARS-CoV infection for more than 14 days after illness onset.[25] In mice infected with SARS-CoV, T cells played an important role in SARS-CoV clearance whereas a reduced T-cell response contributed to severe disease.[26] In another study of mice infected with SARS-CoV, robust virus replication accompanied by delayed type I IFN (IFN-I) signaling was observed orchestrating inflammatory responses and lung immunopathology with reduced survival.[27] Case-control studies have suggested that genetic variants of IL-12 receptor B1 predispose to SARS-CoV infection,[28] whereas Mannose-binding lectin deficiency is a susceptibility factor for acquisition of SARS-CoV infection.[29]

Lung histopathology in patients with severe SARS-CoV infection include DAD, denudation of bronchial epithelia, loss of cilia, squamous metaplasia, and giant cell infiltrate, with a marked increase in macrophages in the alveoli and the interstitium. Hemophagocytosis, atrophy of the white pulp of the spleen, hyaline membranes, and secondary bacterial pneumonia were also noted.[4,5,23,30] Although DAD was the main pulmonary feature,[4,5,23] lesions in subpleural locations resembling bronchiolitis obliterans organizing pneumonia were also seen.[31]

Epidemiology

A 64-year-old nephrologist who came from southern China to HK on February 21, 2003, was the index case causing subsequent outbreaks of SARS-CoV infection in HK, Singapore, and Toronto.[5,6,32,33] Sixteen hotel guests/visitors were infected by the physician while staying or visiting friends on the same floor of the Hotel M, where the physician had stayed. Through international air travel, these visitors spread the infection to 29 countries/regions, with a total of 8098 cases and a mortality rate of 774 (9.6%) by the end of the epidemic in July 2003.[34]

SARS seems to have spread by close person-to-person contact via droplet transmission or contact with fomite.[35] The superspreading event was a hallmark of SARS-CoV infection, as reflected by the nosocomial outbreak at a major teaching hospital in HK where 138 subjects (many HCWs and previously healthy) were infected within 2 weeks after exposure to 1 patient (a visitor of Hotel M), who was hospitalized with community-acquired pneumonia to a general medical ward.[5,36] This superspreading event was likely caused by several factors including the use of a jet nebulizer for delivering bronchodilator to the index case, overcrowding, and poor ventilation in the hospital ward.[5,36] In addition, the temporal-spatial spread of SARS-CoV among inpatients in the index medical ward of the hospital in HK was consistent with airborne transmission.[37] Apart from respiratory secretions, SARS-CoV was detected in feces, urine, and tears of infected individuals.[38]

In addition, SARS-CoV might have spread by opportunistic airborne transmission in a major community outbreak involving more than 300 residents in a private residential complex, Amoy Gardens, in HK.[39,40] Drying up of water inside the U-shaped bathroom floor drain and backflow of contaminated sewage (from a SARS patient with renal failure and diarrhea) related to negative pressure generated by the toilet exhaust fans might have created infectious aerosols that moved upward through the warm airshaft of the building. Based on analysis of the distribution of all confirmed cases, airborne spread was the most likely explanation in the Amoy Gardens outbreak and the SARS-CoV could have spread more than 200 m to nearby residential complexes.[41] Air samples obtained from a hospital room in Toronto occupied by a SARS patient and swab samples taken from frequently touched surfaces in rooms

and in a nurses' station in Toronto were positive by PCR testing.[42] These data suggest the possibility of airborne transmission and stress the importance of taking appropriate respiratory protection apart from strict surface hygiene practices.

Clinical Features

The estimated mean incubation period of SARS was 4.6 days (95% CI, 3.8–5.8 days) whereas the mean time from symptom onset to hospitalization varied between 2 days and 8 days, decreasing over the course of the epidemic. The mean time from onset to death was 23.7 days (95% CI, 22.0–25.3 days).[43]

The major clinical features of SARS-CoV infection on presentation include persistent fever, chills/rigor, myalgia, dry cough, headache, malaise and dyspnea. Sore throat, rhinorrhea, sputum production, nausea and vomiting, and dizziness were less common.[5,6,32,33] Watery diarrhea became prominent in 40% to 70% of patients with SARS one week from illness onset during the clinical course of the illness.[44,45] In 2 patients who presented with status epilepticus, SARS-CoV was detected in the cerebrospinal fluid and serum samples.[46,47] Elderly subjects might not develop fever but present with decrease in general condition, delirium, poor feeding, and fall/fracture.[48] Teenagers tended to follow a clinical course similar to those of adults whereas young children (<12 years of age) often ran a benign clinical course.[49] There was no reported fatality in young children and teenage patients,[49] but SARS in pregnancy carried a significant risk of mortality.[50] Asymptomatic infection seems uncommon because a meta-analysis has shown overall seroprevalence rates of 0.1% for the general population and 0.23% for HCWs, although the true incidence of asymptomatic infection remains unknown.[51]

There was a typical pattern for the clinical course of SARS[5,24,52,53]: phase 1 (viral replication) was associated with increasing SARS-CoV load and characterized by fever, myalgia, and other systemic symptoms that generally improved after a few days; phase 2 (immunopathologic injury) was characterized by recurrence of fever, hypoxemia, and radiologic progression of pneumonia with falls in viral load whereas approximately 20% of patients progressed into acute respiratory distress syndrome (ARDS), necessitating invasive mechanical ventilatory support.[5,53] Because there was peaking of viral load on day 10 of illness followed by progressive decrease in rates of viral shedding from nasopharynx, stool, and urine from day 10 to day 21 after symptom onset, clinical worsening during phase 2 was likely the result of immune-mediated lung injury due to an overex-uberant host response.[24]

Laboratory Features

Lymphopenia, disseminated intravascular coagulation, elevated lactate dehydrogenase, and creatinine kinase were common laboratory features of SARS.[5] The CD4 and CD8 T-lymphocyte counts fell early in the course of SARS, whereas low counts of CD4 and CD8 at presentation were associated with adverse clinical outcome.[54]

Radiologic Features

Although nonspecific, common radiographic features of SARS included the predominant involvement of lung periphery and the lower zone in addition to absence of cavitation, hilar lymphadenopathy, or pleural effusion.[5,55] Radiographic progression from unilateral focal air-space opacity to either multifocal or bilateral involvement occurred during the second phase of the disease, followed by radiographic improvement with treatment.[5,55] In 1 case series, spontaneous pneumomediastinum occurred in 12% of patients whereas 20% of patients developed ARDS over a period of 3 weeks.[24] Common high-resolution CT features included ground-glass opacification, sometimes with consolidation, and interlobular septal and intralobular interstitial thickening, with predominantly a peripheral and lower lobe involvement.[5,55]

Treatment

Ribavirin, a nucleoside analog, was widely used for treating SARS patients in 2003 but ribavirin alone had no significant in vitro activity against SARS-CoV,[56] and it caused significant hemolysis in many patients.[5,33] Lopinavir and ritonavir in combination is a boosted protease inhibitor regimen widely used for treatment HIV infection. In vitro activity against SARS-CoV was demonstrated for lopinavir and ribavirin at 4 µg/mL and 50 µg/mL, respectively, whereas inhibition of in vitro cytopathic effects was achieved down to a concentration of 1 µg/mL of lopinavir combined with 6.25 µg/mL of ribavirin.[57] A retrospective analysis showed that the addition of lopinavir (400 mg)/ritonavir (100 mg) as initial therapy was associated with lower overall death rate (2.3% vs 15.6%) and intubation rate (0% vs 11%) than a matched historical cohort who received ribavirin alone as the initial antiviral therapy.[58] The outcome of a subgroup who had received lopinavir/ritonavir as late rescue therapy after receiving pulsed methylprednisolone for worsening respiratory symptoms, however, was not better than the matched cohort.[57,58]

IFN-Is are produced early as part of the innate immune response to virus infections. There are in vitro and limited animal and observational data that IFN, in particular early use, has efficacy against SARS-CoV.[56,59,60] In experimentally infected cynomolgus macaques, prophylactic treatment with pegylated IFN-α significantly reduced viral replication and excretion, viral antigen (Ag) expression by type I pneumocytes, and lung damage versus untreated macaques, whereas postexposure treatment with pegylated IFN-α yielded intermediate results.[61] Use of IFN-α1 plus systemic corticosteroids was associated with improved oxygen saturation, more rapid resolution of radiographic lung opacities, and lower levels of creatinine kinase than systemic corticosteroids alone in another study of SARS patients.[62]

During the second week of SARS illness, there was evidence of bronchiolitis obliterans organizing pneumonia radiologically[5] and histopathologically in some cases[31] whereas the progression of the pulmonary disease was mediated by the host inflammatory response.[24] Systemic corticosteroids in the form of pulsed methylprednisolone significantly reduced IL-8, MCP-1, and IP-10 concentrations from 5 to 8 days after treatment in 20 adult SARS patients in an uncontrolled study.[25] Induction of IP-10 is thought to be a critical event in the initiation of immune-mediated lung injury and lymphocyte apoptosis.[63] The use of rescue pulsed methylprednisolone during clinical progression was associated with favorable clinical improvement in some patients with resolution of fever and radiographic lung opacities within 2 weeks.[5,64] A retrospective analysis showed, however, that theuse of pulsed methylprednisolone was associated with an increased risk of 30-day mortality (adjusted odds ratio [OR] 26.0; 95% CI, 4.4–154.8).[65] In addition, disseminated fungal disease and avascular osteonecrosis occurred after prolonged systemic corticosteroids therapy.[66,67] A randomized placebo-controlled study showed that plasma SARS-CoV RNA concentrations in the second and third weeks of illness were higher in patients given initial hydrocortisone (n = 10) intravenously than those given normal saline as control (n = 7) during early clinical course of illness. Despite the small sample size, the data suggest that systemic corticosteroid given in the earlier phase might prolong viremia.[68]

Convalescent plasma, donated by patients, including HCWs, who had recovered from SARS, contained high levels of neutralizing antibody and seemed clinically useful for treating other SARS patients. In a study comparing patients with SARS-CoV infection who did and did not receive convalescent plasma, 19 patients who received such therapy had better survival rate (100% vs

56.2%) and discharge rate (77.8% vs 23.0%) compared with 21 controls.[69] Among 80 non-randomized patients with SARS who were given convalescent plasma at the Prince of Wales Hospital (Shatin, Hong Kong) the discharge rate at day 22 was 58.3% for patients (n = 48) treated within 14 days of illness onset versus 15.6% for those (n = 32) treated beyond 14 days.[70] An exploratory post hoc meta-analysis of studies of SARS-CoV infection and severe influenza showed a significant reduction in the pooled odds of mortality after convalescent plasma versus placebo or no treatment (OR 0.25; 95% CI, 0.14–0.45).[71]

Hospital Infection Control Aspects

A case-control study involving 124 medical wards in 26 hospitals in HK and Guangzhou has identified 6 independent factors of superspreading nosocomial outbreaks of SARS-CoV infection: performance of resuscitation, minimum distance between beds less than 1 m, staff working while experience symptoms, and SARS patients requiring oxygen therapy or noninvasive ventilation whereas availability of washing or changing facilities for staff was a protective factor (Box 1).[72] A systematic review has shown that 4 aerosol-generating procedures would increase the risk of nosocomial SARS transmission to HCWs, including tracheal intubation, noninvasive ventilation, tracheotomy, and manual ventilation before intubation (Box 2).[73] Thus it is important for HCWs to take airborne precaution before carrying out aerosol-generating procedures.

MIDDLE EAST RESPIRATORY SYNDROME–CORONAVIRUS INFECTION

MERS-CoV was first reported in September 2012 when a novel βCoV was isolated from a male patient who had died of severe pneumonia and multi-organ failure in Saudi Arabia in June 2012.[74] MERS-CoV infection has spread to 27 countries since its discovery in 2012. Globally, from September 2012 to June 29, 2016, the World Health Organization has been informed of 1769 laboratory-confirmed cases of infection with MERS-CoV, with at least 630 deaths.[75] The case definitions of suspected and confirmed cases of MERS-CoV infection are shown in Box 3.[76]

The Virus and Its Origin

Although the natural reservoir of MERS-CoV is still unclear, bats may be one possible reservoir for the virus. In a study screening fecal specimens of bats from Ghana and 4 European countries for βCoVs, viruses related to the novel human βCoV (EMC/2012, which was later renamed MERS-CoV) were detected in 46 (24.9%) of 185 *Nycteris* bats and 40 (14.7%) of 272 *Pipistrellus* bats.[77] Of 1100 bat samples tested in another study, 1 fragment of MERS-CoV was found in 1 *Taphozous* bat with close matching to a human isolate of MERS-CoV.[78] Their genetic relatedness indicates that MERS-CoV has originated from bats.

Dromedary camels are an important natural host for the maintenance and diversification of

---

Box 1
Independent factors associated with increased risk of superspreading[a] events of severe acute respiratory syndrome–coronavirus infection in the health care setting

Performance of resuscitation (OR 3.81; 95% CI, 1.04–13.87; *P* = .04)

Staff working while experiencing symptoms (OR 10.55; 95% CI, 2.28–48.87; *P* = .003)

SARS patients requiring oxygen therapy at least 6 L/min (OR 4.30; 95% CI, 1.00–18.43; *P* = .05)

SARS patients requiring noninvasive positive pressure ventilation (OR 11.82; 95% CI, 1.97–70.80; *P* = .007)

Minimum distance between beds <1 m (OR 6.94; 95% CI, 1.68–28.75; *P* = .008)

Washing or changing facilities for staff (OR 0.12; 95% CI, 0.02–0.97; *P* = .05)

[a] A superspreading event was defined as 1 patient who could infect at least 3 others.
Data from Yu IT, Xie ZH, Tsoi KK, et al. Why did outbreaks of severe acute respiratory syndrome occur in some hospital wards but not in others? Clin Infect Dis 2007;44:1017–25.

Box 2
Respiratory procedures reported to present an increased risk of transmission of severe acute respiratory syndrome–coronavirus to health care workers (n; pooled OR [95% CI])

Tracheal intubation (n = 4 cohort; 6.6 [2.3, 18.9], and n = 4 case-control; 6.6 [4.1, 10.6])

Noninvasive ventilation (n = 2 cohort; 3.1 [1.4, 6.8]),

Tracheotomy (n = 1 case-control; 4.2 [1.5, 11.5])

Manual ventilation before intubation (n = 1 cohort; 2.8 [1.3, 6.4]).

Data from Tran K, Cimon K, Severn M, et al. Aerosol generating procedures and risk of transmission of acute respiratory infections to healthcare workers: a systematic review. PLoS One 2012;7:e35797.

Box 3
World Health Organization case definitions of the Middle East respiratory syndrome

Confirmed case

A person with laboratory confirmation of MERS-CoV infection,[1] irrespective of clinical signs and symptoms.

Probable case

- A febrile acute respiratory illness with clinical, radiologic, or histopathologic evidence of pulmonary parenchymal disease (eg, pneumonia or ARDS)
  AND
  Direct epidemiologic link[2] with a confirmed MERS-CoV case
  AND
  Testing for MERS-CoV is unavailable, negative on a single inadequate specimen[3] or inconclusive[4]

- A febrile acute respiratory illness with clinical, radiologic, or histopathologic evidence of pulmonary parenchymal disease (eg, pneumonia or ARDS)
  AND
  The person resides or traveled in the Middle East or in countries where MERS-CoV is known to be circulating in dromedary camels or where human infections have recently occurred
  AND
  Testing for MERS-CoV is inconclusive[4]

- An acute febrile respiratory illness of any severity
  AND
  Direct epidemiologic link[2] with a confirmed MERS-CoV case
  AND
  Testing for MERS-CoV is inconclusive[4]

Notes

1 A case may be laboratory confirmed by detection of viral nucleic acid or serology. The presence of viral nucleic acid can be confirmed by either a positive RT-PCR result on at least 2 specific genomic targets or a single positive target with sequencing of a second target. A case confirmed by serology requires demonstration of seroconversion in 2 samples ideally taken at least 14 days apart, by a screening (ELISA or immunofluorescence assay) *and* a neutralization assay.
  The interim recommendations for laboratory testing for MERS-CoV should be consulted, however, for the most recent standard for laboratory confirmation (http://www.who.int/csr/disease/coronavirus_infections/en/).

2 A direct epidemiologic link with a confirmed MERS-CoV patient may include

   - Health care–associated exposure, including providing direct care for MERS-CoV patients, working with HCWs infected with MERS-CoV, visiting patients, or staying in the same close environment of individuals infected with MERS-CoV

   - Working together in close proximity or sharing the same classroom environment with individuals infected with MERS-CoV

   - Traveling together with individuals infected with MERS-CoV in any kind of conveyance

   - Living in the same household as individuals infected with MERS-CoV

   - The epidemiologic link may have occurred within a 14-day period before or after the onset of illness in the case under consideration

3 An inadequate specimen would include a nasopharyngeal swab without an accompanying lower respiratory specimen or a specimen that has had improper handling, is judged to be of poor quality by the testing laboratory, or was taken too late in the course of illness.

4 Inconclusive tests may include

   - A positive screening test on a single rRT-PCR target without further confirmation

   - Evidence of seroreactivity by a single convalescent serum sample ideally taken at least 14 days after exposure by a screening assay (ELISA or immunofluorescence assay) and a neutralization assay, in the absence of molecular confirmation from respiratory specimens.

From WHO. Middle east respiratory syndrome coronavirus case definition for reporting to WHO interim case definition 14 July 2015. Available at: http://www.who.int/csr/disease/coronavirus_infections/case_definition/en/. Accessed July 2, 2016.

MERS-CoV and seem to be the major source of zoonotic human infection. The virus has been isolated from dromedary camels in the Arabian Peninsula and across North Africa, East Africa, West Africa, and Central Africa but is not found in dromedary camels in Kazakhstan[79] or in Bactrian camels in Mongolia[80] or other countries.[81,82] Only a minority of reported MERS human cases, however, have reported direct camel exposure.[83]

Epidemiology

Although MERS-CoV was first described in September 2012,[74] retrospective analysis of a cluster of hospital cases dated back to April 2012 in Jordan confirmed MERS-CoV by RT-PCR and serology as the etiology of the outbreak, which involved at least 10 HCWs.[84] The epidemiology of MERS-CoV is characterized by sporadic zoonotic transmission events, sometimes followed by nosocomial outbreaks within health care settings due to failure in infection control and prevention measures. Saudi Arabia has the largest MERS-CoV caseload, followed by South Korea as the country with the highest caseload outside the Arabic Peninsula.[75]

The risk factors for primary MERS-CoV infection were addressed in a case-control study, consisting of 30 primary MERS-CoV cases reported from March 2014 to November 2014 in Saudi Arabia, with 2 to 4 controls matched by age, gender, and neighborhood for each case patient.[85] Using multivariable analysis, the investigators demonstrated that direct dromedary exposure in the 2 weeks before illness onset was strongly associated with MERS-CoV illness (adjusted OR 7.45; 95% CI, 1.57–35.28), along with having diabetes mellitus (adjusted OR 6.99; 95% CI, 1.89–25.86) or heart disease (adjusted OR 6.87; 95% CI, 1.81–25.99) and current tobacco smoking (adjusted OR 6.84; 95% CI, 1.68–27.94).[85] The risk for secondary transmission from patients to household contacts was estimated at approximately 4%.[86] Risk factors for household transmission included sleeping in an index patient's room and touching respiratory secretions from an index patient whereas casual contact and simple proximity were not associated with transmission.[87]

In a cross-sectional serosurveillance study of 10,009 healthy individuals in Saudi Arabia, 0.15% had evidence of positive MERS-CoV serology, suggesting that the number of mild or asymptomatic infections far exceeds those that are recognized.[88] Seropositivity was more common in men than in women, in central than in coastal provinces, and in camel shepherds (2.3%) and slaughterhouse workers (3.6%) than the general population.[88]

Nosocomial transmission is a hallmark of MERS-CoV infection. Superspreading events of MERS-CoV infection have been reported in Jordan,[84] Al Hasa,[89] Jeddah,[90] and Abu Dhabi,[91] whereas the major outbreak in South Korea in 2015 is characterized by several superspreading events in the hospital settings.[92] Failure in infection control and prevention in health care facilities (HCFs) has resulted in large numbers of secondary cases of MERS-CoV infection involving HCWs, existing patients, and visitors in Saudi Arabia[89,90] and several other countries over the past few years.[84,91,92] Common predisposing factors include exposure to contaminated and overcrowded HCFs, poor compliance with appropriate personal protection equipment (PPE) when assessing patients with febrile respiratory illness, application of potentially aerosol-generating procedures (resuscitation, continuous positive airway pressure, and nebulized medications), and lack of proper isolation room facilities.[84,89–93] The customs of patients seeking care at different HCFs (doctor shopping) and having friends and family members stay with patients as caregivers at already overcrowded HCFs are unique factors in South Korea.[94]

In contrast to SARS, approximately 75% of patients with MERS had at least 1 comorbid illness whereas fatal cases were more likely to have an underlying condition (86% among fatal cases vs 42% among recovered or asymptomatic cases; P<.001). Index/sporadic cases were older (median age 59 years vs 43 years; P<.001) and more likely to suffer from severe disease requiring hospitalization (94% vs 59%; P<.001) in comparison to the secondary cases. Cases specifically reported as "mild disease" or "asymptomatic" occurred only among secondary cases.[89,90] Most (90%) index/sporadic cases had severe disease whereas a higher proportion of patients with renal failure was noted among secondary cases in Saudi Arabia, due to the nosocomial outbreak involving the hemodialysis units in hospitals in Al Hasa.[89] Good infection control measures in reported clusters involving HCS probably limited onward transmission to HCW and hospitalized patients.[89]

Clinical Features

The clinical presentation of MERS-CoV infection ranges from asymptomatic to very severe pneumonia with ARDS, septic shock, and multiorgan failure resulting in death. In contrast to SARS, the clinical course of MERS is more severe in immunocompromised patients and generally mild in individuals without comorbid illness.[95] Few cases have been reported in children less than 5 years of age. Typically, MERS-CoV infection begins with fever, cough, chills, sore throat, myalgia, and arthralgia, followed by dyspnea and rapid progression to pneumonia within the first week (in contrast to SARS), often requiring ventilatory and other organ support.[84,89,96,97] Most patients present with respiratory illness although immunocompromised patients may present with fever, chills, and diarrhea before developing pneumonia due to MERS-CoV.[98] At least one-third of patients also had gastrointestinal symptoms, such as vomiting and diarrhea.[84,89,96–99]

Neurologic complications, such as intracerebral hemorrhage (due to thrombocytopenia, disseminated intravascular coagulation, and platelet dysfunction) and critical illness polyneuropathy, complicating a long ICU stay, have been reported.[100] Pregnant women infected with MERS may develop severe disease and a fatal outcome, including stillbirth.[101–104] Concomitant infections and low albumin were found predictors of severe infection, whereas age greater than or equal to 65 years was the only predictor of increased mortality.[83]

Based on data related to human-to-human transmission in several clusters, the incubation period has been estimated to be more than 5 days but could be as long as 2 weeks (median 5.2 days [95% CI, 1.9–14.7]).[89] The median times from symptom onset of MERS to hospitalization, admission to an ICU, or death were 4.0 (range 0–16, n = 62), 5.0 (1–15, n = 35), and 11.5 days (4–298, n = 40), respectively.[96]

Laboratory Features

Similar to SARS and other severe viral illness, common laboratory findings of MERS include leukopenia, in particular lymphopenia.[74,84,97,99] Reports from several cases found viral RNA in blood, urine, and stool but at much lower viral loads than in the respiratory tract.[98,105] The viral load in upper respiratory tract specimens is generally lower than in the lower respiratory specimens.[106]

Radiologic Features

Radiographic findings of MERS are consistent with viral pneumonitis and ARDS, with bilateral hilar infiltration, unilateral or bilateral patchy densities or infiltrates, segmented or lobar opacities, ground-glass opacities, and small pleural effusions in some cases. Lower lobes are affected more than upper lobes early in the course of illness with more rapid radiographic progression than SARS. The most common CT finding in hospitalized patients with MERS-CoV infection is that of bilateral predominantly subpleural and basilar airspace changes, with more extensive ground-glass opacities than consolidation. The subpleural and peribronchovascular predilection of the abnormalities is suggestive of an organizing pneumonia pattern.[107]

Pathogenesis

The dipeptidyl peptidase 4 (DPP4), also known as CD26, has been identified as the functional cellular receptor for MERS-CoV.[108,109] DPP4 homologues permitting MERS-CoV infection are present in a variety of cell lines.[110,111] Cell-based studies have revealed that MERS-CoV evades innate immune response and this may explain the large number of severe cases.[112–114] Widespread MERS-CoV Ag expression has been observed in type I and type II alveolar cells, ciliated bronchial epithelium, and unciliated cuboid cells of terminal bronchioles. Virus Ag was also found in endothelial cells of pulmonary vessels and rarely in alveolar macrophages[115]

In contrast to a patient who survived nosocomial MERS-CoV infection in France, the index patient with a fatal outcome did not promote type I IFN, especially IFN-α, in response to MERS-CoV. Levels of both mediators IL-12 and IFN-γ that promote viral clearance were much lower in the fatal case than the patient who survived.[116] Lower respiratory tract (LRT) excretion of MERS-CoV could be observed for more than 1 month. The most severely ill patient presented an expression of the virus in blood and urine, consistent with impairment of a type I IFN–mediated immunologic response in the index patient, but such response was developed by the patient who survived.[117]

In a study of 37 adult patients infected with MERS-CoV in Saudi Arabia, viral loads were much higher in the LRT specimens than in the upper respiratory tract; 33% of all 108 serum samples tested yielded viral RNA whereas only 14.6% of stool and 2.4% of urine samples yielded viral RNA. All seroconversions occurred during the first 2 weeks after diagnosis, corresponding to the second and third weeks after symptom onset. All surviving patients, but only slightly more than half of all fatal cases, produced IgG and neutralizing antibodies. The levels of IgG and neutralizing antibodies were weakly and inversely correlated with LRT viral loads. Presence of antibodies did not lead to the elimination of virus from LRT.[106] In most patients in South Korea, robust antibody responses developed by the third week of illness whereas delayed antibody responses with the neutralization test were associated with more severe disease.[118] MERS-CoV antibodies, including neutralizing antibodies, were detectable in 6 (86%) of 7 persons erologically positive or indeterminate for at least 4 months after the nosocomial outbreak in Jordan in 2012.[119]

Autopsy of a 45 year-old man who died of MERS-CoV infection in Abu Dhabi in 2014 revealed DAD. Pneumocytes and epithelial syncytial cells were important targets of MERS-CoV Ag, because DPP4 receptors were found in scattered pneumocytes and syncytial cells but no evidence of extrapulmonary MERS-CoV Ags were detected, including the kidneys.[120] In a renal biopsy, which was performed 8 weeks after the onset of symptoms in a patient infected with MERS-CoV infection in South Korea, acute tubular necrosis was the main finding, whereas proteinaceous cast formation and acute tubule-interstitial nephritis were found. There were no electron dense deposits observed with electron microscopy. The investigators could not verify the virus itself by in situ hybridization and confocal microscopy (MERS-CoV costained with DPP4).[121]

Treatment

MERS-CoV causes cytokine and chemokine dysregulation by inducing significantly higher expression levels of cytokines (IL-12 and IFN-γ) and chemokines (IP-10/C-X-C motif chemokine ligand 10 (CXCL-10), MCP-1/C-C motif chemokine ligand 2 (CCL-2), major intrinsic protein (MIP)-1α/CCL-3, RANTES/CCL-5, and IL-8) than SARS-CoV in human monocyte–derived macrophages.[122] The host innate IFN response is crucial for the control of viral replication after infection because the absence of IFN-α impairs the development of a robust antiviral adaptive TH1 immune response, mediated by IL-12 and IFN-γ that promote viral clearance and bring substantial arguments for the indication of early IFN-α treatment during MERS-CoV infection.[116]

Many compounds have been found to have in vitro inhibitory activity against MERS-CoV infection. Notable are the type I IFNs, with IFN-β showing the strongest inhibitory activity[112,114,123,124] whereas IFN-α2b and ribavirin in combination was superior to individual components in reducing MERS-CoV viral load on Vero cells.[113] In rhesus macaques infected with MERS-CoV, combination therapy with high doses of IFN-α2b with ribavirin modestly reduced viral titers and measures of lung injury[125] but observational studies of clinical use have reported inconsistent findings. A small case series showed 100% mortality in 5 patients who received IFN-α2b plus ribavirin administered at a median of 19 days (range 10–20 days from admission).[126] A study of 32 patients compared outcomes in 13 patients treated with IFN-α2a (180 µg

subcutaneously once weekly) combined with ribavirin (loading dose of 2 g orally followed by 600 mg orally every 12 h) versus 11 patients treated with IFN-β1a (44 µg subcutaneously 3 times weekly) combined with ribavirin and found high mortality in both groups and no significant difference between them, 85% versus 64% (P = .24).[127] Although an earlier study of 20 patients treated with IFN-α2a combined with ribavirin found an improved survival rate at 14 days, these favorable findings were no longer significant by day 28 (70% mortality vs 83% in a comparator group of untreated patients with confirmed MERS-CoV infection; P = .54). The investigators attributed the lack of effectiveness to older age, presence of comorbid conditions, and delay in treatment initiation.[128] One case study described the use of lopinavir as part of triple-therapy regimen (in combination with IFN and ribavirin) in a MERS-CoV infected patient who subsequently died in Greece despite initial resolution of viraemia.[129]

Nitazoxanide is another potent type I IFN inducer that has been used in humans for parasitic infections. It is a synthetic nitrothiazolyl-salicylamide derivative that exhibits broad-spectrum antiviral activities against both RNA and DNA viruses, including canine CoV, influenza viruses, hepatitis B virus, hepatitis C virus, HIV, rotavirus, norovirus, and flaviviruses.[130] The combinational use of these IFN inducers (eg, nitazoxanide and chloroquine) and innate immunomodulators with effective antiviral agents may be synergistic and should be evaluated in animal models.

Systemic corticosteroids have been used empirically in some patients with MERS-CoV infection to dampen immunopathologic host responses, but no survival benefit has been reported.[126,131] A comprehensive review has shown that the use of systemic corticosteroids in patients with severe influenza A(H1N1)pdm09 infection was associated with increased risks of nosocomial pneumonia, higher 90-day mortality, and longer length of stay.[132] Systemic corticosteroids should be used cautiously because their use was associated with worsened outcomes in patients infected with SARS-CoV during the 2003 epidemic,[65] including fatal aspergillosis[66] and osteonecrosis.[67]

The nucleosides/nucleotides are building blocks of viral nucleic acids. Drugs that target nucleosides/nucleotides and/or viral nucleic acids generally have broad-spectrum activities against a wide range of CoVs and other viruses. Mycophenolate mofetil is an antirejection drug that inhibits inosine monophosphate dehydrogenase and guanine monophosphate synthesis. The active compound, mycophenolic acid, exhibits antiviral activity in vitro against various viruses that include hepatitis B virus, hepatitis C virus, and arboviruses. Mycophenolic acid was identified as a potential anti–MERS-CoV drug using high-throughput screening and exhibits potent anti–MERS-CoV activity in vitro.[133] In vitro activity, however, does not necessarily translate to in vivo effectiveness. A follow-up study by the same group of investigators has shown that MERS-CoV–infected common marmosets treated with mycophenolate mofetil had worsened outcome with more severe disease and higher viral loads in necropsied lung and extrapulmonary tissues compared with untreated animals.[134] Renal transplant recipients who were on maintenance mycophenolate mofetil therapy also developed severe or fatal MERS-CoV infection.[116,135] Thus, usual dosages of mycophenolate mofetil monotherapy are unlikely to be useful for either prophylaxis or treatment of CoV infections.

A systematic review and exploratory meta-analysis of patients with SARS-CoV and influenza virus treated with convalescent plasma showed a reduction in mortality[71] and thus should be considered a potential treatment of MER-CoV infection. Convalescent plasma from patients who have fully recovered from MERS-CoV infection with well-defined levels of MERS-CoV neutralizing antibodies, however, is not readily available. There are limiting factors, such as the appropriate window period for plasma retrieval from suitable donors and timely administration to other ill patients with MERS-CoV infection, in addition to the concern that the treatment dose may result in undesired volume expansion in patients with ARDS who require fluid restriction.

Various monoclonal and polyclonal antibody preparations with neutralizing activity inhibiting MERS-CoV are now in preclinical models.[136–140] There are no published human data, however, to date on the use of these preparations or of convalescent plasma for treatment of patients with MERS-CoV infection.

Although there is some concern that challenge of marmosets with MERS-CoV may not consistently lead to severe disease in the marmoset model,[141] more data are needed from suitable animal studies and carefully conducted clinical and virologic studies of priority treatments, such as convalescent plasma and IFNs (ideally in randomized clinical trials if sufficient numbers of patients are available). At present, clinical management of patients with severe disease largely relies on meticulous ICU support and prevention of complications.[142] The more feasible clinical trial options at present include monotherapy or combination therapy with lopinavir/ritonavir, IFN-β1b, passive immunotherapy with convalescent plasma, and human monoclonal or polyclonal antibody. More clinical trial data are needed to assess the role of IFN and ribavirin in

---

Box 4
Treatment modalities for Middle East respiratory syndrome–coronavirus infection

1. Treatment benefits likely to exceed risks

   Convalescent plasma, IFN, lopinavir, and monoclonal and polyclonal neutralizing antibody

2. Treatment data inadequate for assessment

   Interferon and ribavirin combination, nitazoxanide, and chloroquine

3. Risks likely to exceed benefits

   Systemic corticosteroids, ribavirin monotherapy, intravenous gammaglobulin, and mycophenolic acid

Adapted from Treatment of MERS-CoV: information for clinicians. Clinical decision-making support for treatment of MERS-CoV patients. 2015. Version 3.0. Public Health England and ISARIC. Available at: https://www.gov.uk/government/uploads/system/uploads/attachment_data/file/459835/merscov_for_clinicians_sept2015.pdf. Accessed September 5, 2015.

---

combination, nitazoxanide, and chloroquine whereas systemic corticosteroids, ribavirin monotherapy, intravenous gammaglobulin, and mycophenolic acid would pose more harm than benefits (**Box 4**).[143]

SUMMARY

Bats seem the common natural source of both SARS-CoV and MERS-CoV. The clinical features are similar but MERS progresses to respiratory failure much more rapidly than SARS. Although the estimated pandemic potential of MERS-CoV is lower than that of SARS-CoV,[144] the case fatality rate of MERS is much higher and likely related to older age and comorbid illness of the sporadic cases. Lots of knowledge gaps remain since the first discovery of MERS-CoV in 2012.[145] More studies are needed to understand the pathogenesis, viral kinetics, mode of disease transmission, and intermediary source of MERS-CoV to guide public health infection control measures and treatment. It is also important to watch for any emergence and mutation of other SARS-like clusters of circulating CoVs in the bat populations that may threaten human health.[146]

REFERENCES

1. Zumla A, Chan JF, Azhar EI, et al. Coronaviruses - drug discovery and therapeutic options. Nat Rev Drug Discov 2016;15(5):327–47.

2. Drosten C, Gunther S, Preiser W, et al. Identification of a novel coronavirus in patients with severe acute respiratory syndrome. N Engl J Med 2003;348:1967–76.

3. Ksiazek TG, Erdman D, Goldsmith CS, et al, SARS Working Group. A novel coronavirus associated with severe acute respiratory syndrome. N Engl J Med 2003;348:1953–66.

4. Kuiken T, Fouchier RA, Schutten M, et al. Newly discovered coronavirus as the primary cause of severe acute respiratory syndrome. Lancet 2003;362:263–70.

5. Lee N, Hui DS, Wu A, et al. A major outbreak of severe acute respiratory syndrome in Hong Kong. N Engl J Med 2003;348:1986–94.

6. Tsang KW, Ho PL, Ooi GC, et al. A cluster of cases of severe acute respiratory syndrome in Hong Kong. N Engl J Med 2003;348:1977–85.

7. Zhao Z, Zhang F, Xu M, et al. Description and clinical treatment of an early outbreak of severe acute respiratory syndrome (SARS) in Guangzhou, PR China. J Med Microbiol 2003;52:715–20.

8. Xu RH, He JF, Evans MR, et al. Epidemiologic clues to SARS origin in China. Emerg Infect Dis 2004;10:1030–7.

9. Zhong NS, Zheng BJ, Li YM, et al. Epidemiology and cause of severe acute respiratory syndrome in Guangdong, People's Republic of China, in Feb 2003. Lancet 2003;362:1353–8.

10. Du L, Qiu JC, Wang M, et al. Analysis on the characteristics of blood serum Ab-IgG detective result of severe acute respiratory syndrome patients in Guangzhou, China. Zhonghua Liu Xing Bing Xue Za Zhi 2004;25:925–8.

11. Guan Y, Zheng BJ, He YQ, et al. Isolation and characterization of viruses related to the SARS coronavirus from animals in southern China. Science 2003;302:276–8.

12. Wang M, Yan M, Xu H, et al. SARS-CoV infection in a restaurant from palm civet. Emerg Infect Dis 2005;11:1860–5.

13. Song HD, Tu CC, Zhang GW, et al. Cross-host evolution of severe acute respiratory syndrome coronavirus in palm civet and human. Proc Natl Acad Sci U S A 2005;102:2430–5.

14. Lau SK, Woo PC, Li KS, et al. Severe acute respiratory syndrome coronavirus-like virus in Chinese horseshoe bats. Proc Natl Acad Sci 2005;102:14040–5.

15. Li W, Shi Z, Yu M, et al. Bats are natural reservoirs of SARS-like coronaviruses. Science 2005;310:676–9.

16. Shi Z, Hu Z. A review of studies on animal reservoirs of the SARS coronavirus. Virus Res 2008;133:74–87.

17. Chan PK, To KF, Lo AW, et al. Persistent infection of SARS coronavirus in colonic cells in vitro. J Med Virol 2004;74:1–7.

18. Simmons G, Gosalia DN, Rennekamp AJ, et al. Inhibitors of cathepsin L prevent severe acute respiratory syndrome coronavirus entry. Proc Natl Acad Sci 2005;102:11876–81.

19. Li W, Moore MJ, Vasilieva N, et al. Angiotensin-converting enzyme 2 is a functional receptor for the SARS coronavirus. Nature 2003;426:450–4.

20. Imai Y, Kuba K, Rao S, et al. Angiotensin-converting enzyme 2 protects from severe acute lung failure. Nature 2005;436:112–6.

21. Law PT, Wong CH, Au TC, et al. The 3a protein of severe acute respiratory syndrome-associated coronavirus induces apoptosis in Vero E6 cells. J Gen Virol 2005;86:1921–30.

22. Tan YJ, Fielding BC, Goh PY, et al. Over expression of 7a, a protein specifically encoded by the severe acute respiratory syndrome coronavirus, induces apoptosis via a caspase-dependent pathway. J Virol 2004;78:14043–7.

23. Nicholls JM, Poon LL, Lee KC, et al. Lung pathology of fatal severe acute respiratory syndrome. Lancet 2003;361:1773–8.

24. Peiris JS, Chu CM, Cheng VC, et al, HKU/UCH SARS Study Group. Clinical progression and viral load in a community outbreak of coronavirus-associated SARS pneumonia: a prospective study. Lancet 2003;361:1767–72.

25. Wong CK, Lam CWK, Wu AK, et al. Plasma inflammatory cytokines and chemokines in severe acute respiratory syndrome. Clin Exp Immunol 2004;136:95–103.

26. Zhao J, Zhao J, Perlman S. T cell responses are required for protection from clinical disease and for virus clearance in severe acute respiratory syndrome coronavirus-infected mice. J Virol 2010;84(18):9318–25.

27. Channappanavar R, Fehr AR, Vijay R, et al. Dysregulated type I interferon and inflammatory monocyte-macrophage responses cause lethal pneumonia in SARS-CoV-infected mice. Cell Host Microbe 2016;19(2):181–93.

28. Tang F, Liu W, Zhang F, et al. IL-12 RB1 genetic variants contribute to human susceptibility to severe acute respiratory syndrome infection among Chinese. PLoS One 2008;3(5):e2183.

29. Ip WK, Chan KH, Law HK, et al. Mannose-binding lectin in severe acute respiratory syndrome coronavirus infection. J Infect Dis 2005;191(10):1697–704.

30. Franks TJ, Chong PY, Chui P, et al. Lung pathology of severe acute respiratory syndrome (SARS): a study of 8 autopsy cases from Singapore. Hum Pathol 2003;34:743–8.

31. Tse GM, To KF, Chan PK, et al. Pulmonary pathological features in coronavirus associated severe acute respiratory syndrome (SARS). J Clin Pathol 2004;57:260–5.

32. Hsu LY, Lee CC, Green JA, et al. Severe acute respiratory syndrome in Singapore: clinical features of index patient and initial contacts. Emerg Infect Dis 2003;9:713–7.

33. Booth CM, Matukas LM, Tomlinson GA, et al. Clinical features and short-term outcomes of 144 patients with SARS in the greater Toronto area. JAMA 2003;289:2801–9.

34. WHO. Summary of probable SARS cases with onset of illness from 1 November to 31 July 2003. Available at: http://www.who.int/csr/sars/country/table2004_04_21/en/. Accessed July 2, 2016.

35. Peiris JS, Yuen KY, Osterhaus AD, et al. The severe acute respiratory syndrome. N Engl J Med 2003; 349:2431–41.

36. Wong RS, Hui DS. Index patient and SARS outbreak in Hong Kong. Emerg Infect Dis 2004; 10:339–41.

37. Yu IT, Wong TW, Chiu YL, et al. Temporal-spatial analysis of Severe acute respiratory syndrome among hospital inpatients. Clin Infect Dis 2005; 40:1237–43.

38. Loon SC, Teoh SC, Oon LL, et al. The severe acute respiratory syndrome coronavirus in tears. Br J Ophthalmol 2004;88:861–3.

39. Yu IT, Li Y, Wong TW, et al. Evidence of airborne transmission of the severe acute respiratory syndrome virus. N Engl J Med 2004;350:1731–9.

40. Chu CM, Cheng VC, Hung IF, et al. Viral load distribution in SARS outbreak. Emerg Infect Dis 2005; 11:1882–6.

41. Yu IT, Qiu H, Tse LA, et al. Severe acute respiratory syndrome beyond Amoy Gardens: completing the incomplete legacy. Clin Infect Dis 2014;58(5):683–6.

42. Booth TF, Kournikakis B, Bastien N, et al. Detection of airborne Severe acute respiratory syndrome (SARS) coronavirus and environmental contamination in SARS outbreak units. J Infect Dis 2005;191: 1472–7.

43. Leung GM, Hedley AJ, Ho LM, et al. The epidemiology of severe acute respiratory syndrome in the 2003 Hong Kong epidemic: an analysis of all 1755 patients. Ann Intern Med 2004;141:662–73.

44. Peiris JS, Lai ST, Poon LL, et al. Coronavirus as a possible cause of severe acute respiratory syndrome. Lancet 2003;361:1319–25.

45. Leung WK, To KF, Chan PK, et al. Enteric involvement of severe acute respiratory syndrome-associated coronavirus infection. Gastroenterol 2003;125: 1011–7.

46. Hung EC, Chim SS, Chan PK, et al. Detection of SARS coronavirus RNA in the cerebrospinal fluid of a patient with severe acute respiratory syndrome. Clin Chem 2003;49:2108–9.

47. Lau KK, Yu WC, Chu CM, et al. Possible central nervous system infection by SARS coronavirus. Emerg Infect Dis 2004;10:342–4.

48. Wong KC, Leung KS, Hui M. Severe acute respiratory syndrome (SARS) in a geriatric patient with a hip fracture. A case report. J Bone Joint Surg Am 2003;85A:1339–42.

49. Hon KL, Leung CW, Cheng WT, et al. Clinical presentations and outcome of severe acute respiratory syndrome in children. Lancet 2003;561:1701–3.

50. Wong SF, Chow KM, Leung TN, et al. Pregnancy and perinatal outcomes of women with severe acute respiratory syndrome. Am J Obstet Gynecol 2004;191:292–7.

51. Leung GM, Lim WW, Ho LM, et al. Seroprevalence of IgG antibodies to SARS-coronavirus in asymptomatic or subclinical population groups. Epidemiol Infect 2006;134:211–21.

52. Hui DS, Wong KT, Antonio GE, et al. Severe Acute Respiratory Syndrome (SARS): correlation of clinical outcome and radiological features. Radiology 2004;233:579–85.

53. Hui DS, Wong PC, Wang C. Severe acute respiratory syndrome: clinical features and diagnosis. Respirol 2003;8:S20–4.

54. Wong RS, Wu A, To KF, et al. Haematological manifestations in patients with severe acute respiratory syndrome: retrospective analysis. Br Med J 2003; 326:1358–62.

55. Wong KT, Antonio GE, Hui DS, et al. Severe acute respiratory syndrome: radiographic appearances and pattern of progression in 138 patients. Radiology 2003;228:401–6.

56. Stroher U, DiCaro A, Li Y, et al. Severe acute respiratory syndrome-related coronavirus is inhibited by interferon-α. J Infect Dis 2004;189:1164–7.

57. Chu CM, Cheng VC, Hung IF, et al. Role of lopinavir/ritonavir in the treatment of SARS: initial virological and clinical findings. Thorax 2004;59: 252–6.

58. Chan KS, Lai ST, Chu CM, et al. Treatment of severe acute respiratory syndrome with lopinavir/ritonavir: a multicenter retrospective matched cohort study. Hong Kong Med J 2003;9:399–406.

59. Cinatl J, Morgenstern B, Bauer G, et al. Treatment of SARS with human interferons. Lancet 2003; 362:293–4.

60. Hensley LE, Fritz LE, Jahrling PB, et al. Interferon-β 1a and SARS coronavirus replication. Emerg Infect Dis 2004;10:317–9.

61. Haagmans BL, Kuiken T, Martina BE, et al. Pegylated interferon-α protects type 1 pneumocytes against SARS coronavirus infection in macaques. Nat Med 2004;10:290–3.

62. Loutfy MR, Blatt LM, Siminovitch KA, et al. Interferon Alfacon-1 plus corticosteroids in severe acute respiratory syndrome: a preliminary study. JAMA 2003;290:3222–8.

63. Jiang Y, Xu J, Zhou C, et al. Characterization of cytokine/chemokine profiles of severe acute

respiratory syndrome. Am J Respir Crit Care Med 2005;171:850–7.

64. Sung JJ, Wu A, Joynt GM, et al. Severe Acute Respiratory Syndrome: report of treatment and outcome after a major outbreak. Thorax 2004;59: 414–20.

65. Tsang OT, Chau TN, Choi KW, et al. Coronavirus-positive nasopharyngeal aspirate as predictor for severe acute respiratory syndrome mortality. Emerg Infect Dis 2003;9:1381–7.

66. Wang H, Ding Y, Li X, et al. Fatal aspergillosis in a patient with SARS who was treated with corticosteroids. N Engl J Med 2003;349:507–8.

67. Griffith JF, Antonio GE, Kumta SM, et al. Osteonecrosis of hip and knee in patients with severe acute respiratory syndrome treated with steroids. Radiology 2005;235:168–75.

68. Lee N, Allen Chan KC, Hui DS, et al. Effects of early corticosteroid treatment on plasma SARS-associated Coronavirus RNA concentrations in adult patients. J Clin Virol 2004;31:304–9.

69. Soo Y, Cheng Y, Wong R, et al. Retrospective comparison of convalescent plasma with continuing high-dose methylprednisolone treatment in SARS patients. Clin Microbiol Infect 2004;10:676–8.

70. Cheng Y, Wong R, Soo YO, et al. Use of convalescent plasma therapy in SARS patients in Hong Kong. Eur J Clin Microbiol Infect Dis 2005;24:44–6.

71. Mair-Jenkins J, Saavedra-Campos M, Baillie JK, et al, Convalescent Plasma Study Group. The effectiveness of convalescent plasma and hyperimmune immunoglobulin for the treatment of severe acute respiratory infections of viral etiology: a systematic review and exploratory meta-analysis. J Infect Dis 2015;211:80–90.

72. Yu IT, Xie ZH, Tsoi KK, et al. Why did outbreaks of severe acute respiratory syndrome occur in some hospital wards but not in others? Clin Infect Dis 2007;44:1017–25.

73. Tran K, Cimon K, Severn M, et al. Aerosol generating procedures and risk of transmission of acute respiratory infections to healthcare workers: a systematic review. PLoS One 2012;7:e35797.

74. Zaki AM, van Boheemen S, Bestebroer TM, et al. Isolation of a novel coronavirus from a man with pneumonia in Saudi Arabia. N Engl J Med 2012; 367:1814–20.

75. World Health Organization. Middle East Respiratory Syndrome Coronavirus (MERS-CoV) – Qatar. Disease Outbreak News 2016. Available at: http://www.who.int/csr/don/29-june-2016-mers-qatar/en/. Accessed July 2, 2010.

76. WHO. Middle East respiratory syndrome coronavirus case definition for reporting to WHO interim case definition 14 July 2015. Available at: http://www.who.int/csr/disease/coronavirus_infections/case_definition/en/. Accessed July 2, 2016.

77. Annan A, Baldwin HJ, Corman VM, et al. Human betacoronavirus 2c EMC/2012-related viruses in bats, Ghana and Europe. Emerg Infect Dis 2013; 19:456–9.

78. Memish ZA, Mishra N, Olival KJ, et al. Middle East respiratory syndrome coronavirus in bats, Saudi Arabia. Emerg Infect Dis 2013;19:1819–23.

79. Miguel E, Perera RA, Baubekova A, et al. Absence of Middle East respiratory syndrome coronavirus in Camelids, Kazakhstan, 2015. Emerg Infect Dis 2016;22(3):555–7.

80. Chan SM, Damdinjav B, Perera RA, et al. Absence of MERS-coronavirus in bactrian camels, southern Mongolia, November 2014. Emerg Infect Dis 2015;21(7):1269–71.

81. Hemida MG, Perera RA, Al Jassim RA, et al. Seroepidemiology of Middle East Respiratory Syndrome (MERS) coronavirus in Saudi Arabia (1993) and Australia (2014) and characterisation of assay specificity. Euro Surveill 2014;19(23). pii: 20828.

82. Hemida MG, Elmoslemany A, Al-Hizab F, et al. Dromedary camels and the transmission of Middle East Respiratory Syndrome Coronavirus (MERS-CoV). Transbound Emerg Dis 2015. http://dx.doi.org/10.1111/tbed.12401.

83. Saad M, Omrani AS, Baig K, et al. Clinical aspects and outcomes of 70 patients with Middle East respiratory syndrome coronavirus infection: a single-center experience in Saudi Arabia. Int J Infect Dis 2014;29:301–6.

84. Hijawi B, Abdallat M, Sayaydeh A, et al. Novel coronavirus infections in Jordan, April 2012: epidemiological findings from a retrospective investigation. East Mediterr Health J 2013;19(Suppl 1):S12–8.

85. Alraddadi BM, Watson JT, Almarashi A, et al. Risk factors for primary Middle East respiratory syndrome coronavirus illness in humans, Saudi Arabia, 2014. Emerg Infect Dis 2016;22(1):49–55.

86. Drosten C, Meyer B, Müller MA, et al. Transmission of MERS-coronavirus in household contacts. N Engl J Med 2014;371(9):828–35.

87. Arwady MA, Alraddadi B, Basler C, et al. Middle East respiratory syndrome coronavirus transmission in extended family, Saudi Arabia, 2014. Emerg Infect Dis 2016;22(8):1395–402.

88. Müller MA, Meyer B, Corman VM, et al. Presence of Middle East respiratory syndrome coronavirus antibodies in Saudi Arabia: a nationwide, cross-sectional, serological study. Lancet Infect Dis 2015;15(5):559–64.

09. Assiri A, McGeer A, Perl TM, et al. Hospital outbreak of Middle East respiratory syndrome coronavirus. N Engl J Med 2013;369:407–16.

90. Oboho IK, Tomczyk SM, Al-Asmari AM, et al. 2014 MERS-CoV outbreak in Jeddah–a link to health care facilities. N Engl J Med 2015;372:846–54.

91. Hunter JC, Nguyen D, Aden B, et al. Transmission of Middle East respiratory syndrome coronavirus infections in healthcare settings, Abu Dhabi. Emerg Infect Dis 2016;22:647–56.

92. Korea Centers for Disease Control and Prevention. Middle east respiratory syndrome coronavirus outbreak in the Republic of Korea, 2015. Osong Public Health Res Perspect 2015;6(4): 269–78.

93. Oh MD, Choe PG, Oh HS, et al. Middle east respiratory sayndrome coronavirus superspreading event involving 81 persons, Korea 2015. J Korean Med Sci 2015;30(11):1701–5.

94. WHO. WHO recommends continuation of strong disease control measures to bring MERS-CoV outbreak in Republic of Korea to an end. News Release 13 June 2013. Available at: http://www.wpro.who.int/mediacentre/releases/2015/20150613/en/. Accessed June 14, 2015.

95. Zumla A, Hui DS. Infection control and MERS-CoV in health-care workers. Lancet 2014;383(9932): 1869–71.

96. WHO MERS-CoV Research Group. State of knowledge and data gaps of Middle East respiratory syndrome coronavirus (MERS-CoV) in humans. PLoS Curr 2013;5. pii: ecurrents.outbreaks. 0bf719e352e7478f8ad85fa30127ddb8.

97. Assiri A, Al-Tawfiq JA, Al-Rabeeah AA, et al. Epidemiological, demographic, and clinical characteristics of 47 cases of middle east respiratory syndrome coronavirus disease from Saudi Arabia: a descriptive study. Lancet Infect Dis 2013;13: 752–61.

98. Guery B, Poissy J, el Mansouf L, et al. Clinical features and viral diagnosis of two cases of infection with middle east respiratory syndrome coronavirus: a report of nosocomial transmission. Lancet 2013; 381:2265–72.

99. Memish ZA, Zumla AI, Al-Hakeem RF, et al. Family cluster of middle east respiratory syndrome coronavirus infections. N Engl J Med 2013;368: 2487–94.

100. Algahtani H, Subahi A, Shirah B. Neurological complications of middle east respiratory syndrome coronavirus: a report of two cases and review of the literature. Case Rep Neurol Med 2016;2016: 3502683.

101. Assiri A, Abedi GR, Almasry M, et al. Middle east respiratory syndrome coronavirus infection during pregnancy: a report of 5 cases from Saudi Arabia. Clin Infect Dis 2016;63(7):951–3.

102. Alserehi H, Wali G, Alshukairi A, et al. Impact of Middle East Respiratory Syndrome Coronavirus (MERS-CoV) on pregnancy and perinatal outcome. BMC Infect Dis 2016;16:105.

103. Malik A, El Masry KM, Ravi M, et al. Middle east respiratory syndrome- coronavirus during pregnancy, Abu Dhabi, United Arab Emirates, 2013. Emerg Infect Dis 2016;22(3):515–7.

104. Payne DC, Iblan I, Alqasrawi S, et al. Stillbirth during infection with Middle East respiratory syndrome coronavirus. J Infect Dis 2014;209(12):1870–2.

105. Drosten C, Seilmaier M, Corman VM, et al. Clinical features and virological analysis of a case of Middle East respiratory syndrome coronavirus infection. Lancet Infect Dis 2013;13:745–51.

106. Corman VM, Albarrak AM, Omrani AS, et al. Viral shedding and antibody response in 37 patients with Middle East respiratory syndrome coronavirus infection. Clin Infect Dis 2016;62(4):477–83.

107. Ajlan AM, Ahyad RA, Jamjoom LG, et al. Middle East respiratory syndrome coronavirus (MERS-CoV) infection: chest CT findings. AJR Am J Roentgenol 2014;203(4):782–7.

108. Raj VS, Mou H, Smits SL, et al. Dipeptidyl peptidase 4 is a functional receptor for the emerging human coronavirus-EMC. Nature 2013;495:251–4.

109. Lu G, Hu Y, Wang Q, et al. Molecular basis of binding between novel human coronavirus MERS-CoV and its receptor CD26. Nature 2013;500:227–31.

110. Müller MA, Raj VS, Muth D, et al. Human coronavirus EMC does not require the SARS-coronavirus receptor and maintains broad replicative capability in mammalian cell lines. MBio 2012;3(6). pii: e00515–12.

111. Chan JF, Chan KH, Choi GK, et al. Differential cell line susceptibility to the emerging novel human betacoronavirus 2c EMC/2012: implications for disease pathogenesis and clinical manifestation. J Infect Dis 2013;207:1743–52.

112. de Wilde AH, Raj VS, Oudshoorn D, et al. MERS-coronavirus replication induces severe in vitro cytopathology and is strongly inhibited by cyclosporin A or interferon-α treatment. J Gen Virol 2013;94: 1749–60.

113. Falzarano D, de Wit E, Martellaro C, et al. Inhibition of novel β coronavirus replication by a combination of interferon-α2b and ribavirin. Sci Rep 2013;3:1686.

114. Chan RW, Chan MC, Agnihothram S, et al. Tropism of and innate immune responses to the novel human betacoronavirus lineage C virus in human ex vivo respiratory organ cultures. J Virol 2013; 87:6604–14.

115. Hocke AC, Becher A, Knepper J, et al. Emerging human middle east respiratory syndrome coronavirus causes widespread infection and alveolar damage in human lungs. Am J Respir Crit Care Med 2013;188(7):882–6.

116. Faure E, Poissy J, Goffard A, et al. Distinct immune response in two MERS-CoV-infected patients: can we go from bench to bedside? PLoS One 2014; 9(2):e88716.

117. Poissy J, Goffard A, Parmentier-Decrucq E, et al. Kinetics and pattern of viral excretion in biological

specimens of two MERS-CoV cases. J Clin Virol 2014;61(2):275–8.

118. Park WB, Perera RA, Choe PG, et al. Kinetics of serologic responses to MERS coronavirus infection in humans, South Korea. Emerg Infect Dis 2015; 21(12):2186–9.

119. Payne DC, Iblan I, Rha B, et al. Persistence of antibodies against middle east respiratory syndrome coronavirus. Emerg Infect Dis 2016; 22(10):1824–6.

120. Ng DL, Al Hosani F, Keating MK, et al. Clinicopathologic, immunohistochemical, and ultrastructural findings of a fatal case of middle east respiratory syndrome coronavirus infection in the United Arab Emirates, April 2014. Am J Pathol 2016; 186(3):652–8.

121. Cha RH, Yang SH, Moon KC, et al. A case report of a Middle East respiratory syndrome survivor with kidney biopsy results. J Korean Med Sci 2016; 31(4):635–40.

122. Zhou J, Chu H, Li C, et al. Active replication of middle east respiratory syndrome coronavirus and aberrant induction of inflammatory cytokines and chemokines in human macrophages: implications for pathogenesis. J Infect Dis 2014;209(9): 1331–42.

123. Dyall J, Coleman CM, Hart BJ, et al. Repurposing of clinically developed drugs for treatment of Middle East respiratory syndrome coronavirus infection. Antimicrob Agents Chemother 2014;58(8): 4885–93.

124. De Wilde AH, Jochmans D, Posthuma CC, et al. Screening of an FDA-approved compound library identifies four small-molecule inhibitors of Middle East respiratory syndrome coronavirus replication in cell culture. Antimicrob Agents Chemother 2014;58(8):4875–84.

125. Falzarano D, de Wit E, Rasmussen AL, et al. Treatment with interferon-α2b and ribavirin improves outcome in MERS-CoV-infected rhesus macaques. Nat Med 2013;19(10):1313–7.

126. Al-Tawfiq JA, Momattin H, Dib J, et al. Ribavirin and interferon therapy in patients infected with the Middle East respiratory syndrome coronavirus: an observational study. Int J Infect Dis 2014;20: 42–6.

127. Shalhoub S, Farahat F, Al-Jiffri A, et al. IFN-α2a or IFN-β1a in combination with ribavirin to treat Middle East respiratory syndrome coronavirus pneumonia: a retrospective study. J Antimicrob Chemother 2015;70(7):2129–32.

128. Omrani AS, Saad MM, Baig K, et al. Ribavirin and interferon alfa-2a for severe Middle East respiratory syndrome coronavirus infection: a retrospective cohort study. Lancet Infect Dis 2014;14(11):1090–5.

129. Spanakis N, Tsiodras S, Haagmans BL, et al. Virological and serological analysis of a recent Middle East respiratory syndrome coronavirus infection case on a triple combination antiviral regimen. Int J Antimicrob Agents 2014;44(6):528–32.

130. Rossignol JF. Nitazoxanide: a first-in-class broad-spectrum antiviral agent. Antiviral Res 2014;110: 94–103.

131. Arabi Y, Arifi AA, Balkhy HH, et al. Clinical course and outcomes of critically ill patients with Middle East respiratory syndrome coronavirus infection. Ann Intern Med 2014;160(6):389–97.

132. Hui DS, Lee N, Chan PK. Adjunctive therapies and immunomodulatory agents in the management of severe influenza. Antiviral Res 2013;98(3):410–6.

133. Chan JF, Chan KH, Kao RY, et al. Broad-spectrum antivirals for the emerging Middle East respiratory syndrome coronavirus. J Infect 2013;67(6):606–16.

134. Chan JF, Yao Y, Yeung ML, et al. Treatment with lopinavir/ritonavir or interferon-β1b improves outcome of MERS-CoV infection in a nonhuman primate model of common marmoset. J Infect Dis 2015;212(12):1904–13.

135. AlGhamdi M, Mushtaq F, Awn N, et al. MERS CoV infection in two renal transplant recipients: case report. Am J Transplant 2015;15(4):1101–4.

136. Tang XC, Agnihothram SS, Jiao Y, et al. Identification of human neutralizing antibodies against MERS-CoV and their role in virus adaptive evolution. Proc Natl Acad Sci U S A 2014;111(19):E2018–26.

137. Johnson RF, Bagci U, Keith L, et al. 3B11-N, a monoclonal antibody against MERS-CoV, reduces lung pathology in rhesus monkeys following intratracheal inoculation of MERS-CoV Jordan-n3/ 2012. Virology 2016;490:49–58.

138. Corti D, Zhao J, Pedotti M, et al. Prophylactic and postexposure efficacy of a potent human monoclonal antibody against MERS coronavirus. Proc Natl Acad Sci U S A 2015;112(33):10473–8.

139. Jiang L, Wang N, Zuo T, et al. Potent neutralization of MERS-CoV by human neutralizing monoclonal antibodies to the viral spike glycoprotein. Sci Transl Med 2014;6(234):234ra59.

140. Luke T, Wu H, Zhao J, et al. Human polyclonal immunoglobulin G from transchromosomic bovines inhibits MERS-CoV in vivo. Sci Transl Med 2016; 8(326):326ra21.

141. Johnson RF, Via LE, Kumar MR, et al. Intratracheal exposure of common marmosets to MERS-CoV Jordan-n3/2012 or MERS-CoV EMC/2012 isolates does not result in lethal disease. Virology 2015; 485:422–30.

142. WHO. Clinical management of severe acute respiratory infection when Middle East respiratory syndrome coronavirus (MERS-CoV) infection is suspected. Interim guidance. 2015. Available at: http://apps.who.int/iris/bitstream/10665/178529/1/ WHO_MERS_Clinical_15.1_eng.pdf. Accessed July 3, 2015.

143. Version 3.0Treatment of MERS-CoV: information for clinicians. Clinical decision-making support for treatment of MERS-CoV patients. Public Health England and ISARIC; 2015. Available at: https://www.gov.uk/government/uploads/system/uploads/attachment_data/file/459835/merscov_for_clinicians_sept2015.pdf. Accessed September 5, 2015.

144. Breban R, Riou J, Fontanet A. Interhuman transmissibility of middle east respiratory syndrome coronavirus: estimation of pandemic risk. Lancet 2013;382:694–9.

145. Hui DS, Zumla A. Advancing priority research on the middle east respiratory syndrome coronavirus. J Infect Dis 2014;209:173–6.

146. Menachery VD, Yount BL Jr, Sims AC, et al. SARS-like WIV1-CoV poised for human emergence. Proc Natl Acad Sci U S A 2016;113(11):3048–53.

Respiratory Viral Infections in Chronic Lung Diseases

Clemente J. Britto, MD[a,b], Virginia Brady, MD[b],
Seiwon Lee, MD[b], Charles S. Dela Cruz, MD, PhD[b,c],*

KEYWORDS

- Chronic lung diseases • Respiratory viral infections • Chronic obstructive pulmonary disease
- Cystic fibrosis • Interstitial lung diseases • Asthma

KEY POINTS

- Respiratory viruses remain to be important in the pathogenesis of chronic lung diseases.
- Respiratory viruses play an important role in chronic lung diseases, such as chronic obstructive pulmonary disease, asthma, and cystic fibrosis, especially in disease exacerbations.
- There is not much evidence for the association of respiratory viruses with idiopathic pulmonary fibrosis or sarcoidosis.
- Preventive measures are needed to limit such viral infections, with good hand hygiene, avoidance of sick contacts, and viral vaccinations recommended for patients suffering from chronic lung diseases.

INTRODUCTION

Chronic lung diseases, such as chronic obstructive pulmonary disease (COPD), asthma, cystic fibrosis (CF), and interstitial lung diseases (ILD), affect many individuals worldwide. Patients with these chronic lung diseases are susceptible to respiratory lung infections and some of these viral infections can contribute to disease pathogenesis. This review highlights the associations of lung infections and the respective chronic lung diseases and how infection in the different lung diseases affects disease exacerbation and progression.

CHRONIC OBSTRUCTIVE PULMONARY DISEASE

COPD is one of the leading causes of mortality and morbidity worldwide.[1,2] Among several risk factors, cigarette smoking is the most important one. However, smoking alone does not explain all the aspects of COPD. COPD can develop even in nonsmokers, especially in the context of biomass exposure in some parts of the world. More than half of smokers do not develop COPD. A subset of patients with COPD exhibits persistent inflammation despite smoking cessation.[3,4] In addition, accelerated loss of lung function may occur independent of smoking and occur with acute COPD exacerbations.[5] It is important to elucidate additional contributive factors besides smoking to control the disease. COPD is characterized by chronic inflammation of the small airways. Respiratory tract infection is an important cause of acute exacerbation and progression of the disease.[6]

[a] Adult Cystic Fibrosis Program, Section of Pulmonary, Critical Care & Sleep Medicine, Department of Internal Medicine, Yale University, 300 Cedar Street, TAC S419, New Haven, CT 06513, USA; [b] Section of Pulmonary, Critical Care & Sleep Medicine, Department of Internal Medicine, Yale University, 300 Cedar Street, TACS441D, New Haven, CT 06513, USA; [c] Department of Microbial Pathogenesis, Yale University, 300 Cedar Street, TAC S441D, New Haven, CT 06510, USA
* Corresponding author.
E-mail address: charles.delacruz@yale.edu

Clin Chest Med 38 (2017) 87–96
http://dx.doi.org/10.1016/j.ccm.2016.11.014
0272-5231/17/© 2016 Elsevier Inc. All rights reserved.

chestmed.theclinics.com

Common Viral Infections and Chronic Obstructive Pulmonary Disease Exacerbations

Historically, bacteria have been considered the main infectious cause of COPD exacerbations.[7] A growing body of evidence, however, implicates viral upper respiratory tract infections (URIs) as the predominant risk factor associated with exacerbations of COPD.[8] Approximately 40% to 60% of all COPD exacerbations are associated with upper respiratory infections (URIs) and viral infections have been suggested to be important contributors to COPD exacerbations.[9] In fact, it has been shown that respiratory viruses, including rhinovirus, influenza, and respiratory syncytial virus (RSV) cause COPD exacerbations.[10–12] These exacerbations are more severe, last longer, and are associated with more heightened airway and systemic inflammatory responses than exacerbations due to other nonviral causes.[13–15] These differences cannot be attributed solely to pulmonary structural alterations in patients with COPD because healthy smokers also experience exaggerated symptomatic responses after viral infections.[16–18]

Detection rates of virus in COPD exacerbation are variable between approximately 22% and 64%.[9,11,19–27] The detection rates depend on onset to presentation, type of samples, and season. The most commonly identified viruses in exacerbation of COPD include rhinovirus, influenza viruses, RSV, parainfluenza, adenovirus, metapneumovirus, and coronavirus. Among them, rhinovirus and metapneumovirus are the most common viral pathogens in studies using polymerase chain reaction (PCR).[12,13,25] In these studies, rhinovirus was detected in 8% to 44% in the events of COPD acute exacerbation. Influenza vaccination rate can also affect the prevalence. A Hong Kong study showed that influenza was the most common virus in hospitalized patients with COPD; meanwhile, a cohort from a London outpatient clinic showed low prevalence due to relatively high influenza vaccination rate (74%).[11,15] Many COPD exacerbations also include virus and bacteria coinfection. Approximately 25% of the hospitalized patients with COPD exacerbations showed coinfection. The clinical impact of coinfection is longer hospital stay and severe functional impairment.[28]

Symptoms of COPD exacerbation include cough, increased sputum volume and purulence, and dyspnea; however, it is not easy to differentiate viral and nonviral causes of COPD exacerbation by symptoms. Typical "common-cold" symptoms, including fever, nasal congestion, or rhinorrhea, are prevalent in patients with COPD when virus is detected, but those symptoms also can be noted in nonviral exacerbation, so their usefulness in diagnosis remains limited.[13,29] Sputum purulence has been suggested as evidence for bacterial infection in COPD exacerbation, but sputum also can be purulent due to neutrophilia irrespective of causal organism.[30] Furthermore, almost all COPD exacerbations can be marked with change in sputum characteristics.[31] Therefore, the sputum characteristics are not a useful marker to differentiate viral and bacterial infection. On the other hand, sputum purulence may be used to decide the usage of antibiotics.[32] Although neutrophils are the predominantly increased cell type in sputum during COPD exacerbations, one report showed increased eosinophilia during viral exacerbations.[28] Viral exacerbations also are associated with frequent exacerbations, severe exacerbations, and a prolonged time for symptom recovery.[13] Viruses also can be detected in stable COPD. Patients with RSV infection had higher plasma fibrinogen, serum interleukin (IL)-6, and hypercapnia in stable state.[13] This suggests that asymptomatic viral colonization can potentially have a role in chronic inflammation and disease progression of COPD. Another study that supports this showed a relationship between frequent RSV detection and accelerated lung function decline (101.4 mL/y vs 51.2 mL/y, $P = .01$).[33] It has been proposed that the alveolar epithelial cells of smokers and patients with severe emphysema are more frequently latently infected with adenovirus as compared with smokers without airflow obstruction.[34,35] They found COPD lung epithelial cells express adenoviral E1A protein, and that this was associated with specific lung inflammation. The investigators propose such adenoviral infections in patients with COPD contribute to the amplification of the lung inflammatory responses.

PCR of respiratory samples is the main tool to detect causal viruses. Before the widespread use of PCR technique, low virus-detection rates underestimated their role in COPD. The introduction of PCR helped revolutionize viral diagnostics; PCR is far more sensitive and equally specific to the traditional techniques that include culture, antigen-detection tests, and serology.[36,37] Rhinovirus is one of the most common viruses in COPD exacerbation, but it is difficult to culture and serology is not possible due to the presence of more than 100 serotypes. Without PCR, these viruses cannot be identified. As a result, early studies using other diagnostic methods underestimated the prevalence of rhinovirus.[15] Among various methods to obtain samples, such as nasal lavage, throat swab, or induced sputum, it is not yet evident which method is superior. Some viruses, especially RSV, can directly invade the lower respiratory tract; therefore, obtaining a simultaneous lower respiratory tract sample can increase the sensitivity of these assays. The big challenge of this molecular diagnostic approach is that it cannot discriminate causative organisms from colonization.

Antiviral therapy is not necessary in most immunocompetent and asymptomatic patients with COPD. Antiviral therapy is not indicated solely on the basis of a known diagnosis of COPD. Most endemic viral infections are self-limiting, and pharmacologic management is not necessary. In the case of severe and progressive pandemic influenza virus, oseltamivir is indicated when the clinical diagnosis is made.[38] One of the difficult decisions is not to prescribe antibiotics when they are not necessary. When the causative organism is a virus, antibiotics are not usually necessary unless one is concerned about postviral secondary bacterial lung infections. Although sputum characteristics do not indicate the causative organisms, sputum purulence can be suggested to decide the usage of antibiotics.[32] Influenza vaccination is highly recommended in patients with COPD and other chronic lung diseases.

ASTHMA

Asthma is defined as reversible airflow obstruction, bronchial hyperresponsiveness, and underlying inflammation. Asthma continues to be a serious global health problem for all age groups, and its prevalence is still increasing in many countries. Worldwide asthma affects approximately 300 million people, with an increased incidence in the developed world. Through the development of inhaled medications, hospitalization and mortality have decreased, but overall asthma control remains suboptimal. Many studies supported the evidence that viral infection has several important roles in disease development, exacerbation, and progression.

Virus Infection and Asthma Development

The "hygiene hypothesis" proposes that a lower incidence of infections in early childhood explains the rise in allergic diseases such as asthma.[39] The thought is that repeated exposures to infections are associated with a healthier immune system with protection against allergic and autoimmune diseases. Specifically, microbes encountered could elicit a more T-helper type 1 (T_H1) immune response that could downregulate the T-helper type 2 (T_H2) immune responses that favor asthma development. The hygiene hypothesis is focused on a lack of T_H1 stimulation that

caused an overactive T_H2 response and could lead to a more allergic immune response. What role viruses play in the T_H2 response has been long debated and studied. Whether early viral infections set in motion a T_H2-driven immune response or whether a lack of a T_H1 response causes a more symptomatic response to viral infections has been unclear. Similarly, the debate over whether an asthma exacerbation is the result of an immune-deficient response or an exaggerated immune response continues. Many studies supported the evidence that viral infection has several important roles in disease development, exacerbation, and progression.

Common Viral Pathogens in Asthma

Viral infection is closely associated with wheezing episodes, which resembles the manifestations of asthma. Especially in younger groups, these episodes can be related to the later development of asthma. Among viruses causing respiratory infection, RSV and rhinovirus are well-documented to increase the risk of asthma though early adulthood. In an 18-year longitudinal study, severe early RSV bronchiolitis is associated with an increased prevalence of allergic asthma persisting into childhood, and even early adulthood.[40,41] Among viral wheezing illnesses in infancy and early childhood, those caused by RSV infections are the most significant predictors of the subsequent development of asthma.[42] Host factors may also affect the pathogenesis of asthma in connection with viruses. Children with wheezing illness with rhinovirus were associated with asthma development if they had certain variants at chromosome 17q21.[43]

Virus Infection and Exacerbation

Asthma exacerbations may be triggered by respiratory infections as well as by atmospheric and domiciliary environmental factors. Viral infections may cause a loss of asthma control, and most exacerbations, particularly in children with allergic asthma, coincide with respiratory viral infections. Studies of asthma exacerbation showed higher virus-detection rates than those of COPD. PCR showed the presence of viruses in 80% to 85% in children and 60% to 80% in adults.[44–46] The most common viruses included rhinovirus, influenza, RSV, and corona virus, although some seasonal variation is present. In patients with asthma, URI symptoms persisted longer and were more severe than in healthy controls. Like COPD, PCR for respiratory samples is the preferred diagnostic modality. Before the use of PCR technology, the etiology of respiratory infections was established by viral cultures, which are difficult to perform. PCR showed a high sensitivity and specificity, although it may not be quantitative in all cases.

Many studies have attempted to find the pathologic immune response to viruses that cause exacerbations, but the mechanisms for exacerbations remain poorly understood. It is not clear if asthma exacerbations triggered by viruses are a manifestation of impaired or overactive immune responses. There is evidence that the T_H2 pathway causes downregulation of antiviral interferon (IFN)-β and IFN-λ and higher viral loads in vitro; however, this has not been reproducible in in vivo studies. On the other hand, there is evidence to suggest that increased T_H2 cytokines and chemokines produced in response to viral illnesses can activate an inflammatory cascade thought to be associated with asthma exacerbations.

Inhaled corticosteroids (ICS) are commonly used in the treatment of asthma, and this treatment should be continued in the case of viral infection. Pretreatment with the ICS was shown to improve airway hyperresponsiveness and eosinophilic inflammation in patients with atopic asthma experimentally infected with rhinovirus.[47] In acute exacerbation, oral or intravenous (IV) corticosteroids are usually indicated, and the immunosuppressive function of these medications does not preclude their use in viral infectious exacerbation. Most viral infection is self-limiting; therefore, antiviral medications are not necessary except during severe epidemic cases. Influenza vaccination is recommended because influenza can cause asthma exacerbation. However, the available evidence is not sufficient to assert that vaccination can reduce the frequency or severity of asthma exacerbations.[48]

CYSTIC FIBROSIS

CF is the most common fatal genetic disease in the United States, with 28,676 patients living with CF in the United States in 2014.[49] CF is an autosomal recessive disorder caused by mutations in the CF transmembrane conductance regulator gene (CFTR) that lead to abnormalities in epithelial chloride transport, causing multiorgan dysfunction.[50–52] The lungs are particularly affected, with evidence of chronic inflammation, recurrent infections, impaired mucociliary clearance, and innate immune impairments that directly affect host defense against respiratory pathogens.[51,53–55] Pulmonary infections remain the greatest cause of morbidity and mortality leading to premature death in CF.[56]

Common Viral Pathogens in Cystic Fibrosis

Similar to individuals without CF, viral respiratory infections are common in CF. A variety of studies dating to 1981 reported variable incidences of common respiratory pathogens, including influenza A and B (12%–77%), RSV (9%–58%), parainfluenza virus (PIV), rhinovirus, metapneumovirus, coronavirus, and adenovirus.[57–64] In these studies, the incidence of specific viral isolates varied greatly from one study to the next due to multiple factors, including methodology, seasonal variation, geographic location, and different age groups. In a recent study of 100 adults with CF, followed prospectively for 12 months, rhinovirus accounted for 72.5% of confirmed viral infections, followed by metapneumovirus (13.2%), and adenovirus (4.1%). Unlike previous studies, influenza virus A and B, PIV, and RSV together accounted for only 10.6% of viral isolates.[65,66]

Previous studies have shown that individuals with CF are no more susceptible to viral infections than healthy controls. In a prospective study of school-aged individuals with CF compared with age-matched controls, there was no difference in the frequency of culture-documented and seropositive viral infections. Younger patients had a higher incidence of viral infections in both groups; however, this did not translate into accelerated lung function decline in the patients with CF.[59] A later study evaluating the impact of viral infections on pulmonary function in infants with CF similarly showed no difference in the incidence of viral infections. However, infants with CF had an increased frequency of respiratory symptoms. Whereas controls did not demonstrate an association between respiratory illness and lung function, infants with CF who suffered an RSV infection and developed respiratory symptoms had a reduction in lung function.[67] A prospective study examining the impact of RSV infection on lung function in a pediatric population demonstrated again that subjects with CF had an increased frequency of respiratory symptoms despite similar rates of viral isolation from cultures and serology in healthy controls. The investigators demonstrated clear associations between RSV infection and worsening clinical severity score, lung function measurements, and rates and duration of hospitalizations for respiratory exacerbations.[68]

Viruses, Exacerbations, and Clinical Deterioration in Cystic Fibrosis

CF respiratory exacerbations are acute clinical deteriorations in a patient's clinical condition characterized by increased respiratory symptoms and sputum production, and declines in lung function. Exacerbations are commonly precipitated by acquisition of new organisms or changes in respiratory flora.[69–71] CF pulmonary exacerbation rates are increased during winter and have been linked to the influenza season.[72,73] The viruses most frequently implicated in causing respiratory symptoms in CF include rhinovirus, RSV, adenovirus, PIV, influenza A and B, and metapneumovirus.[57–61,66,67] Viral infections are frequently detected during CF exacerbations and viral detection has improved with significant leaps in diagnostic technologies. The implementation of quantitative real-time PCR studies for viral detection in the CF population achieved the highest detection rate of 46% compared with existing literature that previously relied on serologic testing or viral isolation.[61]

Identification of a respiratory virus during exacerbation purports clinical deterioration and increased duration of IV antibiotic compared with virus-negative exacerbations.[60] In a study of 103 children with CF respiratory exacerbations, 61.3% had a positive viral isolation.[74] Two studies in adult patients with CF reported viral isolation rates during exacerbation of 30.5% (n = 100) and 50% (n = 30).[66,75] Although virus-positive exacerbations were associated with higher respiratory symptom scores and serum biomarkers of inflammation, viral infection did not increase rates of lung function decline compared with virus-negative exacerbation. Similarly, there was no significant association between viral infection and accelerated lung function decline in long-term follow-up.[66] A recent study combining pediatric and adult populations reported even higher incidence of virus-positive exacerbations, with 68% in adults and 72% in children.[76]

RSV is the most common cause of lower respiratory tract infection in young children.[77] In children with CF, RSV and influenza have been shown to have the most significant effect in lung function. In infants with CF, RSV infection accounted for up to one-third of hospitalizations, respiratory failure, and chronic supplemental oxygen requirement when followed for more than 2 years.[78] In addition to RSV, influenza A and B infection has been detected in 12% to 23% of CF exacerbations.[61,79,80] Influenza also has been associated with acute and sustained declines in lung function, as well as respiratory failure, and subsequent supplemental oxygen requirement. In a study of 54 pediatric patients, those with an influenza virus–positive exacerbation had larger declines in lung function (26% vs 6% with other viruses). In addition, influenza infection was more frequently associated with larger drops in forced expiratory volume in 1 second (FEV$_1$) than the other viral infections.[81]

According to data from the European Cystic Fibrosis Society, the influenza A (H1N1) pandemic in 2009 had a severe impact on adult and pediatric patients with CF. The prevalence of infection among 25 centers in multiple countries ranged from 0% to 9.4%. Among the 110 cases reported, the incidence of exacerbations was 53%; 48% of these patients required hospitalization, and 31% required supplemental oxygen. There were 6 incidences of respiratory failure and 3 fatalities. Patients with advanced lung disease were more likely to suffer a severe clinical course. Interestingly, most of the patients recovered lung function to preinfection values.[82,83] Rhinovirus is increasingly reported as a significant pathogen in the CF population. Rhinovirus has now been associated with increased respiratory symptoms, lung function decline, and frequency of exacerbations.[66,74,76] This may be due to improvements in detection techniques and inclusion of a more recently detected species, rhinovirus C.[74]

Interactions Between Viruses and Bacteria

The clinical significance of viral infections in CF extends beyond their immediate morbidity, as viral infections have been proposed to play a role new bacterial acquisition and worsening clinical outcomes. The new acquisition of *Pseudomonas aeruginosa* in CF has been associated with the winter months, coinciding with the peak of respiratory viral infections.[84] Some have proposed that RSV could facilitate the initial infection of the CF airway by *P aeruginosa*[64]; however, a study of 35 adults with CF showed no change in sputum density of *P aeruginosa* when concurrent viral infection was present.[75] A retrospective study in older patients with chronic *P aeruginosa* infection reported an acute deterioration in clinical status in association with influenza A virus infection.[85] Punch and colleagues[86] used a multiplex reverse-transcriptase PCR (RT-PCR) assay combined with an enzyme-linked amplicon hybridization assay (ELAHA) for the identification of 7 common respiratory viruses in the sputum of 38 patients with CF. Fifty-three sputum samples were collected over 2 seasons and 12 (23%) samples from 12 patients were positive for a respiratory virus (4 for influenza B, 3 for parainfluenza type 1, 3 for influenza A, and 2 for RSV). There were no statistical associations between virus status and demographics, clinical variables, or isolation rates for *P aeruginosa*, *Staphylococcus aureus* or *Aspergillus fumigatus*. Retrospective study in older patients with chronic *P aeruginosa* infection reported an acute deterioration in clinical status in association with influenza virus infection.[85]

PULMONARY FIBROSIS

Pulmonary fibrosis is the end stage of several diffuse parenchymal lung diseases characterized by excessive matrix deposition, lung parenchymal destruction, and progressive respiratory insufficiency.[87] Idiopathic pulmonary fibrosis (IPF) is a form of pulmonary fibrosis with overall poor survival rate and its etiology remains poorly understood. Several risk and predisposing factors of pulmonary fibrosis include environmental, tobacco smoking, viral infections, family history, and genetics. Pulmonary fibrosis is characterized by progressive lung decline over time, with many patients experiencing disease stability punctuated by episodes of acute worsening of clinical symptoms and radiographic changes on chest imaging.

Acute exacerbation of pulmonary fibrosis has been defined to be when no obvious identifiable cause is found for the pulmonary worsening.[88,89] Up to 10% of patients with IPF develop acute exacerbations each year with some resulting in deaths. However, it is unclear if these exacerbations truly accelerate the underlying fibrotic and proliferative process in pulmonary fibrosis or if it is due to complications such as infections, given IPF exacerbations are often accompanied by cough and fever. Initially it has been suspected that respiratory viruses are likely causes of IPF exacerbations. Compared with the strong association between viruses and exacerbations of obstructive lung diseases, such as asthma and COPD, there is currently very little research to suggest possible cause for exacerbations in IPF.

There have been several investigations on the role of pulmonary viruses in acute exacerbations that have resulted, however, in mixed results.[90] Gene expression analyses of stable IPF versus exacerbation in patients with IPF did find evidence of infectious or overwhelming inflammatory etiology. Although the antimicrobial peptide, alpha defensing, was found to be increased in the epithelium and the peripheral blood,[91] using multiplex PCR and pan-viral microarray discovery platform and next-generation deep sequencing to increase viral detection sensitivity, viral infection was not detected in most cases of acute IPF exacerbations. Four of 43 patients with IPF acute exacerbations had evidence of common respiratory viral infections (2 rhinovirus, 1 coronavirus, 1 parainfluenza), whereas no viruses were detected in bronchoalveolar lavage fluid from stable patients.[92] Interestingly, torque teno virus (TTV), a relatively new single-stranded DNA virus, was found to be more common in patients with acute exacerbations than in stable controls. However, TTV also can be detected in patients with acute respiratory distress syndrome, suggesting that this virus is not specific to IPF. Deep sequencing of the lungs from patients with acute exacerbation of IPF did not reveal any evidence for viral pathogens.

Whether viral infections truly have no major role in IPF pathogenesis remains unclear, although evidence suggests this is the case given the studies thus far. It is still possible viral associations have not been clearly proven due to the timing of sampling of IPF patients during their exacerbations or possible incorrect compartment sampling to identify viruses (bronchoalveolar fluid vs interstitial disease). Gene expression studies of lung tissues show suggestive of type II alveolar epithelial cell injury or proliferation, endothelial cell injury, and coagulation in patients with acute exacerbation of IPF that is distinct from patients with acute lung injury.[93] It is possible there are no major associations with conventional respiratory viruses with IPF. However, there have been reports of the presence of certain human herpesviruses, such as Epstein-Barr virus (EBV), in patients with IPF and animal models of fibrosis.[94] Another study showed patients with IPF who underwent lung transplantation were found to be positive for EBV (11/12) and human herpesvirus (HHV)-6B (10/12) compared with control lung samples that were positive for HHV-6B (3/10) and negative for EBV (0/10).[95] They suggest that herpesviruses could contribute to the lung epithelial injury that initiates profibrotic responses in IPF. Whether or not IPF acute exacerbation represents reactivation of latent herpesviruses remains unknown and requires further explorations.

It is interesting the evidence associating respiratory viruses with IPF is rather weak, whereas it is quite clear that respiratory viral infections are important in the pathogenesis of obstructive lung diseases, such as COPD and asthma. Is this difference in association of respiratory virus and chronic lung disease due to the involvement of different cell types in the lung, such as airway epithelium versus alveolar epithelium? Understanding the mechanism behind these differences will be important to determine.

SARCOIDOSIS

Sarcoidosis is a systemic inflammatory disease characterized by noncaseating epithelioid granulomatous inflammation in affected sites, including the lung.[96] Although many patients experience disease remission within the first few years, more than 30% to 50% of patients develop chronic disease requiring treatment to prevent progression of organ dysfunction and fibrotic changes. Epidemiologic studies and basic research suggest that sarcoidosis represents an immune response to an exogenous agent in a genetically susceptible individual. A definitive exogenous agent responsible for sarcoidosis remains elusive. Some investigators have speculated that a transmissible or infectious agent may cause sarcoidosis.[97] There has been an increasing body of evidence to suggest a link between infection and sarcoidosis, especially with regard to *Mycobacteria* and *Propionibacteria*. The thought is that maybe persistent antigenic stimulation from microbial agents at sites of inflammation results in sarcoidosis. However, to date, identifying the etiology of sarcoidosis has remained elusive. A variety of viruses have been proposed as etiologic agents or triggers for sarcoidosis; yet, this association has been difficult to define. The viruses associated with sarcoidosis based on serology include EBV, cytomegalovirus, herpes simplex, HHV-6 and HHV-8, and coxsackie virus.[96,98] Data supporting an increased frequency of these viral respiratory infections in sarcoidosis have been lacking.

SUMMARY

Respiratory viruses remain to be important in the pathogenesis of chronic lung diseases. Recent data with the use of more sensitive nucleic acid–based viral diagnostics highlight the underappreciation of prevalence of respiratory viruses and their role in lung diseases. Evidence for their contribution in disease pathogenesis and exacerbation is more compelling in chronic lung diseases, such as COPD, asthma, and CF, in which viruses are commonly found and associated with disease exacerbations. There is much less compelling evidence for the association of viruses with IPF or sarcoidosis. Measures to better understand how respiratory viral infections contribute to disease pathogenesis of many of the chronic lung diseases are needed. Preventive measures to limit such viral infections with good hand hygiene, avoidance of sick contacts, and viral vaccinations are recommended for patients suffering from chronic lung diseases.

REFERENCES

1. Vestbo J, Hurd SS, Agusti AG, et al. Global strategy for the diagnosis, management, and prevention of chronic obstructive pulmonary disease: GOLD executive summary. Am J Respir Crit Care Med 2013;187:347–65.

2. Mathers CD, Loncar D. Projections of global mortality and burden of disease from 2002 to 2030. PLoS Med 2006;3:e442.

3. Rutgers SR, Postma DS, ten Hacken NH, et al. Ongoing airway inflammation in patients with COPD who do not currently smoke. Thorax 2000;55:12–8.

4. Willemse BW, ten Hacken NH, Rutgers B, et al. Effect of 1-year smoking cessation on airway inflammation in COPD and asymptomatic smokers. Eur Respir J 2005;26:835–45.

5. Camilli AE, Burrows B, Knudson RJ, et al. Longitudinal changes in forced expiratory volume in one second in adults. Effects of smoking and smoking cessation. Am Rev Respir Dis 1987;135:794–9.

6. Sethi S. Bacterial infection and the pathogenesis of COPD. Chest 2000;117:286S–91S.

7. Mallia P, Johnston SL. How viral infections cause exacerbation of airway diseases. Chest 2006;130: 1203–10.

8. Proud D, Chow CW. Role of viral infections in asthma and chronic obstructive pulmonary disease. Am J Respir Cell Mol Biol 2006;35:513–8.

9. Tan WC, Xiang X, Qiu D, et al. Epidemiology of respiratory viruses in patients hospitalized with near-fatal asthma, acute exacerbations of asthma, or chronic obstructive pulmonary disease. Am J Med 2003;115:272–7.

10. Mallia P, Contoli M, Caramori G, et al. Exacerbations of asthma and chronic obstructive pulmonary disease (COPD): focus on virus induced exacerbations. Curr Pharm Des 2007;13:73–97.

11. Ko FW, Ip M, Chan PK, et al. Viral etiology of acute exacerbations of COPD in Hong Kong. Chest 2007;132:900–8.

12. Martinello RA, Esper F, Weibel C, et al. Human metapneumovirus and exacerbations of chronic obstructive pulmonary disease. J Infect 2006;53:248–54.

13. Seemungal T, Harper-Owen R, Bhowmik A, et al. Respiratory viruses, symptoms, and inflammatory markers in acute exacerbations and stable chronic obstructive pulmonary disease. Am J Respir Crit Care Med 2001;164:1618–23.

14. Bhowmik A, Seemungal T, Sapsford R, et al. Relation of sputum inflammatory markers to symptoms and lung function changes in COPD exacerbations. Thorax 2000;55:114–20.

15. Wedzicha JA. Role of viruses in exacerbations of chronic obstructive pulmonary disease. Proc Am Thorac Soc 2004;1:115–20.

16. Arcavi L, Benowitz NL. Cigarette smoking and infection. Arch Intern Med 2004;164:2206–16.

17. Kark J, Lebiush M. Smoking and epidemic influenza-like illness in female military recruits: a brief survey. Am J Public Health 1981;71:530–2.

18. Kark J, Lebiush M, Rannon L. Cigarette smoking as a risk factor for epidemic A(H1N1) influenza in young men. N Engl J Med 1982;307:1042–6.

19. Camargo CA Jr, Ginde AA, Clark S, et al. Viral pathogens in acute exacerbations of chronic obstructive pulmonary disease. Intern Emerg Med 2008;3:355–9.

20. Hutchinson AF, Ghimire AK, Thompson MA, et al. A community-based, time-matched, case-control study of respiratory viruses and exacerbations of COPD. Respir Med 2007;101:2472–81.

21. Bozinovski S, Hutchinson A, Thompson M, et al. Serum amyloid a is a biomarker of acute exacerbations of chronic obstructive pulmonary disease. Am J Respir Crit Care Med 2008;177:269–78.

22. Almansa R, Sanchez-Garcia M, Herrero A, et al. Host response cytokine signatures in viral and nonviral acute exacerbations of chronic obstructive pulmonary disease. J Interferon Cytokine Res 2011;31:409–13.

23. Pant S, Walters EH, Griffiths A, et al. Airway inflammation and anti-protease defences rapidly improve during treatment of an acute exacerbation of COPD. Respirology 2009;14:495–503.

24. Kherad O, Kaiser L, Bridevaux PO, et al. Upper-respiratory viral infection, biomarkers, and COPD exacerbations. Chest 2010;138:896–904.

25. Perotin JM, Dury S, Renois F, et al. Detection of multiple viral and bacterial infections in acute exacerbation of chronic obstructive pulmonary disease: a pilot prospective study. J Med Virol 2013;85:866–73.

26. Bafadhel M, McKenna S, Terry S, et al. Acute exacerbations of chronic obstructive pulmonary disease: identification of biologic clusters and their biomarkers. Am J Respir Crit Care Med 2011;184: 662–71.

27. Dimopoulos G, Lerikou M, Tsiodras S, et al. Viral epidemiology of acute exacerbations of chronic obstructive pulmonary disease. Pulm Pharmacol Ther 2012;25:12–8.

28. Papi A, Bellettato CM, Braccioni F, et al. Infections and airway inflammation in chronic obstructive pulmonary disease severe exacerbations. Am J Respir Crit Care Med 2006;173:1114–21.

29. Rohde G, Wiethege A, Borg I, et al. Respiratory viruses in exacerbations of chronic obstructive pulmonary disease requiring hospitalisation: a case-control study. Thorax 2003;58:37–42.

30. Stockley RA, O'Brien C, Pye A, et al. Relationship of sputum color to nature and outpatient management of acute exacerbations of COPD. Chest 2000;117: 1638–45.

31. Celli BR, Barnes PJ. Exacerbations of chronic obstructive pulmonary disease. Eur Respir J 2007; 29:1224–38.

32. Soler N, Esperatti M, Ewig S, et al. Sputum purulence-guided antibiotic use in hospitalised patients with exacerbations of COPD. Eur Respir J 2012;40:1344–53.

33. Wilkinson TM, Donaldson GC, Johnston SL, et al. Respiratory syncytial virus, airway inflammation, and FEV1 decline in patients with chronic obstructive pulmonary disease. Am J Respir Crit Care Med 2006;173:871–6.

34. Meshi B, Vitalis TZ, Ionescu D, et al. Emphysematous lung destruction by cigarette smoke. The effects of latent adenoviral infection on the lung inflammatory response. Am J Respir Cell Mol Biol 2002;26:52–7.

35. Retamales I, Elliott WM, Meshi B, et al. Amplification of inflammation in emphysema and its association with latent adenoviral infection. Am J Respir Crit Care Med 2001;164:469–73.

36. Magnard C, Valette M, Aymard M, et al. Comparison of two nested PCR, cell culture, and antigen detection for the diagnosis of upper respiratory tract infections due to influenza viruses. J Med Virol 1999;59: 215–20.

37. Raty R, Kleemola M, Melen K, et al. Efficacy of PCR and other diagnostic methods for the detection of respiratory adenoviral infections. J Med Virol 1999; 59:66–72.

38. WHO guidelines for pharmacological management of pandemic influenza A(H1N1) 2009 and other influenza viruses. Geneva (Switzerland); 2010. Available at: http://www.who.int/csr/resources/publications/ swineflu/h1n1_guidelines_pharmaceutical_mngt.pdf. Accessed December 14, 2016.

39. Strachan DP. Family size, infection and atopy: the first decade of the "hygiene hypothesis". Thorax 2000;55(Suppl 1):S2–10.

40. Sigurs N, Bjarnason R, Sigurbergsson F, et al. Respiratory syncytial virus bronchiolitis in infancy is an important risk factor for asthma and allergy at age 7. Am J Respir Crit Care Med 2000;161:1501–7.

41. Sigurs N, Aljassim F, Kjellman B, et al. Asthma and allergy patterns over 18 years after severe RSV bronchiolitis in the first year of life. Thorax 2010;65: 1045–52.

42. Jackson DJ, Gangnon RE, Evans MD, et al. Wheezing rhinovirus illnesses in early life predict asthma development in high-risk children. Am J Respir Crit Care Med 2008;178:667–72.

43. Caliskan M, Bochkov YA, Kreiner-Moller E, et al. Rhinovirus wheezing illness and genetic risk of childhood-onset asthma. N Engl J Med 2013;368: 1398–407.

44. Arden KE, Chang AB, Lambert SB, et al. Newly identified respiratory viruses in children with asthma exacerbation not requiring admission to hospital. J Med Virol 2010;82:1458–61.

45. Grissell TV, Powell H, Shafren DR, et al. Interleukin-10 gene expression in acute virus-induced asthma. Am J Respir Crit Care Med 2005;172:433–9.

46. Johnston SL, Pattemore PK, Sanderson G, et al. Community study of role of viral infections in exacerbations of asthma in 9-11 year old children. BMJ 1995;310:1225–9.

57. Grunberg K, Sharon RF, Sont JK, et al. Rhinovirus-induced airway inflammation in asthma: effect of treatment with inhaled corticosteroids before and during experimental infection. Am J Respir Crit Care Med 2001;164:1816–22.

58. Cates CJ, Rowe BH. Vaccines for preventing influenza in people with asthma. Cochrane Database Syst Rev 2013;(2):CD000364.

59. 2014 annual data report. In cystic fibrosis foundation patient registry. Bethesda (MD): Cystic Fibrosis Foundation; 2015 . Available at: https://www.cff.org/Our-Research/CF-Patient-Registry/2015-Patient-Registry-Annual-Data-Report.pdf. Accessed December 14, 2016.

60. Riordan JR, Rommens JM, Kerem B, et al. Identification of the cystic fibrosis gene: cloning and characterization of complementary DNA. Science 1989; 245:1066–73.

61. Rowe SM, Miller S, Sorscher EJ. Cystic fibrosis. N Engl J Med 2005;352:1992–2001.

62. Ratjen F, Doring G. Cystic fibrosis. Lancet 2003;361: 681–9.

63. Hartl D, Gaggar A, Bruscia E, et al. Innate immunity in cystic fibrosis lung disease. J Cyst Fibros 2012; 11:363–82.

64. Stoltz DA, Meyerholz DK, Welsh MJ. Origins of cystic fibrosis lung disease. N Engl J Med 2015; 372:351–62.

65. Saiman L, Siegel J. Infection control in cystic fibrosis. Clin Microbiol Rev 2004;17:57–71.

66. Rajan S, Saiman L. Pulmonary infections in patients with cystic fibrosis. Semin Respir Infect 2002;17: 47–56.

57. Collinson J, Nicholson KG, Cancio E, et al. Effects of upper respiratory tract infections in patients with cystic fibrosis. Thorax 1996;51:1115–22.

58. Garcia DF, Hiatt PW, Jewell A, et al. Human metapneumovirus and respiratory syncytial virus infections in older children with cystic fibrosis. Pediatr Pulmonol 2007;42:66–74.

59. Ramsey BW, Gore EJ, Smith AL, et al. The effect of respiratory viral infections on patients with cystic fibrosis. Am J Dis Child 1989;143:662–8.

60. Smyth AR, Smyth RL, Tong CY, et al. Effect of respiratory virus infections including rhinovirus on clinical status in cystic fibrosis. Arch Dis Child 1995;73: 117–20.

61. Wat D, Gelder C, Hibbitts S, et al. The role of respiratory viruses in cystic fibrosis. J Cyst Fibros 2008;7: 320–8.

62. Armstrong D, Grimwood K, Carlin JB, et al. Severe viral respiratory infections in infants with cystic fibrosis. Pediatr Pulmonol 1998;26:371–9.

63. Hordvik NL, Konig P, Hamory B, et al. Effects of acute viral respiratory tract infections in patients with cystic fibrosis. Pediatr Pulmonol 1989;7: 217–22.

64. Petersen NT, Hoiby N, Mordhorst CH, et al. Respiratory infections in cystic fibrosis patients caused by virus, chlamydia and mycoplasma–possible synergism with Pseudomonas aeruginosa. Acta Paediatr Scand 1981;70:623–8.

65. Flight WG, Bright-Thomas RJ, Sarran C, et al. The effect of the weather on pulmonary exacerbations and viral infections among adults with cystic fibrosis. Int J Biometeorol 2014;58:1845–51.

66. Flight WG, Bright-Thomas RJ, Tilston P, et al. Incidence and clinical impact of respiratory viruses in adults with cystic fibrosis. Thorax 2014;69:247–53.

67. Hiatt PW, Grace SC, Kozinetz CA, et al. Effects of viral lower respiratory tract infection on lung function in infants with cystic fibrosis. Pediatrics 1999;103: 619–26.

68. Wang EE, Prober CG, Manson B, et al. Association of respiratory viral infections with pulmonary deterioration in patients with cystic fibrosis. N Engl J Med 1984;311:1653–8.

69. Goss CH, Burns JL. Exacerbations in cystic fibrosis. 1: epidemiology and pathogenesis. Thorax 2007;62: 360–7.

70. Wood RE, Leigh MW. What is a "pulmonary exacerbation" in cystic fibrosis? J Pediatr 1987;111: 841–2.

71. Aaron SD, Ramotar K, Ferris W, et al. Adult cystic fibrosis exacerbations and new strains of Pseudomonas aeruginosa. Am J Respir Crit Care Med 2004;169:811–5.

72. Ortiz JR, Neuzil KM, Victor JC, et al. Predictors of influenza vaccination in the Cystic Fibrosis Foundation patient registry, 2006 through 2007. Chest 2010;138:1448–55.

73. Ortiz JR, Neuzil KM, Victor JC, et al. Influenza-associated cystic fibrosis pulmonary exacerbations. Chest 2010;137:852–60.

74. de Almeida MB, Zerbinati RM, Tateno AF, et al. Rhinovirus C and respiratory exacerbations in children with cystic fibrosis. Emerg Infect Dis 2010;16: 996–9.

75. Chin M, De Zoysa M, Slinger R, et al. Acute effects of viral respiratory tract infections on sputum bacterial density during CF pulmonary exacerbations. J Cyst Fibros 2015;14:482–9.

76. Wark PA, Tooze M, Cheese L, et al. Viral infections trigger exacerbations of cystic fibrosis in adults and children. Eur Respir J 2012;40:510–2.

77. Muller-Pebody B, Edmunds WJ, Zambon MC, et al. Contribution of RSV to bronchiolitis and pneumonia-associated hospitalizations in English children, April 1995-March 1998. Epidemiol Infect 2002;129: 99–106.

78. Abman SH, Ogle JW, Harbeck RJ, et al. Early bacteriologic, immunologic, and clinical courses of young infants with cystic fibrosis identified by neonatal screening. J Pediatr 1991;119:211–7.

79. Colombo C, Battezzati PM, Lucidi V, et al. Influenza A/H1N1 in patients with cystic fibrosis in Italy: a multicentre cohort study. Thorax 2011;66:260–1.

80. Nash EF, Whitmill R, Barker B, et al. Clinical outcomes of pandemic (H1N1) 2009 influenza (swine flu) in adults with cystic fibrosis. Thorax 2011;66:259.

81. Pribble CG, Black PG, Bosso JA, et al. Clinical manifestations of exacerbations of cystic fibrosis associated with nonbacterial infections. J Pediatr 1990; 117:200–4.

82. Renk H, Regamey N, Hartl D. Influenza A(H1N1) pdm09 and cystic fibrosis lung disease: a systematic meta-analysis. PLoS One 2014;9:e78583.

83. Viviani L, Assael BM, Kerem E, ECFS (A) H1N1 study group. Impact of the A (H1N1) pandemic influenza (season 2009-2010) on patients with cystic fibrosis. J cyst Fibros 2011;10:370–6.

84. Johansen HK, Høiby N. Seasonal onset of initial colonisation and chronic infection with *Pseudomonas aeruginosa* in patients with cystic fibrosis in Denmark. Thorax 1992;47:109–11.

85. Conway SP, Simmonds EJ, Littlewood JM. Acute severe deterioration in cystic fibrosis associated with influenza A virus infection. Thorax 1992;47:112–4.

86. Punch G, Syrmis MW, Rose BR, et al. Method for detection of respiratory viruses in the sputa of patients with cystic fibrosis. Eur J Clin Microbiol Infect Dis 2005;24:54–7.

87. Raghu G, Rochwerg B, Zhang Y, et al, American Thoracic Society, European Respiratory society, Japanese Respiratory Society, Latin American Thoracic Association. An official ATS/ERS/JRS/ALAT clinical practice guideline: treatment of idiopathic pulmonary fibrosis. An update of the 2011 clinical practice guideline. Am J Respir Crit Care Med 2015;192:e3–19.

88. Song JW, Hong SB, Lim CM, et al. Acute exacerbation of idiopathic pulmonary fibrosis: incidence, risk factors and outcome. Eur Respir J 2011;37: 356–63.

89. Collard HR, Moore BB, Flaherty KR, et al, Idiopathic Pulmonary Fibrosis Clinical Research Network Investigators. Acute exacerbations of idiopathic pulmonary fibrosis. Am J Respir Crit Care Med 2007; 176:636–43.

90. Huie TJ, Olson AL, Cosgrove GP, et al. A detailed evaluation of acute respiratory decline in patients with fibrotic lung disease: aetiology and outcomes. Respirology 2010;15:909–17.

91. Konishi K, Gibson KF, Lindell KO, et al. Gene expression profiles of acute exacerbations of idiopathic pulmonary fibrosis. Am J Respir Crit Care Med 2009;180:167–75.

92. Wootton SC, Kim DS, Kondoh Y, et al. Viral infection in acute exacerbation of idiopathic pulmonary fibrosis. Am J Respir Crit Care Med 2011;183:1698–702.

93. Kolb MR, Richeldi L. Viruses and acute exacerbations of idiopathic pulmonary fibrosis: rest in peace? Am J Respir Crit Care Med 2011;183:1583–4.

94. Egan JJ, Woodcock AA, Stewart JP. Viruses and idiopathic pulmonary fibrosis. Eur Respir J 1997; 10:1433–7.

95. Pulkkinen V, Salmenkivi K, Kinnula VL, et al. A novel screening method detects herpesviral DNA in the idiopathic pulmonary fibrosis lung. Ann Med 2012; 44:178–86.

96. Chen ES, Moller DR. Etiologies of sarcoidosis. Clin Rev Allergy Immunol 2015;49:6–18.

97. Mandel J, Weinberger SE. Clinical insights and basic science correlates in sarcoidosis. Am J Med Sci 2001;321:99–107.

98. Chen ES, Moller DR. Etiologic role of infectious agents. Semin Respir Crit Care Med 2014;35:285–95.

Viral Pneumonia in Patients with Hematologic Malignancy or Hematopoietic Stem Cell Transplantation

Erik Vakil, MD[a],*, Scott E. Evans, MD[b],*

KEYWORDS

- Viral pneumonia • Hematologic malignancy • Stem cell transplant
- Immunocompromised host pneumonia

KEY POINTS

- Viral pneumonias in patients with hematologic malignancies and recipients of hematopoietic stem cell transplantation cause significant morbidity and mortality.
- Advances in diagnostic techniques have enabled rapid identification of respiratory viral pathogens from upper and lower respiratory tract samples.
- Lymphopenia, myeloablative and T-cell–depleting chemotherapy, graft-versus-host disease, and other factors increase the risk of developing life-threatening viral pneumonia.
- Chest imaging is often nonspecific but may aid in diagnoses. Bronchoscopy with bronchoalveolar lavage is recommended in those at high risk for viral pneumonia who have new infiltrates on chest imaging.
- Early initiation of antiviral therapy in patients with influenza or respiratory syncytial virus is recommended.

POPULATION AND DEFINITIONS

This review focuses on common community-acquired respiratory viruses transmitted via aerosolized droplets or direct contact to patients with hematologic malignancy (HM) and hematopoietic stem cell transplant (HSCT) recipients. These viruses include influenza virus, respiratory syncytial virus (RSV), parainfluenza virus (PIV), human enterovirus (HEV), human rhinovirus (HRV), coronavirus (CoV), and human metapneumovirus (hMPV). Cytomegalovirus (CMV) has also been included, because CMV pneumonia plays an important role among immunocompromised patients. Other latent endogenous viruses associated with viral pneumonia in this population are less prevalent and are beyond the scope of this article.

Disclosures: E. Vakil declares no relevant conflicts of interest. S.E. Evans is an author of US patent 8,883,174 entitled, "Stimulation of Innate Resistance of the Lungs to Infection with Synthetic Ligands." S.E. Evans owns stock in Pulmotect, which holds the commercial options on these patent disclosures.
[a] Division of Internal Medicine, Department of Pulmonary, Critical Care and Sleep Medicine, The University of Texas Health Sciences Center, 6431 Fannin Street, MSB 1.434, Houston, TX 77030, USA; [b] Division of Internal Medicine, Department of Pulmonary Medicine, The University of Texas MD Anderson Cancer Center, 1515 Holcombe Boulevard, Unit 1100, Houston, TX 77030, USA
* Corresponding author.
E-mail addresses: erik.vakil@uth.tmc.edu; seevans@mdanderson.org

Clin Chest Med 38 (2017) 97–111
http://dx.doi.org/10.1016/j.ccm.2016.11.002
0272-5231/17/© 2016 Elsevier Inc. All rights reserved.

No standard definition for viral pneumonia is accepted. A distinction is generally made between viral upper respiratory tract infection (URTI) and lower respiratory tract infection (LRTI). Viral LRTI includes viral tracheitis, bronchitis, bronchiolitis, and alveolitis. Viral pneumonia is typically understood to describe an infectious syndrome with (1) symptoms consistent with a respiratory infection (eg, cough, rhinorrhea, dyspnea); (2) isolation of a viral pathogen known to cause respiratory infections from either nasal, oropharyngeal, tracheal, or bronchoalveolar secretions; and (3) new infiltrates on chest radiograph (CXR) or computed tomography (CT).

CMV pneumonia is considered separately, but similarly lacks a uniform definition. In a recent review of CMV infection and disease, Ljungman and colleagues[1] defined CMV pneumonia in HSCT patients as "the presence of signs and/or symptoms of pulmonary disease combined with the detection of CMV in bronchoalveolar lavage fluid or lung tissue sample." However, the updated International Consensus Guidelines on the Management of Cytomegalovirus in Solid-Organ Transplantation published in 2013 recommends histologic or immunohistochemical demonstration of tissue invasive disease, because bronchoalveolar lavage (BAL) culture or quantitative polymerase chain reaction (PCR) may not consistently correlate with disease.[2] CMV infection is an umbrella term to describe detection of CMV in a blood sample. CMV antigenemia indicates blood samples positive for CMV antigens (usually pp65). CMV disease refers to tissue-invasive disease.

SCOPE OF THE PROBLEM

Pneumonia is a major cause of morbidity and mortality in patients with HM/HSCT. Bacteria and fungi account for most of the documented pathogens, but advances in DNA-based diagnostic tools highlight the larger role of respiratory viruses as a cause of pneumonia. A recent epidemiologic study of community-acquired pneumonia in US adults, irrespective of immune status, isolated viral pathogens in 23% of patients.[3] Studies of patients with HM/HSCT suggest that viral URTIs progress to pneumonia 35% to 58% of the time, depending on the center, virus, underlying condition, and transmission patterns.[4–8] The incidence of respiratory viral infections among HM/HSCT patients mirrors the incidence observed among immunocompetent patients, although the HM/HSCT population frequently demonstrates more severe disease.[9] The incidence of CMV pneumonia in allogeneic HSCT recipients has decreased following widespread use of posttransplant chemoprophylaxis but remains around 1% to 8% in both the early and the posttransplant periods[10–12] and remains low in patients with autologous HSCT[13–15] and HM without transplant.[16]

RISK FACTORS
Patient Risk Factors

A limited number of characteristics have been identified as risk factors for developing viral pneumonia in HM/HSCT patients. The best established is severe lymphopenia (absolute lymphocyte count <200 cells/μL). Chemaly and colleagues[8] retrospectively found that 52% of patients with HM/HSCT with a viral URTI and severe lymphopenia progressed to viral pneumonia compared with 31% for patients with absolute lymphocyte count greater than 200 cells/μL. Studies by Martino and colleagues[7] and Ljungman and colleagues[17] prospectively corroborated these findings, and similar observations were made in smaller studies involving influenza,[18] PIV,[19,20] and HEV/HRV.[21] A single-center prospective HSCT case-control autopsy study also identified lymphopenia as an independent risk factor for CMV pneumonia.[11,22]

Patients who receive more intensely myeloablative conditioning regimens before HSCT face higher risk of progression to viral pneumonia, although this is controversial for CMV. Data from a large retrospective study of HSCT recipients and a smaller case-control study failed to detect a difference in the incidence of CMV disease following myeloablative therapy.[23,24]

Patients receiving T-cell–depleting chemotherapeutic agents (eg, alemtuzumab, fludarabine, or antithymocyte globulin) appear to remain at elevated risk both during treatment and, in some cases, for years after treatment has been completed.[25,26] The use of these agents appears especially important for the risk of developing CMV disease in HSCT recipients.[11,27–29] Furthermore, because infection with viruses such as influenza and RSV can directly impair lymphocyte function in previously healthy patients,[30] even moderate chemotherapy-induced lymphopenia and/or lymphocyte dysfunction may place HM/HSCT patients at elevated risk of viral pneumonia.

In a large single-center study, 44% of HSCT patients with acute graft-versus-host disease (GVHD) developed viral pneumonia, compared with 22% among patients without GVHD.[7] Similar findings are described for HSCT patients who develop CMV disease[12,31–33] and other individual respiratory viruses.[10,11,34–37]

CMV pneumonia principally arises from disease reactivation. HSCT recipients who are seropositive for CMV (R+) before transplant, irrespective of donor status, are at the highest risk for reactivation of latent virus.[33] Alternately, as seronegative recipients (R−) face limited reactivation risk, their rate of CMV pneumonia is lower than R+ recipients, even with seropositive donors (D+).[38]

Additional risk factors for the progression of viral URTI to viral pneumonia identified by multivariate analyses include age greater than 65 years,[8] hypoalbuminemia,[39] and cumulative dose of corticosteroids.[20,37,40,41]

Environmental Risk Factors

Exposure to viruses is prominently driven by seasonal variation in viral carriage. In general, influenza, RSV, and hMPV infections peak in late autumn and continue through winter. HRV demonstrates biphasic peaks in autumn and spring. Parainfluenza rates are highest in spring and summer, although certain subtypes are present all year. Pandemics and localized outbreaks further increase risk.

Although most viruses are acquired through community or household contacts, nosocomial outbreaks also result in significant morbidity and mortality due to intensive exposures to the health care environment coupled with disease-related susceptibility to viral infections. Careful molecular typing of viral isolates has demonstrated that nosocomial outbreaks persist in the outpatient and inpatient settings despite established infection control practices.[42–49]

CLINICAL PRESENTATION

Rhinorrhea, sore throat, cough, and fever are characteristic of most respiratory viral infections and thus cannot be used to reliably distinguish viral URTI, viral pneumonia, or other infections.

The acute febrile illness that typically characterizes influenza infections in the general population is less consistently observed in HM/HSCT patients.[18] In a study by Claus and colleagues,[50] the Centers for Disease Control and Prevention (CDC) influenza-like illness criteria (fever ≥100°F with cough and/or sore throat) was applied to patients with solid organ transplant or HSCT who presented with influenza. They found a positive predictive value of only 50% and a negative predictive value of 82% using these criteria. Ferguson and colleagues[51] applied a clinical prediction score using URTI and LRTI symptoms to HSCT recipients and found a positive predictive value of 28.7% and a negative predictive value of 84.5%. These studies suggest that symptoms common to viral infections in immunocompetent patients are moderately sensitive but poorly specific in patients with HM/HSCT.

In RSV pneumonia, fever, cough, dyspnea, and wheezing are common, whereas rhinorrhea and sore throat are less frequently observed.[52] In a large retrospective study of patients with HSCT and PIV, 87% of patients presented with upper respiratory tract symptoms and 6% presented with both upper and lower respiratory tract symptoms.[53] HRV infections usually exacerbate symptoms associated with an underlying chronic lung disease and include dyspnea, chest tightness, and wheezing.[54–57] HEV presents frequently with cough, even when lower respiratory involvement is not suspected.[58] Limited information is available for hMPV, but cough, wheeze, and fever predominate.[36,59] Symptoms of CMV pneumonia are nonspecific but are usually consistent with a non-suppurative pneumonitis, including nonproductive cough, dyspnea, and hypoxia. The presence of fever is variable.[60] Because CMV pneumonia may also be coincident with CMV viremia, symptoms of fever, malaise, arthralgia, cytopenias, and elevation of liver associated enzymes may also occur.

DIAGNOSTIC CONSIDERATIONS

Patients with HM/HSCT have many potential causes of respiratory symptoms, pulmonary infiltrates, and fevers. Thus, a high degree of suspicion is essential for diagnosing viral pneumonia in a patient with nonspecific symptoms. The clinician must remain vigilant in consideration of patient risk factors, time of year, and exposure history, and those suspected of having a viral infection should be promptly referred for laboratory and radiographic evaluation. **Fig. 1** presents an algorithmic approach to patients presenting with syndromes suggestive of viral respiratory infections.

Virus Isolation

Viral nucleic acid amplification techniques using PCR, microarray, or DNA chip technologies have largely supplanted direct fluorescent antibody stains and conventional viral culture for the diagnosis of respiratory viruses. These techniques have been specifically validated in patients with HM/HSCT.[61–63] Samples for nucleic acid assays are commonly obtained from the nasopharynx using sterile swabs or washings. Similar test performance is observed when analyzing sputum samples, tracheal aspirates, and BAL fluid.

Radiographic Characteristics

Although plain CXR can demonstrate lower respiratory tract involvement of viral infections, they

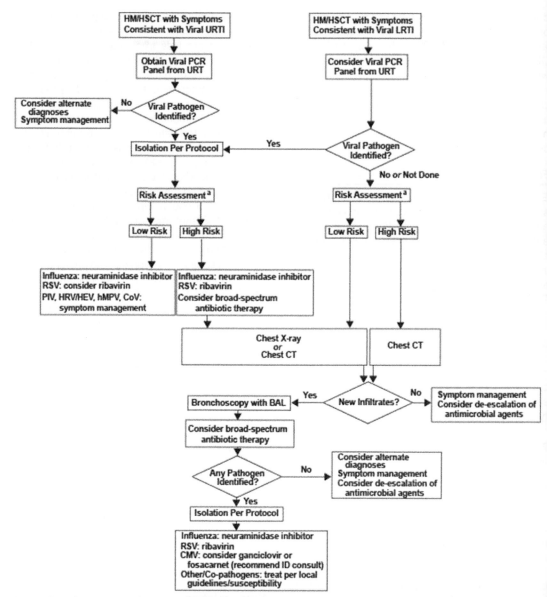

Fig. 1. Algorithmic approach to the HM/HSCT patient with suspected viral infection. ID consult, consultation with infectious disease expert; PCR Panel, PCR-base viral nucleic acid detection panel. [a] High-risk patient characteristics: lymphopenia, neutropenia, active GVHD, T-cell–depleting regimens, myeloablative conditioning, high-dose corticosteroids, age >65 years, hypoalbuminemia.

are nonspecific and have a poor negative predictive value, particularly in HM/HSCT patients. In a study by Logan and colleagues,[64] radiologist-interpreted CXR predicted the correct type of infection in immunocompromised patients with pneumonia only 34% of the time. Heussel and colleagues[65] compared CXR with chest CT in adult patients presenting with febrile neutropenia. Forty-eight percent of patients whose chest CT was suggestive of pneumonia were found to have a CXR that was interpreted as normal.

As shown in **Fig. 2**, the CT patterns most commonly observed in viral pneumonias are ground glass opacities (GGOs), nodules, interlobular septal thickening, bronchial wall thickening, and subtle changes in attenuation. Although it is widely presumed that these distinct radiographic patterns relate to unique histopathologic injury caused by different viruses, there is considerable histopathologic and radiographic overlap between respiratory viruses, rendering the findings nonspecific.[66] Furthermore, patients with HM/HSCT and

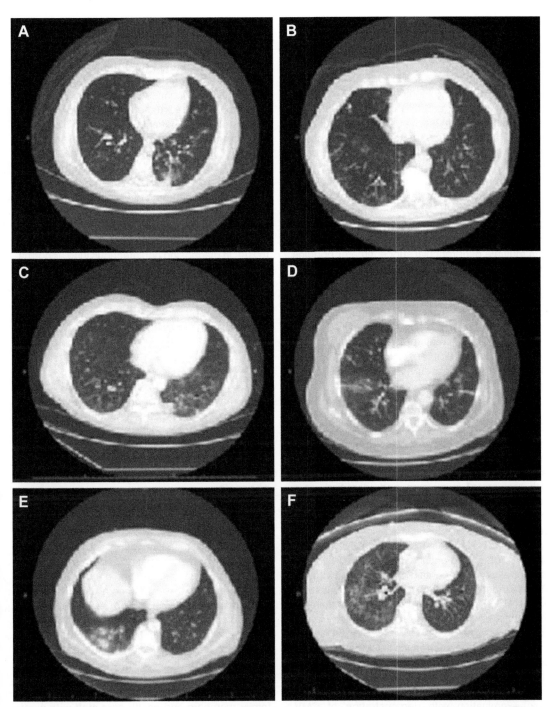

Fig. 2. Radiographic presentations of BAL-documented viral pneumonia. (*A*) Mucus plugging and consolidative opacities in a patient with hMPV and multiple myeloma following autologous HSCT. (*B*) Mucus plugging and GGOs in a patient with RSV and acute myelogenous leukemia following allogeneic HSCT. (*C*) Bronchial wall thickening and consolidative opacities in a patient with rhinovirus and chronic lymphocytic leukemia following allogeneic HSCT. (*D*) Multifocal GGO and micronodules in a patient with PIV and acute myelogenous leukemia receiving clofarabine. (*E*) Focal consolidative opacity in a patient with influenza A and untreated acute myelogenous leukemia. (*F*) Diffuse GGOs and micronodules in a patient with CMV pneumonitis and acute myelogenous leukemia following matched-unrelated donor allogeneic HSCT.

viral pneumonia frequently have coinfection with bacterial or fungal pathogens, and their radiographic patterns may be further confounded by noninfectious conditions.

Influenza virus is associated with bronchial thickening, mucus plugging of the terminal bronchioles, GGOs, and nodules that may evolve into confluent opacities.[67,68] Severe influenza may be associated with secondary infections and/or the acute respiratory distress syndrome, potentially presenting with consolidative opacities. In a case series of adult patients with HM/HSCT with RSV pneumonia, the most common patterns were centrilobular subcentimeter nodules, airspace consolidation, GGOs, and bronchial wall thickening.[69] PIV manifests most often with multiple peribronchial subcentimeter nodules and GGOs.[70] The predominant pattern in hMPV is a mixture of bilateral GGOs and subcentimeter nodular opacities without a predilection for lung zones.[71] Little data are available for HRV viral pneumonia, but bilateral diffuse GGOs are described.[72] CMV may present with a miliary pattern or a diffuse interstitial pneumonitis with GGOs, small centrilobular nodules, and air space opacities.[73–75]

Bronchoscopy

In order to assess progression to the lower respiratory tract and to detect additional pathogens, BAL is frequently recommended in HM/HSCT patients with respiratory symptoms and identified virus from an upper respiratory sample, particularly in the setting of an abnormal CXR or CT. A meta-analysis of BAL and lung biopsy in patients with cancer and HSCT demonstrated an overall yield of 43% for any infectious cause by BAL, with 13% of all samples containing identifiable virus.[76] The diagnostic yield of BAL is reduced substantially in HSCT patients if bronchoscopy is delayed more than 4 days after presentation for any infectious cause.[77]

BAL diagnostic performance in CMV pneumonia depends on the analytical modality chosen. Shell vial culture has high sensitivity but poor specificity for diagnosing tissue-invasive disease.[78] Cytologic examination with demonstration of CMV intracytoplasmic inclusions is highly specific but poorly sensitive.[79] PCR is highly sensitive and specific if the pretest clinical suspicion for CMV pneumonia is high.[80–82] In patients without respiratory symptoms, PCR-based results may result in false positives because pulmonary shedding of virus is common in patients with CMV infection without tissue-invasive disease.[83,84] In theory, false positives could be mitigated with quantitative PCR

techniques, but a viral DNA threshold has not been established.[85–87]

The prognostic value of isolating virus from the lower respiratory tract by BAL has been the subject of recent investigation. Seo and colleagues[88] found that HSCT patients with new pulmonary infiltrates and BAL-detected PIV had worse 90-day survival than did patients with new infiltrates and PIV detected only in the upper respiratory tract (45% vs 85%). Alternatively, a study by Campbell and colleagues[89] evaluated the prognostic value of quantitative PCR in BAL samples but found high viral copy numbers of PIV was not a predictor of outcome.

The role of lung biopsy, either surgical or endoscopic, is unclear. Although lung biopsy is superior to BAL in diagnosing noninfectious lung abnormality, it is associated with significant complications and procedure-related mortality.[76] High clinical suspicion for a diagnosis other than viral pneumonia would be needed to justify tissue biopsy in HM/HSCT patients with new pulmonary infiltrates.

PREVENTION AND TREATMENT
Prevention

Three main principles of preventing respiratory virus infections in HM/HSCT patients are infection control, chemoprophylaxis, and vaccination. Given the high attendant mortality and the variable efficacy of antiviral treatments, effective prevention likely offers the greatest potential for a mortality benefit.

Standard infection control practices should be instituted for all patients with suspected respiratory viral infection. These infection control practices include the use of personal protective equipment, patient isolation, and frequent hand hygiene. A systemic review demonstrated that these practices are a low, cost-effective way of reducing transmission.[90] The American Society for Blood and Marrow Transplant published extensive guidelines on infection prevention in transplant recipients.[91] Additional measures include early and aggressive testing for respiratory viral infections with rapid diagnostic methods, reverse isolation with face mask, and strict policies for family members and health care staff with symptoms of a respiratory infection.

Despite these practices, nosocomial transmission remains high. A likely contributor is noncompliance with infection control practices by staff members, visitors, and patients. Maziarz and colleagues[48] described successfully curtailing a nosocomial outbreak of PIV in the outpatient setting by establishing a rigorous 7-step protocol. During an RSV outbreak, Lehners and colleagues[45] described isolation of contacts for up to 8 days, routinely swabbing to monitor viral shedding and requiring 3 consecutive negative throat swabs before lifting isolation. These extra precautions, along with strict compliance with routine measures, are likely required for effective prevention and management of outbreaks.

The CDC recommends annual influenza vaccination for all persons aged 6 months or older who do not have contraindications.[92] Vaccination in patients with HSCT is complicated by impaired immunologic response. If vaccination is given before 6 months after transplant, vaccine efficacy is significantly impaired.[93–95] The addition of a second dose has little effect.[96] Vaccination before transplant has theoretic advantages, although HSCT candidates with HM also often have an impaired immunologic response to vaccination, especially while receiving highly myelosuppressive chemotherapy.[97–100] If vaccination is performed, only the intramuscular preparation with inactivated influenza should be used. Vaccinations for other respiratory viruses are under investigation.

Chemoprophylaxis with antiviral therapy can limit the spread of infection during outbreaks or high-risk seasons. Higa and colleagues[101] demonstrated that neuraminidase (NA) inhibitors may be effective at preventing nosocomial transmission of influenza in hospitalized patients. In a study of HSCT recipients who reside in an outpatient residential facility while undergoing treatment, oseltamivir was provided to all residents after several patients were diagnosed with influenza.[102] After initiation, no new cases of influenza were diagnosed for the duration of the influenza season, which compared favorably with matched controls in previous years.

The humanized monoclonal antibody palivizumab (PVZ) is effective at reducing the rate of RSV transmission in children with HSCT. In a study by Kassis and colleagues,[103] 16 children with HSCT on an inpatient ward who were considered high risk for contracting RSV during an outbreak received PZV, and none contracted RSV.

Chemoprophylaxis against CMV in recipients of HSCT is critically important in preventing tissue-invasive disease. Prevention strategies are multimodal with a focus on preventing primary CMV infection when possible, preventing CMV reactivation in seropositive HSCT recipients, and preemptive therapy in patients with early indications of CMV reactivation.

Chemoprophylaxis is not yet available for other respiratory viral infections. Given unpredictable virus exposure patterns, profound immune defects in HM/HSCT patients, and narrow specificity of available chemopreventive agents, broad

stimulation of antiviral responses via host-directed therapies may provide an opportunity to enhance survival in these populations. Several groups are focused on stimulating antiviral protection through manipulation of pattern recognition receptors.[104–108]

Approved Therapies

There are 2 classes of antiviral agents approved for the treatment of influenza. M2 proton channel inhibitors amantadine and rimantadine have antiviral activity against influenza A virus. NA inhibitors oseltamivir (oral), zanamivir (inhaled), and peramivir (intravenous) have activity against influenza A and B virus. Given high levels of resistance (in some series reported as >99%) to M2 inhibitors in influenza A H1N1 and H5N3, the CDC now recommends empiric therapy with an NA inhibitor in high-risk patients.[109] All patients with HM/HSCT are considered high risk, and NA inhibitors should be started without delay in those with confirmed or suspected influenza infection, because this confers a mortality benefit in HM[110] and HSCT[111] in both inpatient and outpatient settings.[112] For most studies, the average duration of NA therapy was 5 days; however, the optimal duration is unknown because patients with HM/HSCT frequently demonstrate prolonged viral shedding.

Aerosolized ribavirin, delivered via facemask in a scavenging tent, is approved for the treatment of RSV infection in children and is used frequently in high-risk adults. Data supporting its use in adults with HM/HSCT are mainly from retrospective studies that demonstrate improved mortality but no reduction in the progression to pneumonia.[8,113,114] Combination therapy with intravenous immunoglobulin (IVIG)[114,115] or PVZ[116–118] also seems to reduce mortality, but similarly does not clearly reduce progression to pneumonia.[119] Duration of therapy is usually 5 to 7 days but may be longer in severe disease. Aerosolized ribavirin can cause bronchospasm in patients with asthma or chronic obstructive pulmonary disease (COPD). It is also associated with high treatment cost, especially when combined with IVIG or PVZ.

Compassionate use of ribavirin and IVIG in patients with PIV and hMPV pneumonia has been described, but no mortality benefit or reduction in the rate of progression to pneumonia was demonstrated.[34,36,120]

CMV pneumonia is generally treated with intravenous ganciclovir or foscarnet in combination with IVIG or CMV-specific immunoglobulin (CMV-Ig),[121–124] with an intensive induction phase followed by maintenance therapy. Duration of treatment depends on patient risk factors, viral burden, response to treatment, and institutional preference. Although generally considered the first-line agent, treatment with ganciclovir is limited by myelosuppression and is considered contraindicated in the pre-engraftment phase of transplant and in neutropenic patients. Ganciclovir resistance is also a significant concern. Foscarnet use is limited by nephrotoxicity. Combination therapy has been described in CMV-antigenemia and may play a role in select cases.[125] The oral valine esters valganciclovir and valacyclovir are not recommended. No randomized trials comparing antiviral therapy with or without immunoglobulins are available, and the benefit of immunoglobulins is debatable.[126,127] However, given the high mortality associated with CMV pneumonia and the limited toxicity profile of IVG and CMV-Ig,

combination therapy is favored. The choice of immunoglobulin is based on cost, availability, and institutional preference.

Future Therapies

Several novel therapies are under development for a variety of respiratory viruses in HM/HSCT patients. **Table 1** presents an annotated list of promising antiviral therapies.

Coinfection and Underlying Disease

Rates of bacterial, fungal, and viral copathogen infection are high in HM/HSCT patients with viral infections. Exact rates are difficult to estimate due to confounding elements of related studies, but when identified, prompt treatment of copathogens is imperative. Patients with HM/HSCT and comorbid

Table 1
Select antiviral agents in development for use in hematologic malignancy/hematopoietic stem cell transplant populations

Name	Target	Mechanism of Action	Stage
DAS181	Parainfluenza	Sialidase fusion protein that enzymatically cleaves sialic acids on respiratory epithelium preventing viral binding	Phase II ongoing to determine efficacy in immunocompromised patients (NCT01644877)
BCX2798 BCX2855	Parainfluenza	Selective inhibitors of hemagglutinin-NA glycoprotein	Preclinical animals studies completed[140,141]
PUL-042	Broad antiviral	Toll-like receptor–mediated stimulation of lung epithelial cells to activate antiviral responses in target cells of respiratory viruses	Phase I completed in health volunteers (NCT02124278); phase II in HSCT recipients planned
Presatovir	RSV	Small molecule inhibitor of RSV F protein preventing viral-envelop fusion with host-cell membrane	Phase II ongoing to determine efficacy in HSCT recipients (NCT02254408, NCT02254421)
ALN-RSVO1	RSV	Small interfering RNA directed against nucleocapsid gene required for replication	Phase IIb completed for bronchiolitis obliterans (BO) in lung transplant recipients[142]
Maribavir	CMV	Selective inhibitor of viral encapsidation and nuclear egress of viral particles from infected cells through binding of CMV protein kinase UL97	Phase III completed for prophylaxis in HSCT recipients[143]
Brincidofovir	CMV	Lipid conjugate prodrug of cidofovir, which is a selective inhibitor of viral DNA polymerase	Phase II completed for prophylaxis in HSCT recipients[144] Phase III ongoing for prophylaxis in HSCT recipients (NCT01769170)
Letermovir	CMV	Selective inhibitor of viral terminase subunit pUL56	Phase II completed for prophylaxis in HSCT recipients[145] Phase III ongoing for prophylaxis in HSCT recipients (NCT02137772)

underlying lung disease, particularly asthma and COPD, are at increased risk of respiratory failure, especially with HRV infection. Appropriate therapy for bronchospasm and airway inflammation should be part of the treatment algorithm.

PROGNOSIS

There is significant heterogeneity reported for studies of mortality caused by respiratory viral infections in HM/HSCT patients, and most are based on single-center experience. Published mortalities for influenza pneumonia vary depending on the center, use of NA inhibitors, and influenza strain. Data from a large cancer center during the 1991 to 1992 influenza A epidemic demonstrated a 17% mortality from influenza A pneumonia in HSCT patients who had not received NA inhibitors or influenza prophylaxis.[128] Prospective data from several European centers between 1997 and 1998 demonstrated an all-cause mortality in patients with HSCT and influenza of 25%.[17] In a study with early initiation of oseltamivir in HSCT patients with influenza A or B in Brazil, mortality was 0% in 39 patients studied.[111] During the 2009 H1N1 outbreak, a prospective survey of HSCT recipients at several European centers reported an H1N1-attributable mortality of 6.3%.[129]

Mortality from RSV pneumonia is high, with rates reported between 29% and 88%.[5,6,17,52,130] Mortality from HRV-associated pneumonia is commonly associated with coinfection and is between 38% and 83%.[21,39,131] Overall mortality in patients with PIV who developed pneumonia in 2 large retrospective studies was 17%[20] and 35%[53] at 30 days. Very limited data are available for hMPV but mortalities of 0%,[59,132] 12.5%,[36] and 43%[133] have been reported. Risk of mortality from HEV and nonepidemic CoV appears low, but more data are needed.[35,58] Overall 6-month mortality from CMV-pneumonitis in patients with HSCT was 30% in a large transplant center.[134]

Respiratory virus infection may also result in progressive loss of lung function, particularly in patients with HSCT. Erard and colleagues[134] retrospectively studied 132 patients with HSCT over a 12-year period and found that 58% of patients developed airflow limitations that did not improve following resolution of their infection. Viral infections were also independently associated with bronchiolitis obliterans syndrome and idiopathic pulmonary syndrome in HSCT.[135,136]

Viral infections may also impact graft function. Toupin and colleagues[137] described 3 patients with HSCT and severe PIV pneumonia who developed engraftment failure. Grewal and colleagues[138] described 2 patients with Hurler

syndrome who underwent HSCT that had secondary marrow failure coincident with PIV infection. CMV has also been shown to alter gene expression in the stromal environment of bone marrow transplant recipient and inhibit engraftment.[139]

SUMMARY

Respiratory viruses are increasingly recognized as a cause of pneumonia in patients with HM/HSCT and are associated with notable morbidity. Modern molecular diagnostic tools coupled with a high index of suspicion can assist identification of patients with viral pneumonia. CXR or CT scans should be considered in all patients with symptoms and signs of lower respiratory tract involvement, and referral to bronchoscopy should not be delayed. Prompt empiric antivirals followed by tailored therapy should be administered when treatments are available, and careful management of copathogens and comorbid pulmonary disease is critical. Patients with HM/HSCT should receive yearly influenza vaccination. Patients, families, and health care workers should be routinely educated on hand hygiene and isolation practices while institutional policies for infection control should be strictly enforced. Much remains understudied and large prospective studies are needed to improve the understanding of the role respiratory virus play in patients with HM and HSCT.

REFERENCES

1. Ljungman P, Griffiths P, Paya C. Definitions of cytomegalovirus infection and disease in transplant recipients. Clin Infect Dis 2002;34:1094–7.
2. Kotton CN, Kumar D, Caliendo AM, et al. Updated international consensus guidelines on the management of cytomegalovirus in solid-organ transplantation. Transplantation 2013;96:333–60.
3. Jain S, Williams DJ, Arnold SR, et al. Community-acquired pneumonia requiring hospitalization among U.S. children. N Engl J Med 2015;372:835–45.
4. Whimbey E, Champlin RE, Couch RB, et al. Community respiratory virus infections among hospitalized adult bone marrow transplant recipients. Clin Infect Dis 1996;22:778–82.
5. Ljungman P. Respiratory virus infections in bone marrow transplant recipients: the European perspective. Am J Med 1997;102:44–7.
6. Bowden RA. Respiratory virus infections after marrow transplant: the Fred Hutchinson Cancer Research Center experience. Am J Med 1997;102:27–30.
7. Martino R, Porras RP, Rabella N, et al. Prospective study of the incidence, clinical features, and outcome of symptomatic upper and lower respiratory tract

infections by respiratory viruses in adult recipients of hematopoietic stem cell transplants for hematologic malignancies. Biol Blood Marrow Transplant 2005; 11:781–96.

8. Chemaly RF, Ghosh S, Bodey GP, et al. Respiratory viral infections in adults with hematologic malignancies and human stem cell transplantation recipients: a retrospective study at a major cancer center. Medicine 2006;85:278–87.

9. Boeckh M. The challenge of respiratory virus infections in hematopoietic cell transplant recipients. Br J Haematol 2008;143:455–67.

10. Boeckh M, Nichols WG, Papanicolaou G, et al. Cytomegalovirus in hematopoietic stem cell transplant recipients: current status, known challenges, and future strategies. Biol Blood Marrow Transplant 2003;9:543–58.

11. Boeckh M, Leisenring W, Riddell SR, et al. Late cytomegalovirus disease and mortality in recipients of allogeneic hematopoietic stem cell transplants: importance of viral load and T-cell immunity. Blood 2003;101:407–14.

12. Ljungman P, Perez-Bercoff L, Jonsson J, et al. Risk factors for the development of cytomegalovirus disease after allogeneic stem cell transplantation. Haematologica 2006;91:78–83.

13. Ljungman P, Biron P, Bosi A, et al. Cytomegalovirus interstitial pneumonia in autologous bone marrow transplant recipients. Infectious Disease Working Party of the European Group for Bone Marrow Transplantation. Bone Marrow Transplant 1994;13: 209–12.

14. Fassas AB, Bolanos-Meade J, Buddharaju LN, et al. Cytomegalovirus infection and non-neutropenic fever after autologous stem cell transplantation: high rates of reactivation in patients with multiple myeloma and lymphoma. Br J Haematol 2001;112: 237–41.

15. Marchesi F, Pimpinelli F, Gumenyuk S, et al. Cytomegalovirus reactivation after autologous stem cell transplantation in myeloma and lymphoma patients: a single-center study. World J Transplant 2015;5:129–36.

16. Chang H, Tang TC, Hung YS, et al. Cytomegalovirus infection in non-transplant patients with hematologic neoplasms: a case series. Chang Gung Med J 2011;34:65–74.

17. Ljungman P, Ward KN, Crooks BN, et al. Respiratory virus infections after stem cell transplantation: a prospective study from the infectious diseases working party of the European Group for Blood and Marrow Transplantation. Bone Marrow Transplant 2001;28:479–84.

18. Nichols WG, Guthrie KA, Corey L, et al. Influenza infections after hematopoietic stem cell transplantation: risk factors, mortality, and the effect of antiviral therapy. Clin Infect Dis 2004;39:1300–6.

19. Marcolini JA, Malik S, Suki D, et al. Respiratory disease due to parainfluenza virus in adult leukemia patients. Eur J Clin Microbiol Infect Dis 2003;22:79–84.

20. Chemaly RF, Hanmod SS, Rathod DB, et al. The characteristics and outcomes of parainfluenza virus infections in 200 patients with leukemia or recipients of hematopoietic stem cell transplantation. Blood 2012;119:2738–45.

21. Ferguson PE, Gilroy NM, Faux CE, et al. Human rhinovirus C in adult haematopoietic stem cell transplant recipients with respiratory illness. J Clin Virol 2013;56:339–43.

22. Torres HA, Aguilera E, Safdar A, et al. Fatal cytomegalovirus pneumonia in patients with haematological malignancies: an autopsy-based case-control study. Clin Microbiol Infect 2008;14:1160–6.

23. Junghanss C, Boeckh M, Carter RA, et al. Incidence and outcome of cytomegalovirus infections following nonmyeloablative compared with myeloablative allogeneic stem cell transplantation, a matched control study. Blood 2002;99:1978–85.

24. Nakamae H, Kirby KA, Sandmaier BM, et al. Effect of conditioning regimen intensity on CMV infection in allogeneic hematopoietic cell transplantation. Biol Blood Marrow Transplant 2009;15:694–703.

25. Schiffer JT, Kirby K, Sandmaier B, et al. Timing and severity of community acquired respiratory virus infections after myeloablative versus nonmyeloablative hematopoietic stem cell transplantation. Haematologica 2009;94(8):1101–8.

26. Chakrabarti S, Avivi I, Mackinnon S, et al. Respiratory virus infections in transplant recipients after reduced-intensity conditioning with Campath-1H: high incidence but low mortality. Br J Haematol 2002;119:1125–32.

27. Dodero A, Carrabba M, Milani R, et al. Reduced-intensity conditioning containing low-dose alemtuzumab before allogeneic peripheral blood stem cell transplantation: graft-versus-host disease is decreased but T-cell reconstitution is delayed. Exp Hematol 2005;33:920–7.

28. van Burik J-AH, Carter SL, Freifeld AG, et al. Higher risk of cytomegalovirus and aspergillus infections in recipients of T cell–depleted unrelated bone marrow: analysis of infectious complications in patients treated with T cell depletion versus immunosuppressive therapy to prevent graft-versus-host disease. Biol Blood Marrow Transplant 2007;13: 1487–98.

29. Chakrabarti S, Mackinnon S, Chopra R, et al. High incidence of cytomegalovirus infection after nonmyeloablative stem cell transplantation: potential role of Campath-1H in delaying immune reconstitution. Blood 2002;99:4357–63.

30. Welliver TP, Garofalo RP, Hosakote Y, et al. Severe human lower respiratory tract illness caused by respiratory syncytial virus and influenza virus is

characterized by the absence of pulmonary cytotoxic lymphocyte responses. J Infect Dis 2007; 195:1126–36.

31. Asano-Mori Y, Kanda Y, Oshima K, et al. Clinical features of late cytomegalovirus infection after hematopoietic stem cell transplantation. Int J Hematol 2008;87:310–8.

32. Miller W, Flynn P, McCullough J, et al. Cytomegalovirus infection after bone marrow transplantation: an association with acute graft-v-host disease. Blood 1986;67:1162–7.

33. George B, Pati N, Gilroy N, et al. Pre-transplant cytomegalovirus (CMV) serostatus remains the most important determinant of CMV reactivation after allogeneic hematopoietic stem cell transplantation in the era of surveillance and preemptive therapy. Transpl Infect Dis 2010;12:322–9.

34. Ustun C, Slabý J, Shanley RM, et al. Human parainfluenza virus infection after hematopoietic stem cell transplantation: risk factors, management, mortality, and changes over time. Biol Blood Marrow Transplant 2012;18:1580–8.

35. Hakki M, Rattray RM, Press RD. The clinical impact of coronavirus infection in patients with hematologic malignancies and hematopoietic stem cell transplant recipients. J Clin Virol 2015;68:1–5.

36. Egli A, Bucher C, Dumoulin A, et al. Human metapneumovirus infection after allogeneic hematopoietic stem cell transplantation. Infection 2012;40:677–84.

37. George B, Kerridge I, Gilroy N, et al. A risk score for early cytomegalovirus reactivation after allogeneic stem cell transplantation identifies low-, intermediate-, and high-risk groups: reactivation risk is increased by graft-versus-host disease only in the intermediate-risk group. Transpl Infect Dis 2012; 14:141–8.

38. Pergam SA, Xie H, Sandhu R, et al. Efficiency and risk factors for CMV transmission in seronegative hematopoietic stem cell recipients. Biol Blood Marrow Transplant 2012;18:1391–400.

39. Jacobs S, Soave R, Shore T, et al. Human rhinovirus infections of the lower respiratory tract in hematopoietic stem cell transplant recipients. Transpl Infect Dis 2013;15:474–86.

40. Nichols WG, Gooley T, Boeckh M. Community-acquired respiratory syncytial virus and parainfluenza virus infections after hematopoietic stem cell transplantation: the Fred Hutchinson Cancer Research Center experience. Biol Blood Marrow Transplant 2001;7:11S–5S.

41. Kim Y-J, Guthrie KA, Waghmare A, et al. Respiratory syncytial virus in hematopoietic cell transplant recipients: factors determining progression to lower respiratory tract disease. J Infect Dis 2014; 209:1195–204.

42. Jalal H, Bibby DF, Bennett J, et al. Molecular investigations of an outbreak of parainfluenza virus type 3 and respiratory syncytial virus infections in a hematology unit. J Clin Microbiol 2007;45:1690–6.

43. Lee A, Bibby D, Oakervee H, et al. Nosocomial transmission of parainfluenza 3 virus in hematological patients characterized by molecular epidemiology. Transpl Infect Dis 2011;13:433–7.

44. Harvala H, Gaunt E, McIntyre C, et al. Epidemiology and clinical characteristics of parainfluenza virus 3 outbreak in a Haemato-oncology unit. J Infect 2012;65:246–54.

45. Lehners N, Schnitzler P, Geis S, et al. Risk factors and containment of respiratory syncytial virus outbreak in a hematology and transplant unit. Bone Marrow Transplant 2013;48:1548–53.

46. Nichols WG, Erdman DD, Han A, et al. Prolonged outbreak of human parainfluenza virus 3 infection in a stem cell transplant outpatient department: insights from molecular epidemiologic analysis. Biol Blood Marrow Transplant 2004;10:58–64.

47. Cortez KJ, Erdman DD, Peret TC, et al. Outbreak of human parainfluenza virus 3 infections in a hematopoietic stem cell transplant population. J Infect Dis 2001;184:1093–7.

48. Maziarz RT, Sridharan P, Slater S, et al. Control of an outbreak of human parainfluenza virus 3 in hematopoietic stem cell transplant recipients. Biol Blood Marrow Transplant 2010;16:192–8.

49. Chu HY, Englund JA, Podczervinski S, et al. Nosocomial transmission of respiratory syncytial virus in an outpatient cancer center. Biol Blood Marrow Transplant 2014;20:844–51.

50. Claus J, Hodowanec A, Singh K. Poor positive predictive value of influenza-like illness criteria in adult transplant patients: a case for multiplex respiratory virus PCR testing. Clin Transplant 2015;29(10): 938–43.

51. Ferguson P, Gilroy N, Sloots T, et al. Evaluation of a clinical scoring system and directed laboratory testing for respiratory virus infection in hematopoietic stem cell transplant recipients. Transpl Infect Dis 2011;13:448–55.

52. Ebbert JO, Limper AH. Respiratory syncytial virus pneumonitis in immunocompromised adults: clinical features and outcome. Respiration 2005;72:263–9.

53. Nichols WG, Corey L, Gooley T, et al. Parainfluenza virus infections after hematopoietic stem cell transplantation: risk factors, response to antiviral therapy, and effect on transplant outcome. Blood 2001;98:573–8.

54. Folkerts G, Busse WW, Nijkamp FP, et al. Virus-induced airway hyperresponsiveness and asthma. Am J Respir Crit Care Med 1998;157:1708–20.

55. Nicholson KG, Kent J, Ireland DC. Respiratory viruses and exacerbations of asthma in adults. BMJ 1993;307:982–6.

56. Nicholson KG, Kent J, Hammersley V, et al. Risk factors for lower respiratory complications of

rhinovirus infections in elderly people living in the community: prospective cohort study. BMJ 1996; 313:1119–23.

57. Papadopoulos NG, Bates PJ, Bardin PG, et al. Rhinoviruses infect the lower airways. J Infect Dis 2000;181:1875–84.

58. Waghmare A, Pergam SA, Jerome KR, et al. Clinical disease due to enterovirus D68 in adult hematologic malignancy patients and hematopoietic cell transplant recipients. Blood 2015;125:1724–9.

59. Debur M, Vidal L, Stroparo E, et al. Human metapneumovirus infection in hematopoietic stem cell transplant recipients. Transpl Infect Dis 2010;12: 173–9.

60. Travi G, Pergam SA. Cytomegalovirus pneumonia in hematopoietic stem cell recipients. J Intensive Care Med 2014;29:200–12.

61. van Elden LJR, van Kraaij MGJ, Nijhuis M, et al. Polymerase chain reaction is more sensitive than viral culture and antigen testing for the detection of respiratory viruses in adults with hematological cancer and pneumonia. Clin Infect Dis 2002;34:177–83.

62. Murali S, Langston AA, Nolte FS, et al. Detection of respiratory viruses with a multiplex polymerase chain reaction assay (MultiCode-PLx Respiratory Virus Panel) in patients with hematologic malignancies. Leuk Lymphoma 2009;50:619–24.

63. van Kraaij MGJ, van Elden LJR, van Loon AM, et al. Frequent detection of respiratory viruses in adult recipients of stem cell transplants with the use of real-time polymerase chain reaction, compared with viral culture. Clin Infect Dis 2005;40:662–9.

64. Logan PM, Primack SL, Staples C, et al. Acute lung disease in the immunocompromised host: diagnostic accuracy of the chest radiograph. Chest 1995;108:1283–7.

65. Heussel CP, Kauczor HU, Heussel G, et al. Early detection of pneumonia in febrile neutropenic patients: use of thin-section CT. AJR Am J Roentgenol 1997;169:1347–53.

66. Franquet T. Imaging of pulmonary viral pneumonia. Radiology 2011;260(1):18–23.

67. Oikonomou A, Muller NL, Nantel S. Radiographic and high-resolution CT findings of influenza virus pneumonia in patients with hematologic malignancies. AJR Am J Roentgenol 2003;181:507–11.

68. Kim EA, Lee KS, Primack SL, et al. Viral pneumonias in adults: radiologic and pathologic findings. Radiographics 2002;22:S137–49.

69. Gasparetto EL, Escuissato DL, Marchiori E, et al. High-resolution CT findings of respiratory syncytial virus pneumonia after bone marrow transplantation. Am J Roentgenol 2004;182:1133–7.

70. Ferguson PE, Sorrell TC, Bradstock KF, et al. Parainfluenza virus type 3 pneumonia in bone marrow transplant recipients: multiple small nodules in high-resolution lung computed tomography scans provide a radiological clue to diagnosis. Clin Infect Dis 2009;48:905–9.

71. Franquet T, Rodríguez S, Martino R, et al. Human metapneumovirus infection in hematopoietic stem cell transplant recipients: high-resolution computed tomography findings. J Comput Assist Tomogr 2005;29:223–7.

72. Gutman JA, Peck AJ, Kuypers J, et al. Rhinovirus as a cause of fatal lower respiratory tract infection in adult stem cell transplantation patients: a report of two cases. Bone Marrow Transplant 2007;40: 809–11.

73. Beschorner WE, Hutchins GM, Burns WH, et al. Cytomegalovirus pneumonia in bone marrow transplant recipients: miliary and diffuse patterns. Am Rev Respir Dis 1980;122:107–14.

74. Gasparetto EL, Ono SE, Escuissato D, et al. Cytomegalovirus pneumonia after bone marrow transplantation: high resolution CT findings. Br J Radiol 2004;77:724–7.

75. Franquet T, Lee KS, Müller NL. Thin-section CT findings in 32 immunocompromised patients with cytomegalovirus pneumonia who do not have AIDS. Am J Roentgenol 2003;181:1059–63.

76. Chellapandian D, Lehrnbecher T, Phillips B, et al. Bronchoalveolar lavage and lung biopsy in patients with cancer and hematopoietic stem-cell transplantation recipients: a systematic review and meta-analysis. J Clin Oncol 2015;33:501–9.

77. Shannon VR, Andersson BS, Lei X, et al. Utility of early versus late fiberoptic bronchoscopy in the evaluation of new pulmonary infiltrates following hematopoietic stem cell transplantation. Bone Marrow Transplant 2010;45:647–55.

78. Tamm M, Traenkle P, Solèr M, et al. Pulmonary cytomegalovirus infection in immunocompromised patients. Chest 2001;119:838–43.

79. Paradis IL, Grgurich WF, Dummer JS, et al. Rapid detection of cytomegalovirus pneumonia from lung lavage cells. Am Rev Respir Dis 1988;138: 697–702.

80. Bewig B, Haacke TC, Tiroke A, et al. Detection of CMV pneumonitis after lung transplantation using PCR of DNA from bronchoalveolar lavage cells. Respiration 2000;67:166–72.

81. Liesnard C, De Wit L, Motte S, et al. Rapid diagnosis of cytomegalovirus lung infection by DNA amplification in bronchoalveolar lavages. Mol Cell Probes 1994;8:273–83.

82. Honda J, Yonemitsu J, Kitajima H, et al. Clinical utility of capillary polymerase chain reaction for diagnosis of Cytomegalovirus pneumonia. Scand J Infect Dis 2001;33:702–5.

83. Schmidt GM, Horak DA, Niland JC, et al. A randomized, controlled trial of prophylactic ganciclovir for cytomegalovirus pulmonary infection in recipients of allogeneic bone marrow transplants;

the City of Hope-Stanford-Syntex CMV Study Group. N Engl J Med 1991;324:1005–11.

84. Lee HY, Choi JY, Lee HY, et al. Clinical utility of quantitative cytomegalovirus detection in bronchial washing fluid in patients with hematologic malignancies. Eur Respir J 2015;46(59):PA572.

85. Boivin G, Olson CA, Quirk MR, et al. Quantitation of cytomegalovirus DNA and characterization of viral gene expression in bronchoalveolar cells of infected patients with and without pneumonitis. J Infect Dis 1996;173:1304–12.

86. Westall GP, Michaelides A, Williams TJ, et al. Human cytomegalovirus load in plasma and bronchoalveolar lavage fluid: a longitudinal study of lung transplant recipients. J Infect Dis 2004;190: 1076–83.

87. Chemaly RF, Yen-Lieberman B, Chapman J, et al. Clinical utility of cytomegalovirus viral load in bronchoalveolar lavage in lung transplant recipients. Am J Transplant 2005;5:544–8.

88. Seo S, Xie H, Campbell AP, et al. Parainfluenza virus lower respiratory tract disease after hematopoietic cell transplant: viral detection in the lung predicts outcome. Clin Infect Dis 2014;58:1357–68.

89. Campbell AP, Chien JW, Kuypers J, et al. Respiratory virus pneumonia after hematopoietic cell transplantation (HCT): associations between viral load in bronchoalveolar lavage samples, viral RNA detection in serum samples, and clinical outcomes of HCT. J Infect Dis 2010;201:1404–13.

90. Jefferson T, Foxlee R, Mar CD, et al. Physical interventions to interrupt or reduce the spread of respiratory viruses: systematic review. BMJ 2009;339: b3675.

91. Tomblyn M, Chiller T, Einsele H, et al. Guidelines for preventing infectious complications among hematopoietic cell transplantation recipients: a global perspective. Biol Blood Marrow Transplant 2009; 15:1143–238.

92. Grohskopf LA, Sokolow LZ, Olsen SJ, et al. Prevention and control of influenza with vaccines: recommendations of the Advisory Committee on Immunization Practices, United States, 2015-16 influenza season. Am J Transplant 2015;15(10):2767–75.

93. Engelhard D, Nagler A, Hardan I, et al. Antibody response to a two-dose regimen of influenza vaccine in allogeneic T cell-depleted and autologous BMT recipients. Bone Marrow Transplant 1993;11:1–5.

94. Avetisyan G, Aschan J, Hassan M, et al. Evaluation of immune responses to seasonal influenza vaccination in healthy volunteers and in patients after stem cell transplantation. Transplantation 2008;86: 257–63.

95. Machado CM, Cardoso MR, da Rocha IF, et al. The benefit of influenza vaccination after bone marrow transplantation. Bone Marrow Transplant 2005;36: 897–900.

96. Karras NA, Weeres M, Sessions W, et al. A randomized trial of one versus two doses of influenza vaccine after allogeneic transplantation. Biol Blood Marrow Transplant 2013;19:109–16.

97. Mazza JJ, Yale SH, Arrowood JR, et al. Efficacy of the influenza vaccine in patients with malignant lymphoma. Clin Med Res 2005;3:214–20.

98. Lo W, Whimbey E, Elting L, et al. Antibody response to a two-dose influenza vaccine regimen in adult lymphoma patients on chemotherapy. Eur J Clin Microbiol Infect Dis 1993;12:778–82.

99. Ljungman P, Nahi H, Linde A. Vaccination of patients with haematological malignancies with one or two doses of influenza vaccine: a randomised study. Br J Haematol 2005;130:96–8.

100. van der Velden AM, Mulder AH, Hartkamp A, et al. Influenza virus vaccination and booster in B-cell chronic lymphocytic leukaemia patients. Eur J Intern Med 2001;12:420–4.

101. Higa F, Tateyama M, Tomishima M, et al. Role of neuraminidase inhibitor chemoprophylaxis in controlling nosocomial influenza: an observational study. Influenza Other Respir Viruses 2012;6: 299–303.

102. Vu D, Peck AJ, Nichols WG, et al. Safety and tolerability of oseltamivir prophylaxis in hematopoietic stem cell transplant recipients: a retrospective case-control study. Clin Infect Dis 2007; 45:187–93.

103. Kassis C, Champlin RE, Hachem RY, et al. Detection and control of a nosocomial respiratory syncytial virus outbreak in a stem cell transplantation unit: the role of palivizumab. Biol Blood Marrow Transplant 2010;16:1265–71.

104. Cleaver JO, You D, Michaud DR, et al. Lung epithelial cells are essential effectors of inducible resistance to pneumonia. Mucosal Immunol 2014;7: 78–88.

105. Duggan JM, You D, Cleaver JO, et al. Synergistic interactions of TLR2/6 and TLR9 induce a high level of resistance to lung infection in mice. J Immunol 2011;186:5916–26.

106. Shirey KA, Lai W, Scott AJ, et al. The TLR4 antagonist Eritoran protects mice from lethal influenza infection. Nature 2013;497:498–502.

107. Wu CC, Hayashi T, Takabayashi K, et al. Immunotherapeutic activity of a conjugate of a Toll-like receptor 7 ligand. Proc Natl Acad Sci U S A 2007; 104:3990–5.

108. Wong JP, Christopher ME, Viswanathan S, et al. Activation of toll-like receptor signaling pathway for protection against influenza virus infection. Vaccine 2009;27:3481–3.

109. Fiore AE, Fry A, Shay D, et al. Antiviral agents for the treatment and chemoprophylaxis of influenza: recommendations of the advisory committee on immunization practices (ACIP). Atlanta (GA):

Centers for Disease Control and Prevention; 2011. Available at: http://www.cdc.gov./mmwr/preview/mmwrhtml/rr6001a1.htm. Accessed December 22, 2015.

110. Chemaly RF, Torres HA, Aguilera EA, et al. Neuraminidase inhibitors improve outcome of patients with leukemia and influenza: an observational study. Clin Infect Dis 2007;44:964–7.

111. Machado CM, Boas LS, Mendes AV, et al. Use of Oseltamivir to control influenza complications after bone marrow transplantation. Bone Marrow Transplant 2004;34:111–4.

112. Khanna N, Steffen I, Studt JD, et al. Outcome of influenza infections in outpatients after allogeneic hematopoietic stem cell transplantation. Transpl Infect Dis 2009;11:100–5.

113. McColl MD, Corser RB, Bremner J, et al. Respiratory syncytial virus infection in adult BMT recipients: effective therapy with short duration nebulised ribavirin. Bone Marrow Transplant 1998; 21:423–5.

114. Torres HA, Aguilera EA, Mattiuzzi GN, et al. Characteristics and outcome of respiratory syncytial virus infection in patients with leukemia. Haematologica 2007;92:1216–23.

115. Ghosh S, Champlin RE, Englund J, et al. Respiratory syncytial virus upper respiratory tract illnesses in adult blood and marrow transplant recipients: combination therapy with aerosolized ribavirin and intravenous immunoglobulin. Bone Marrow Transplant 2000;25:751–5.

116. Boeckh M, Berrey MM, Bowden RA, et al. Phase 1 evaluation of the respiratory syncytial virus-specific monoclonal antibody palivizumab in recipients of hematopoietic stem cell transplants. J Infect Dis 2001;184:350–4.

117. de Fontbrune FS, Robin M, Porcher R, et al. Palivizumab treatment of respiratory syncytial virus infection after allogeneic hematopoietic stem cell transplantation. Clin Infect Dis 2007;45:1019–24.

118. Khanna N, Widmer AF, Decker M, et al. Respiratory syncytial virus infection in patients with hematological diseases: single-center study and review of the literature. Clin Infect Dis 2008;46:402–12.

119. Shah JN, Chemaly RF. Management of RSV infections in adult recipients of hematopoietic stem cell transplantation. Blood 2011;117:2755–63.

120. Shah DP, Shah PK, Azzi JM, et al. Parainfluenza virus infections in hematopoietic cell transplant recipients and hematologic malignancy patients: a systematic review. Cancer Lett 2016;370:358–64.

121. Schmidt GM, Kovacs A, Zaia JA, et al. Ganciclovir/immunoglobulin combination therapy for the treatment of human cytomegalovirus-associated interstitial pneumonia in bone marrow allograft recipients. Transplantation 1988;46:905–7.

122. Reed EC, Bowden RA, Dandliker PS, et al. Treatment of cytomegalovirus pneumonia with ganciclovir and intravenous cytomegalovirus immunoglobulin in patients with bone marrow transplants. Ann Intern Med 1988;109:783–8.

123. Emanuel D, Cunningham I, Jules-Elysee K, et al. Cytomegalovirus pneumonia after bone marrow transplantation successfully treated with the combination of ganciclovir and high-dose intravenous immune globulin. Ann Intern Med 1988;109:777–82.

124. Boeckh M, Ljungman P. How we treat cytomegalovirus in hematopoietic cell transplant recipients. Blood 2009;113:5711–9.

125. Bacigalupo A, Bregante S, Tedone E, et al. Combined foscarnet-ganciclovir treatment for cytomegalovirus infections after allogeneic hemopoietic stem cell transplantation (Hsct). Bone Marrow Transplant 1996;18(Suppl 2):110–4.

126. Ljungman P, Engelhard D, Link H, et al. Treatment of interstitial pneumonitis due to cytomegalovirus with ganciclovir and intravenous immune globulin: experience of European Bone Marrow Transplant Group. Clin Infect Dis 1992;14:831–5.

127. Machado CM, Dulley FL, Boas LS, et al. CMV pneumonia in allogeneic BMT recipients undergoing early treatment of pre-emptive ganciclovir therapy. Bone Marrow Transplant 2000;26:413–7.

128. Whimbey E, Elting LS, Couch RB, et al. Influenza A virus infections among hospitalized adult bone marrow transplant recipients. Bone Marrow Transplant 1994;13:437–40.

129. Ljungman P, de la Camara R, Perez-Bercoff L, et al. Outcome of pandemic H1N1 infections in hematopoietic stem cell transplant recipients. Haematologica 2011;96:1231–5.

130. Harrington RD, Hooton TM, Hackman RC, et al. An outbreak of respiratory syncytial virus in a bone marrow transplant center. J Infect Dis 1992;165:987–93.

131. Ison MG, Hayden FG, Kaiser L, et al. Rhinovirus infections in hematopoietic stem cell transplant recipients with pneumonia. Clin Infect Dis 2003;36:1139–43.

132. Kamboj M, Gerbin M, Huang C-K, et al. Clinical characterization of human metapneumovirus infection among patients with cancer. J Infect 2008;57:464–71.

133. Williams JV, Martino R, Rabella N, et al. A prospective study comparing human metapneumovirus with other respiratory viruses in adults with hematologic malignancies and respiratory tract infections. J Infect Dis 2005;192:1061–5.

134. Erard V, Chien JW, Kim HW, et al. Airflow decline after myeloablative allogeneic hematopoietic cell transplantation: the role of community respiratory viruses. J Infect Dis 2006;193:1619–25.

35. Versluys AB, Rossen JWA, van Ewijk B, et al. Strong association between respiratory viral infection early after hematopoietic stem cell transplantation and the development of life-threatening acute and chronic alloimmune lung syndromes. Biol Blood Marrow Transplant 2010;16:782–91.

36. Xu J, Chen G, Song T, et al. Study on the correlation between CMV reactivation and bronchiolitis obliteans after allogeneic hematopoietic stem cell transplantation. Zhonghua Xue Ye Xue Za Zhi 2015;36:389–92 [in Chinese].

37. Toupin M, Hamadah A, Madore S, et al. Impact of parainfluenza virus type 3 infection on engraftment after hematopoietic SCT. Bone Marrow Transplant 2012;47:451–2.

38. Grewal S, van Burik JH, Peters C. Secondary graft failure associated with parainfluenza virus infection following hematopoietic cell transplantation. Bone Marrow Transplant 2005;35:425.

39. Steffens H-P, Podlech J, Kurz S, et al. Cytomegalovirus inhibits the engraftment of donor bone marrow cells by downregulation of hemopoietin gene expression in recipient stroma. J Virol 1998; 72:5006–15.

40. Alymova IV, Taylor G, Takimoto T, et al. Efficacy of novel hemagglutinin-neuraminidase inhibitors BCX 2798 and BCX 2855 against human parainfluenza viruses in vitro and in vivo. Antimicrobial Agents Chemother 2004;48:1495–502.

141. Watanabe M, Mishin VP, Brown SA, et al. Effect of hemagglutinin-neuraminidase inhibitors BCX 2798 and BCX 2855 on growth and pathogenicity of Sendai/human parainfluenza type 3 chimera virus in mice. Antimicrobial Agents Chemother 2009;53: 3942–51.

142. Clayton C. Alnylam presents complete results from Phase IIb trial with ALN-RSV0[1], an inhaled Rnai therapeutic for the treatment of respiratory syncytial virus (RSV) infection. Cambridge, MA: Alnylam Pharmaceuticals; 2012.

143. Marty FM, Ljungman P, Papanicolaou GA, et al. Maribavir prophylaxis for prevention of cytomegalovirus disease in recipients of allogeneic stem-cell transplants: a phase 3, double-blind, placebo-controlled, randomised trial. Lancet Infect Dis 2011;11:284–92.

144. Marty FM, Winston DJ, Rowley SD, et al. CMX001 to prevent cytomegalovirus disease in hematopoietic-cell transplantation. N Engl J Med 2013;369: 1227–36.

145. Chemaly RF, Ullmann AJ, Stoelben S, et al. Letermovir for cytomegalovirus prophylaxis in hematopoietic-cell transplantation. N Engl J Med 2014;370:1781–9.

Viral Pneumonia and Acute Respiratory Distress Syndrome

Raj D. Shah, MD, Richard G. Wunderink, MD*

KEYWORDS

- Acute respiratory distress syndrome • Respiratory virus • Community-acquired pneumonia

KEY POINTS

- Respiratory viruses are increasingly recognized in patients with severe community-acquired pneumonia and acute respiratory distress syndrome (ARDS).
- Pandemic and seasonal respiratory viral infections have been implicated in the pathogenesis of ARDS in adults.
- Supportive care for adults with ARDS caused by respiratory viruses is similar to the care of patients with ARDS from other causes.
- Antiviral therapy is available for some respiratory viral infections; however, further research is needed to determine which groups of patients would benefit.

INTRODUCTION

Acute respiratory distress syndrome (ARDS) is a severe form of inflammatory lung injury characterized by increased vascular permeability in the lung.[1] Clinically, ARDS is defined by the presence of severe hypoxemia and bilateral opacities on chest imaging that are not explained by the presence of cardiac failure or volume overload.[2,3] Community-acquired pneumonia (CAP) is the most common cause of ARDS that develops outside of the hospital.[4] Respiratory viruses are increasingly recognized in patients with severe CAP and ARDS.[5,6] This article reviews the epidemiology, diagnosis, and management of adult patients with severe pneumonia and ARDS caused by viral respiratory pathogens.

EPIDEMIOLOGY

Improved diagnostic testing, particularly multiplex reverse transcription polymerase chain reaction (RT-PCR) assays, have increased recognition that respiratory viruses cause critical illness in adults.[7–9] Although no studies have reported the incidence of ARDS specifically caused by viral pneumonia, epidemiologic surveys of adults admitted to the intensive care unit (ICU) with pneumonia and respiratory failure suggest that respiratory viruses are a common cause of severe pneumonia.[10,11] In the Etiology of Pneumonia in the Community (EPIC) study, a population-based surveillance for CAP, respiratory viruses were identified in 22% of adults admitted to the ICU with radiographically proven pneumonia.[12] In a prospective, observational study of consecutive patients admitted to an ICU with CAP in 6 hospitals in Kentucky, respiratory viruses were identified in 23% of adults.[13] In a retrospective study of 198 patients with pneumonia admitted to a single ICU in South Korea, 36.4% had evidence of viral pneumonia, including 23 patients with a virus identified in bronchoalveolar lavage (BAL).[5] In

Disclosure: None.
Division of Pulmonary and Critical Care Medicine, Northwestern University Feinberg School of Medicine, 676 North St. Clair Street, Arkes 14-045, Chicago, IL 60611, USA
* Corresponding author.
E-mail address: r-wunderink@northwestern.edu

Clin Chest Med 38 (2017) 113–125
http://dx.doi.org/10.1016/j.ccm.2016.11.013
0272-5231/17/© 2016 Elsevier Inc. All rights reserved.

these series, influenza virus and rhinovirus were the most commonly detected respiratory viruses, identified in approximately 6% and 8% of cases of viral pneumonia respectively. The prevalence of identified bacterial coinfection was low, and in 1 series[5] the mortalities related to bacterial and viral pneumonia were comparable.

Epidemiologic studies have shown that respiratory viruses are an underappreciated cause of severe CAP. However, the results of these studies should be interpreted with caution for several reasons. First, the viruses most commonly detected in patients with CAP vary across reports, which likely reflects differences in patient populations, season, and geographic location. Although respiratory viruses are commonly detected in critically ill patients using RT-PCR, their role in the pathogenesis of severe pneumonia and ARDS is less clear.[14,15] Respiratory viruses may be the sole cause of CAP and ARDS in some patients, or may be a risk factor predisposing patients to infections with other organisms, or may also represent concurrent upper respiratory tract infection, colonization, or prolonged viral shedding.[16–20]

PATHOGENESIS

The pathogenesis of ARDS in patients infected with respiratory viruses is incompletely understood. Most adults with respiratory viral infections have mild symptoms. However, viral strains associated with ARDS, such as the 2009 pandemic influenza A virus strain, are the identical to those seen in mild cases.[21,22] A combination of variable host factors and the host immune response therefore likely leads to the development of severe pneumonia and ARDS. Detailed review of the pathologic mechanisms implicated in the development of ARDS caused by respiratory viruses is beyond the scope of this article, but several excellent reviews on this topic exist.[23–26] Respiratory viruses initially infect the nasal and bronchial epithelium. This point of entry leads to respiratory airway and alveolar endothelial injury, elaboration of cytokines and chemokines, and recruitment of both innate and adaptive immune cells.[27] Specific cytokine profiles vary by virus, but converge on a common end pathway, resulting in the pathologic hallmark of ARDS, diffuse alveolar damage.[28–30] The mechanisms of acute lung injury caused by viral pathogens have important clinical implications; if ARDS results from the inflammatory host response rather than viral-mediated injury, then antiviral therapy alone may not be central to resolution of lung injury.[31]

GENERAL APPROACH TO VIRAL PNEUMONIA AND ACUTE RESPIRATORY DISTRESS SYNDROME
Diagnosis

The diagnosis of ARDS should be considered in all patients with respiratory viral infection, hypoxemia, and bilateral opacities on chest radiography unless there is strong clinical suspicion for cardiogenic pulmonary edema or volume overload. Criteria for diagnosing ARDS, referred to as the Berlin criteria,[2] are listed in **Box 1**. In resource-limited settings, diagnostic testing to ensure that patients meet each criterion, such as echocardiography or arterial blood gas analysis, may not be possible. In such situations, any patient with hypoxemia and bilateral opacities on chest radiography should be considered to have ARDS unless strong clinical suspicion for cardiogenic pulmonary edema or volume overload is present.[32]

Diagnosis of respiratory viruses can be made using isolation of intact virus particles from cell culture, viral antigen detection by immunofluorescence, or multiplex RT-PCR. When available, multiplex RT-PCR provides more rapid diagnosis with equal or better sensitivity and specificity compared with viral culture and immunofluorescence testing.[33,34] Multiplex RT-PCR testing using specimens collected from nasopharyngeal (NP)

Box 1
Definition of acute respiratory distress syndrome, Berlin criteria

Within 1 week of known clinical insult or new or worsening respiratory symptoms.

Bilateral opacities on chest imaging not fully explained by effusions, lobar/lung collapse, or nodules.

Respiratory failure not explained by cardiac failure or fluid overload. Need objective assessment such as echocardiography to exclude hydrostatic edema if no risk factor present.

Impaired oxygenation:

   Mild: $200 < P_aO_2/FiO_2 \leq 300$ with PEEP or CPAP ≥ 5 cm H_2O

   Moderate: $100 < P_aO_2/FiO_2 \leq 200$ with PEEP ≥ 5 cm H_2O

   Severe: $P_aO_2/FiO_2 \leq 100$ with PEEP ≥ 5 cm H_2O

Abbreviations: CPAP, continuous positive airway pressure; FiO_2, fraction of inspired oxygen; PEEP, positive end-expiratory pressure.
   Adapted from Force ADT, Ranieri VM, Rubenfeld GD, et al. Acute respiratory distress syndrome: the Berlin Definition. JAMA 2012;307:2526–33.

spirate or BAL have higher sensitivity compared with nasal swab.[35] Studies comparing BAL and NP aspirate have not shown one method to be superior to the other.[36] The optimal site of sampling depends on the particular respiratory virus, incubation time, and the duration of symptoms. For patients with viral pneumonia in whom bronchoscopy can safely be performed, the combination of RT-PCR testing from NP plus BAL specimens may increase the diagnostic yield compared with NP testing alone.[37,38]

Treatment

In additional antiviral therapy, special attention should be paid to ventilator management and other supportive care. Similar to ARDS of any other cause, patients who require invasive mechanical ventilation should be treated with a low-tidal-volume strategy targeting 6 mL/kg of ideal body weight.[39–41] In cases of severe ARDS, consideration should be given to salvage therapies, including prone positioning and paralytic therapy for the first 48 hours following intubation.[42–44] Although noninvasive positive pressure ventilation has been tried in patients with ARDS,[45,46] reports from the 2009 H1N1 pandemic suggest that this strategy is not effective in patients with ARDS caused by influenza.[47] Patients with severe viral infection are at risk for secondary bacterial pneumonia, because of both the effects of the virus alone and the risk of ventilator-associated pneumonia from prolonged mechanical ventilation.[48,49] Invasive tests, such as bronchoscopy, may be helpful to differentiate bacterial coinfection from viral pneumonia alone.[5,50] In general, the empiric use of antibiotic therapy in patients with viral pneumonia should be avoided and may increase the risk of antibiotic resistance and subsequent nosocomial infection.[51,52] The use of intravenous corticosteroids in the treatment of ARDS has generally not improved outcomes.[53,54] In patients with ARDS related to influenza and severe acute respiratory syndrome (SARS), adjunctive corticosteroids have not improved outcomes and may increase the risk subsequent nosocomial infection.[55,56]

Extracorporeal membrane oxygenation (ECMO) gained attention during the 2009 H1N1 influenza pandemic after several studies reported low mortality in patients with viral ARDS treated with this modality.[57,58] The only randomized clinical trial that compared ARDS treatment with ECMO with conventional care, the CESAR trial, enrolled a significant proportion of patients with influenza.[59] However, this trial had several significant methodological limitations; in particular, more patients in the ECMO arm were treated with a low-tidal-volume ventilation strategy compared with patients in the conventional arm. In a retrospective matched cohort study of patients with influenza A (H1N1) and ARDS, the mortality in patients treated with ECMO was similar to propensity score–matched controls not treated with ECMO.[60]

PANDEMIC VIRUSES

Over the past 15 years, 3 respiratory viruses have attracted special attention because of the high proportion of affected patients who develop critical illness and ARDS: influenza, particularly influenza A H1N1 2009; and 2 novel coronaviruses, Middle Eastern respiratory syndrome coronavirus (MERS-CoV) and SARS coronavirus (SARS-CoV).

Influenza Virus

Influenza A virus is the most frequently described cause of viral pneumonia and ARDS in adult patients.[26,61] Influenza A virus has a wide variety of hosts and antigenic subtypes; this genetic diversity allows the virus to cause annual epidemics, as well as occasional pandemics. By contrast, humans are the primary host for influenza B and the virus relies mainly on genetic drift to propagate epidemics.[62]

Influenza causes seasonal epidemics during the winter months in the northern and south hemispheres, and year-round in the tropics.[63] Seasonal influenza is a self-limited infection in the general population, with an average annual mortality of 1.4 to 16.7 deaths per 100,000 persons. In the United States, seasonal influenza accounts for an estimated 18,491 to 95,390 ICU admissions yearly.[64] Adults greater than 65 years of age, residents of nursing homes and chronic care facilities, pregnant women, patients with chronic medical conditions, immune-compromised individuals, and obese patients are at higher risk for more severe disease and death.[65,66]

In 2009, a novel H1N1 strain of influenza A virus was detected in the western United States and Mexico, and quickly spread globally, triggering the first influenza pandemic since 1968.[67] The new strain caused a range of clinical syndromes in humans, ranging from mild self-limited illness to fulminant pneumonia and ARDS.[47,68,69] During the 2009 pandemic in the United States, approximately 275,000 hospitalizations and in excess of 12,000 deaths were attributed to the 2009 H1N1 virus.[70] ICU admission occurred in 9% to 31% of hospitalized adults, and 14% to 47% of critically ill adults died.[71] Risk factors for poor outcomes in hospitalized patients with H1N1 were age less than 5 years, pregnancy (especially during the third trimester), chronic medical illness, morbid obesity, and immune suppression.[72]

In adults with influenza virus, the principal clinical syndrome leading to ARDS is viral pneumonitis and severe hypoxemic respiratory failure, sometimes accompanied by shock and acute renal failure.[28,67] This syndrome accounted for most of the ICU admissions during the 2009 pandemic.[47,69,73] The radiographic presentation of influenza-induced ARDS is similar to ARDS of any other causes. On computed tomography scan of the chest, influenza classically presents with bilateral ground glass opacities, but areas of the alveolar consolidation and air bronchograms are also common.[74] Bacterial and viral coinfection is common, particularly in patients greater than 65 years of age, and can complicate up to 34% of cases.[75] Radiographic findings typical of bacterial pneumonia, such as alveolar consolidation or air bronchograms, are not specific enough to confirm or exclude the presence of secondary bacterial pnuemonia.[76] Other important complications of influenza in critically ill patients include venous thromboembolism, myocarditis, rhabdomyolysis, and neurologic manifestations (confusion, seizures, unconsciousness, encephalopathy, quadriparesis, and encephalitis).[77,78]

The neuraminidase inhibitors, oseltamivir and zanamivir, are the mainstay of treatment of patients with influenza. Early administration of antiviral therapy may decrease progression to critical illness in hospitalized patients.[71]

Typical dosing of oseltamivir is 75 mg twice daily; however, optimal dosing and duration of oseltamivir therapy in patients with ARDS is not known. Treatment failure, as shown by persistent influenza detection in BAL samples of critically ill adults, was frequently reported during the H1N1 pandemic with standard-dose oseltamivir.[67] Two clinical trials comparing oseltamivir 75 mg twice a day with 150 mg twice a day did not show any significant difference in clinical outcomes, but the proportion of critically ill subjects enrolled in each trial was low.[79,80] The authors recommend administration of a higher dose of oseltamivir of 150 mg twice daily for up to 10 days for treatment of H1N1 or H5N1 influenza, and this dose should be considered for patients with ARDS related to seasonal influenza virus.

Zanamivir is available as an inhaled powder or intravenous therapy.[81] Zanamivir is generally well tolerated but has not been extensively studied in critically ill adults. The inhaled powder should be avoided in patients with obstructive airways disease because it may provoke bronchospasm. The use of nebulized zanamivir in mechanically ventilated patients has been associated with ventilator dysfunction caused by the lactose carrier.[82] During the 2009 H1N1 pandemic, sporadic reports of oseltamivir resistance were reported caused by a mutation in viral neuraminidase; these cases can be treated with intravenous zanamivir.[83]

Evidence for the use of adjuvant corticosteroid therapy in patients with influenza infection and ARDS is largely based on retrospective studies form the H1N1 pandemic, and is conflicting. Several studies have shown an increased risk of nosocomial infection and mortality.[55,84,85] However, 1 study showed a reduction in the need for mechanical ventilation in patients with hematopoietic stem cell transplant hospitalized with H1N1 influenza.[86] The authors recommend against the routine use of corticosteroid therapy in patients with influenza pneumonia and ARDS.

Middle Eastern respiratory syndrome coronavirus

MERS-CoV is a novel lineage B coronavirus first identified in Saudi Arabia in 2012.[87,88] Since then, sporadic cases and outbreaks have been reported in people living in or recently traveling to the Arabian Peninsula.[89] MERS-CoV infects both humans and camels via the CD26 receptor present on nonciliated bronchial epithelial cells found in the lower respiratory tract.[90,91] Median incubation time of the virus is 5 to 6 days, but can be as long as 14 days.[92] MERS-CoV should be suspected in patients with an acute febrile respiratory illness or CAP who live in or have recently traveled to the Arabian Peninsula. Clinically, patients with MERS-CoV can present with a range of symptoms from mild upper respiratory symptoms to severe pneumonia, acute renal failure, and ARDS.[93] Gastrointestinal complaints, including diarrhea and abdominal pain, are common and may precede the onset of respiratory symptoms.[94] In one case series of 47 hospitalized patients with laboratory-confirmed cases of MERS-CoV, 42 (89%) needed intensive care and 34 (72%) required mechanical ventilation.[95] The reported mortality in most case series exceeds 50%.[95,96]

Most hospitalized patients with MERS-CoV have abnormal chest radiograph (CXR) or computed tomography findings consistent with infectious pneumonia, most commonly bilateral and subpleural ground-glass opacities, although lobular consolidation has also been described.[97] In one series, microbiologic evidence from blood and respiratory samples of bacterial, viral, or fungal coinfection was not found in any patient, suggesting that MERS-CoV was the sole organism responsible for respiratory failure and ARDS.[95] Diagnosis is made using RT-PCR obtained from an NP, lower respiratory, or serum specimen.[98] In patients presenting with lower respiratory symptoms or severe illness, RT-PCR testing from a lower respiratory source, such as sputum, endotracheal aspirate, or BAL, is more sensitive than testing from an upper respiratory source.[99]

Treatment of SARS-CoV is supportive, and to date there are no prospective clinical trials of any specific treatment intervention. Glucocorticoids have been used as adjuvant therapy in patients with severe MERS-CoV; however, there is no clear evidence that this practice improves outcomes.[100] Combination antiviral therapy with high-dose interferon alfa-2b and ribavirin administered shortly after inoculation of MERS-CoV in rhesus macaques showed a decrease in viral replication and radiographic evidence of pneumonia. A retrospective cohort study of 20 patients with MERS-CoV treated with combination interferon alfa-2b and ribavirin initiated a median of 3 days after diagnosis found reduced 14-day mortality compared with 24 patients treated with supportive care alone.[101] In 2015, a MERS-CoV antibody, LCA60, was isolated from memory B cells of a human patient previously infected with the virus.[102] This antibody has the potential to be used for postexposure prophylaxis and treatment of MERS-CoV, but data for its efficacy in human patients are lacking.

Severe acute respiratory syndrome coronavirus

SARS-CoV was discovered in 2002 during an outbreak of 300 cases of rapidly progressive pneumonia in the Guoduong Province of China.[103] Between 2002 and mid-2004, a total of 8096 cases of SARS were reported, with a case fatality rate of 9.6%.[104] The animal reservoir for SARS is not known, although both palm civets and bats have been implicated.[105] During epidemics, SARS spread from person to person by respiratory droplets, and to a lesser extent by airborne and fecal-oral transmission.[106] Because of increased transmission by close physical proximity, SARS was frequently contracted by health care workers caring for hospitalized patients.

The pathogenesis of SARS is incompletely understood, but is likely related to both viral infection and immunopathologic injury. The functional receptors for SARS coronavirus are angiotensin receptor enzyme 2 (ACE-2) and CD209L.[107,108] Autopsy studies of patient who have died of SARS show that the lung and intestinal tract are the primary sites of infection.[109] Lung histology often shows diffuse alveolar damage with varying degrees of organization.[110] Downregulation of ACE-2 caused by viral replication, which plays a protective role in acute lung injury, has been implicated in the development of ARDS in patients with SARS.[111]

Clinical manifestations of SARS are a mild prodrome of fever and myalgias lasting 3 to 7 days, during which viral replication occurs. Respiratory symptoms, usually cough followed by dyspnea and hypoxemia, occur during the second week of the illness. Clinical worsening occurs during a time of decreasing viral load, and may be caused by immunopathologic injury rather than direct injury from the virus.[112] Dyspnea may progress to respiratory failure, ARDS, and need for mechanical ventilation.[113] The radiographic pattern of SARS is nonspecific, but it most commonly presents as ill-defined airspace opacities or ground-glass opacities, with progression to multifocal airspace opacities in patients who develop ARDS.[114,115] The diagnosis of SARS is made from the presence of symptoms along with radiographic abnormalities or autopsy consistent with pneumonia and/or ARDS, and detection of virus by RT-PCR from 2 body-fluid samples, cell culture from a single sample, or detection of viral antibodies by enzyme-linked immunosorbent assay and/or immunofluorescent assays.[116]

During the SARS pandemic approximately 20% of hospitalized patients developed ARDS.[117,118] The management of patients with SARS and ARDS is primarily supportive with low-tidal-volume ventilation and other rescue therapies as indicated. Strict infection control measures should be instituted, including the isolation of affected patients, and the rigorous use of masks, gloves, and gowns by health care workers to prevent human-to-human transmission. During 2003, the most severely ill patients with SARS were treated with high-dose ribavirin, corticosteroids, or both. However, most experts agree that these therapies were of little or no benefit, and adverse effects of these therapies were common.[119,120] SARS-CoV has been dormant since the end of the outbreak in 2004. Vaccine development has been ongoing, but the best approach remains an area of debate.[121]

Seasonal Viruses

Seasonal respiratory viruses are identified in 22% to 36% of adults with community-acquired-pneumonia who require ICU admission.[5,12,122] Influenza and rhinoviruses (human rhinoviruses [HRVs]) are the most frequently detected viruses, but respiratory syncytial virus (RSV), coronaviruses, parainfluenza virus (PIV), human metapneumovirus (hMPV), and adenovirus are also commonly reported. Whether these viruses are the sole cause of pneumonia or ARDS is controversial; however, bacteria are less commonly identified than viruses even when invasive methods such as bronchoscopy are routinely used to test for the cause of pneumonia.[5] Although the precise frequency of ARDS caused by seasonal respiratory viruses is unknown, the overall frequency is probably very low.

Rhinovirus

HRV, a single-stranded RNA virus of the Picornaviridae family, is the most common cause of upper respiratory tract infections in adults and children.[123] HRV is also one of the most commonly identified viruses in adults admitted to hospital and ICU with CAP. Whether rhinovirus is the sole cause of pneumonia, an incidental finding, a risk factor for bacterial or viral coinfection, or asymptomatic carriage, is controversial.[15] In adults with radiographically proven CAP, rhinovirus is identified more frequently in patients with CAP compared with asymptomatic controls.[14,124] HRV has been shown to trigger cytokine release in both the lower respiratory epithelium and blood, suggesting a potential pathogenic link to both pneumonia and ARDS.[125,126]

Rhinovirus has been reported as a cause of ARDS most frequently in elderly and immunocompromised adults.[127] Autopsy findings of 4 bone marrow transplant patients with suspected HRV pneumonia showed findings consistent with viral pneumonia, including acute and chronic interstitial pneumonitis and diffuse alveolar damage with hyaline membrane consistent with ARDS.[128] Among patients with pneumonia admitted to an ICU at a single center in South Korea, 96.2% of patients with HRV pneumonia required mechanical ventilation, and 59.3% had diffuse abnormalities on CXR suggestive of ARDS.[129] In another retrospective analysis of 80 hospitalized adults with HRV infection, 27.4% of whom were immunocompromised, 50% had radiographic evidence of pneumonia and 11.3% required ICU admission.[130] In these cohorts, mortality related to HRV ranged from 2.3% to 55.7% and was highest among patients with an underlying immunocompromised state.

There is no clear role for antiviral therapy in critically ill adults with HRV pneumonia. The capsid-binding anti-HRV agent pleconaril reduces the duration of uncomplicated HRV upper respiratory infections by 1 day; however, the drug was not approved for clinical use because of concern for drug-drug interactions.[131] Intranasal recombinant interferon alfa-2b is effective in preventing HRV colds when used for postexposure prophylaxis but is not effective for treatment of established HRV infection.[132,133] Further studies of antiviral therapy in patients with HRV and critical illness are needed.

Respiratory Syncytial Virus

RSV, an enveloped paramyxovirus, is an important cause of lower respiratory tract infection in children but can infect people at all ages. RSV subtypes A and B are responsible for most human disease. RSV epidemics occur during the winter months and overlap with seasonal influenza.[134] In adults, RSV causes a range of clinical syndromes, including upper respiratory tract infection, bronchitis, respiratory failure, and ARDS.[135] Adults with underlying cardiopulmonary disease, immunocompromised state, hematopoietic bone marrow transplant, and those more than 65 years of age are at risk for severe infection.[136,137] In one study of elderly and hospitalized adults with RSV infection, 15% were admitted to the ICU, 13% required mechanical ventilation, and 8% died.[138]

Antiviral therapy with ribavirin, in combination with human intravenous immunoglobulin (IVIG) or corticosteroids, may be beneficial in immunocompromised adults with severe pneumonia caused by RSV.[139] A small case series suggested that both oral and inhaled ribavirin may improve morbidity and mortality in hematopoietic cell transplant recipients.[140,141] Nonrandomized studies of adult lung transplant recipients with RSV infection suggested that combination therapy with corticosteroids and ribavirin is effective.[142,143] Ribavirin should be used with caution in some patient populations. The inhaled formulation of ribavirin can provoke bronchospasm. Both inhaled and oral ribavirin are potential teratogens that should be used with caution in pregnant patients, and pregnant health care providers should avoid contact with patients receiving aerosolized ribavirin.

Parainfluenza Virus

PIVs are single-stranded, enveloped RNA viruses of the Paramyxoviridae family. Three serotypes cause clinical disease: PIV 1 and 2 are seen primarily in the fall and winter months, whereas PIV3 is seen in the spring and summer seasons. Although PIV infections are generally self-limited, hospitalization, ICU admission, and ARDS can occur.[12,144] Patients with underlying obstructive lung disease and immunocompromised hosts may be more susceptible. In a retrospective cohort study of 253 hematopoietic cell transplant patients with PIV infection, 24.1% developed pneumonia and the associated mortality was 35%.[145]

No antiviral agents have shown efficacy against PIV. Use of inhaled, oral, or intravenous ribavirin for the treatment of PIV has been described in case reports.[146] However, a retrospective study of hematopoietic cell transplant recipients with parainfluenza who received inhaled ribavirin combined with IVIG or corticosteroids showed no benefit in terms of either viral shedding or mortality.[145] DAS181, an investigational sialidase fusion protein, has in vitro activity against PIV but the efficacy of this drug in humans is not known.[147,148]

Human Metapneumovirus

hMPV is an enveloped negative-sense RNA virus of the Paramyxoviridae family, discovered in 2001.[149] hMPV infections show the seasonal variation typical of RSV and are usually mild and self-limiting. hMPV is difficult to culture in vitro, and the diagnosis is more readily made using RT-PCR from an NP or lower respiratory tract specimen.[150] Respiratory failure and ARDS caused by hMPV have been reported in adults, including residents of long-term care facilities[151,152] and severely immunocompromised patients, such as those with bone marrow transplant[153] and acquired human deficiency syndrome.[28] In a case series of 128 hospitalized adults with hMPV infection, 31% required ICU admission and 14.8% developed ARDS.[154]

Animal models show that hMPV infects bronchial epithelial cells, leading to bronchial hyperresponsiveness, and induces proinflammatory cytokines, including interleukin (IL)-2, IL-8, IL-4, and interferon alfa.[155,156] Histopathologic changes suggestive of ARDS, including hyaline membrane formation and organizing pneumonia–like reaction, have been described in open-lung or transbronchial biopsy specimens of immunocompromised patients with hMPV identified on BAL.[157] Murine models have also shown that hMPV increases the risk of severe secondary pneumococcal infection similar to influenza A virus.[158]

Antiviral therapy for hMPV is not well established, but several antiviral agents for severe hMPV are under investigation. Ribavirin limits viral replication and downregulates cytokine production in in vivo and mouse modelsl[159]; however, uncontrolled case series of patients with hMPV infection treated with ribavirin have not shown a consistent improvement in outcomes.[160,161] A monoclonal antibody against the hMPV fusion protein seems to have both prophylactic and therapeutic benefit in mouse models[162] but studies in human subjects are currently lacking.

Adenovirus

The adenovirus is part of the nonenveloped family of viruses with a double-stranded DNA genome. The true incidence of adenovirus in adults is difficult to estimate because testing for this virus is not routinely done; in most series, adenovirus is found in 1% of ICU patients.[5,12,13] In addition to typical lower respiratory symptoms, adults with adenovirus pneumonia may also present with abdominal complaints, such as diarrhea, and neurologic manifestations, such as encephalitis and seizures. Outbreaks of severe adenovirus pneumonia have been reported in military recruits,[163] residents of long-term care facilities,[164] and immunocompromised individuals.[165,166] Although rare, ARDS has been reported in immunocompetent adults.[167,168] Adenovirus can be detected by RT-PCR from an NP, lower respiratory, or stool sample, but the diagnosis should be confirmed by PCR or cell culture detection from a sterile site such as blood, cerebrospinal fluid, or tissue biopsy.

In addition to supportive care, patients with severe adenovirus pneumonia and ARDS may benefit from antiviral therapy. Cidofovir, a mononucleotide analog of cytosine, reduces viral load and improves clinical symptoms in patients with hematopoietic stem cell transplant and invasive adenoviral disease compared with historical controls.[169] In a case series of 7 immunocompetent adults with adenovirus pneumonia who were administered cidofovir within 48 hours of diagnosis, all survived and had radiographic resolution of pneumonia by 21 days.[170] Brincidofovir, a lipid-linked derivative of cidofovir, is currently under phase III clinical trials in hematopoietic stem cell transplant patients.[171] Pooled human IVIG has high levels of neutralizing antibodies against adenoviruses and can be used as adjunctive therapy.[169] In a retrospective review, the use of corticosteroids in immunocompetent patients with adenovirus pneumonia did not show any benefit.[172]

SUMMARY

Respiratory viruses are a common cause of severe pneumonia and ARDS in adults. The advent of new diagnostic technologies, particularly multiplex reaction-PCR, have increased the recognition of viral respiratory infections in critically ill adults. Supportive care for adults with ARDS caused by respiratory viruses is similar to the care of patients with ARDS from other causes. Although antiviral therapy is available for some respiratory viral infections, further research is needed to determine which groups of patients would benefit.

REFERENCES

1. Ashbaugh DG, Bigelow DB, Petty TL, et al. Acute respiratory distress in adults. Lancet 1967;2:319–23.
2. Force ADT, Ranieri VM, Rubenfeld GD, et al. Acute respiratory distress syndrome: the Berlin Definition. JAMA 2012;307:2526–33.
3. Bernard GR, Artigas A, Brigham KL, et al. Report of the American-European Consensus Conference on Acute Respiratory Distress Syndrome: definitions, mechanisms, relevant outcomes, and clinical trial coordination. Consensus Committee 1994;9:72–81.
4. Torres A, Serra-Batlles J, Ferrer A, et al. Severe community-acquired pneumonia. Epidemiology and prognostic factors. Am Rev Respir Dis 1991; 144:312–8.
5. Choi SH, Hong SB, Ko GB, et al. Viral infection in patients with severe pneumonia requiring intensive care unit admission. Am J Respir Crit Care Med 2012;186:325–32.
6. Nguyen C, Kaku S, Tutera D, et al. Viral respiratory infections of adults in the intensive care unit. J Intensive Care Med 2015;31(7):427–41.
7. Legoff J, Guerot E, Ndjoyi-Mbiguino A, et al. High prevalence of respiratory viral infections in patients hospitalized in an intensive care unit for acute respiratory infections as detected by nucleic acid-based assays. J Clin Microbiol 2005;43:455–7.
8. Wu X, Wang Q, Wang M, et al. Incidence of respiratory viral infections detected by PCR and real-time PCR in adult patients with community-acquired pneumonia: a meta-analysis. Respiration 2015;89:343–52.
9. Karhu J, Ala-Kokko TI, Vuorinen T, et al. Lower respiratory tract virus findings in mechanically ventilated patients with severe community-acquired pneumonia. Clin Infect Dis 2014;59:62–70.
10. Garg S, Jain S, Dawood FS, et al. Pneumonia among adults hospitalized with laboratory-confirmed seasonal influenza virus infection–United States, 2005–2008. BMC Infect Dis 2015; 15:369.
11. Hong HL, Hong SB, Ko GB, et al. Viral infection is not uncommon in adult patients with severe hospital-acquired pneumonia. PLoS One 2014;9: e95865.
12. Jain S, Self WH, Wunderink RG. Community-acquired pneumonia requiring hospitalization. N Engl J Med 2015;373:2382.
13. Wiemken T, Peyrani P, Bryant K, et al. Incidence of respiratory viruses in patients with community-acquired pneumonia admitted to the intensive care unit: results from the Severe Influenza Pneumonia Surveillance (SIPS) project. Eur J Clin Microbiol Infect Dis 2013;32:705–10.
14. Self WH, Williams DJ, Zhu Y, et al. Respiratory viral detection in children and adults: comparing asymptomatic controls and patients with community-acquired pneumonia. J Infect Dis 2016;213:584–91.
15. Pavia AT. What is the role of respiratory viruses in community-acquired pneumonia? What is the best therapy for influenza and other viral causes of community-acquired pneumonia? Infect Dis Clin North Am 2013;27:157–75.
16. Gadsby NJ, Russell CD, McHugh MP, et al. Comprehensive molecular testing for respiratory pathogens in community-acquired pneumonia. Clin Infect Dis 2016;62:817–23.
17. Loffler B, Niemann S, Ehrhardt C, et al. Pathogenesis of *Staphylococcus aureus* necrotizing pneumonia: the role of PVL and an influenza coinfection. Expert Rev Anti Infect Ther 2013;11: 1041–51.
18. Zhan Y, Yang Z, Chen R, et al. Respiratory virus is a real pathogen in immunocompetent community-acquired pneumonia: comparing to influenza like illness and volunteer controls. BMC Pulm Med 2014;14:144.
19. Campbell AP, Guthrie KA, Englund JA, et al. Clinical outcomes associated with respiratory virus detection before allogeneic hematopoietic stem cell transplant. Clin Infect Dis 2015;61:192–202.
20. Zlateva KT, de Vries JJ, Coenjaerts FE, et al. Prolonged shedding of rhinovirus and re-infection in adults with respiratory tract illness. Eur Respir J 2014;44:169–77.
21. Dawood FS, Jain S, Finelli L, et al. Emergence of a novel swine-origin influenza A (H1N1) virus in humans. N Engl J Med 2009;360:2605–15.
22. Garten RJ, Davis CT, Russell CA, et al. Antigenic and genetic characteristics of swine-origin 2009 A(H1N1) influenza viruses circulating in humans. Science 2009;325:197–201.
23. Howard WA, Peiris M, Hayden FG. Report of the 'mechanisms of lung injury and immunomodulator interventions in influenza' workshop, 21 March 2010, Ventura, California, USA. Influenza Other Respir Viruses 2011;5:453–4. e458–75.
24. Hendrickson CM, Matthay MA. Viral pathogens and acute lung injury: investigations inspired by the SARS epidemic and the 2009 H1N1 influenza pandemic. Semin Respir Crit Care Med 2013;34: 475–86.
25. Gralinski LE, Baric RS. Molecular pathology of emerging coronavirus infections. J Pathol 2015; 235:185–95.
26. Herold S, Becker C, Ridge KM, et al. Influenza virus-induced lung injury: pathogenesis and implications for treatment. Eur Respir J 2015;45: 1463–78.
27. Itoh Y, Shinya K, Kiso M, et al. In vitro and in vivo characterization of new swine-origin H1N1 influenza viruses. Nature 2009;460:1021–5.

28. Shieh WJ, Blau DM, Denison AM, et al. 2009 pandemic influenza A (H1N1): pathology and pathogenesis of 100 fatal cases in the United States. Am J Pathol 2010;177:166–75.

29. Fujita J, Ohtsuki Y, Higa H, et al. Clinicopathological findings of four cases of pure influenza virus A pneumonia. Intern Med 2014;53:1333–42.

30. Wang R, Xiao H, Guo R, et al. The role of C5a in acute lung injury induced by highly pathogenic viral infections. Emerg Microbes Infect 2015;4:e28.

31. To KK, Hung IF, Li IW, et al. Delayed clearance of viral load and marked cytokine activation in severe cases of pandemic H1N1 2009 influenza virus infection. Clin Infect Dis 2010;50:850–9.

32. Luks AM. Ventilatory strategies and supportive care in acute respiratory distress syndrome. Influenza other Respir viruses 2013;7(Suppl 3):8–17.

33. Liolios L, Jenney A, Spelman D, et al. Comparison of a multiplex reverse transcription-PCR-enzyme hybridization assay with conventional viral culture and immunofluorescence techniques for the detection of seven viral respiratory pathogens. J Clin Microbiol 2001;39:2779–83.

34. Puppe W, Weigl JA, Aron G, et al. Evaluation of a multiplex reverse transcriptase PCR ELISA for the detection of nine respiratory tract pathogens. J Clin Virol 2004;30:165–74.

35. Meerhoff TJ, Houben ML, Coenjaerts FE, et al. Detection of multiple respiratory pathogens during primary respiratory infection: nasal swab versus nasopharyngeal aspirate using real-time polymerase chain reaction. Eur J Clin Microbiol Infect Dis 2010;29:365–71.

36. Wurzel DF, Marchant JM, Clark JE, et al. Respiratory virus detection in nasopharyngeal aspirate versus bronchoalveolar lavage is dependent on virus type in children with chronic respiratory symptoms. J Clin Virol 2013;58:683–8.

37. Azadeh N, Sakata KK, Brighton AM, et al. FilmArray respiratory panel assay: comparison of nasopharyngeal swabs and bronchoalveolar lavage samples. J Clin Microbiol 2015;53:3784–7.

38. Hakki M, Strasfeld LM, Townes JM. Predictive value of testing nasopharyngeal samples for respiratory viruses in the setting of lower respiratory tract disease. J Clin Microbiol 2014;52:4020–2.

39. Ventilation with lower tidal volumes as compared with traditional tidal volumes for acute lung injury and the acute respiratory distress syndrome. The Acute Respiratory Distress Syndrome Network. N Engl J Med 2000;342:1301–8.

40. Brochard L, Roudot-Thoraval F, Roupie E, et al. Tidal volume reduction for prevention of ventilator-induced lung injury in acute respiratory distress syndrome. The Multicenter Trail Group on Tidal Volume reduction in ARDS. Am J Respir Crit Care Med 1998;158:1831–8.

41. Amato MB, Barbas CS, Medeiros DM, et al. Effect of a protective-ventilation strategy on mortality in the acute respiratory distress syndrome. N Engl J Med 1998;338:347–54.

42. Guerin C, Reignier J, Richard JC, et al. Prone positioning in severe acute respiratory distress syndrome. N Engl J Med 2013;368:2159–68.

43. Papazian L, Forel JM, Gacouin A, et al. Neuromuscular blockers in early acute respiratory distress syndrome. N Engl J Med 2010;363:1107–16.

44. Al-Dorzi HM, Alsolamy S, Arabi YM. Critically ill patients with Middle East respiratory syndrome coronavirus infection. Crit Care 2016;20:65.

45. Rana S, Jenad H, Gay PC, et al. Failure of noninvasive ventilation in patients with acute lung injury: observational cohort study. Crit Care 2006;10:R79.

46. Correa TD, Sanches PR, de Morais LC, et al. Performance of noninvasive ventilation in acute respiratory failure in critically ill patients: a prospective, observational, cohort study. BMC Pulm Med 2015;15:144.

47. Rello J, Rodriguez A, Ibanez P, et al. Intensive care adult patients with severe respiratory failure caused by Influenza A (H1N1)v in Spain. Crit Care (London, England) 2009;13:R148.

48. Viasus D, Pano-Pardo JR, Pachon J, et al. Pneumonia complicating pandemic (H1N1) 2009: risk factors, clinical features, and outcomes. Medicine 2011;90:328–36.

49. Palacios G, Hornig M, Cisterna D, et al. *Streptococcus pneumoniae* coinfection is correlated with the severity of H1N1 pandemic influenza. PLoS One 2009;4:e8540.

50. Choi SH, Hong SB, Hong HL, et al. Usefulness of cellular analysis of bronchoalveolar lavage fluid for predicting the etiology of pneumonia in critically ill patients. PLoS One 2014;9:e97346.

51. Barlow G, Moss P. A/H1N1 flu... as does policy on antibiotics. BMJ 2009;339:b2738.

52. Crotty MP, Meyers S, Hampton N, et al. Impact of antibacterials on subsequent resistance and clinical outcomes in adult patients with viral pneumonia: an opportunity for stewardship. Crit Care (London, England) 2015;19:404.

53. Bernard GR, Luce JM, Sprung CL, et al. High-dose corticosteroids in patients with the adult respiratory distress syndrome. N Engl J Med 1987;317:1565–70.

54. Steinberg KP, Hudson LD, Goodman RB, et al. Efficacy and safety of corticosteroids for persistent acute respiratory distress syndrome. N Engl J Med 2006;354:1671–84.

55. Brun-Buisson C, Richard JC, Mercat A, et al. Early corticosteroids in severe influenza A/H1N1 pneumonia and acute respiratory distress syndrome. Am J Respir Crit Care Med 2011;183:1200–6.

56. Auyeung TW, Lee JS, Lai WK, et al. The use of corticosteroid as treatment in SARS was associated with adverse outcomes: a retrospective cohort study. J Infect 2005;51:98–102.

57. Combes A, Pellegrino V. Extracorporeal membrane oxygenation for 2009 influenza A (H1N1)-associated acute respiratory distress syndrome. Semin Respir Crit Care Med 2011;32:188–94.

58. Davies A, Jones D, Bailey M, et al. Extracorporeal membrane oxygenation for 2009 influenza A(H1N1) acute respiratory distress syndrome. JAMA 2009;302:1888–95.

59. Peek GJ, Mugford M, Tiruvoipati R, et al. Efficacy and economic assessment of conventional ventilatory support versus extracorporeal membrane oxygenation for severe adult respiratory failure (CESAR): a multicentre randomised controlled trial. Lancet 2009;374:1351–63.

60. Pham T, Combes A, Roze H, et al. Extracorporeal membrane oxygenation for pandemic influenza A(H1N1)-induced acute respiratory distress syndrome: a cohort study and propensity-matched analysis. Am J Respir Crit Care Med 2013;187: 276–85.

61. Ortiz JR, Neuzil KM, Shay DK, et al. The burden of influenza-associated critical illness hospitalizations. Crit Care Med 2014;42:2325–32.

62. Webster RG, Sharp GB, Claas EC. Interspecies transmission of influenza viruses. Am J Respir Crit Care Med 1995;152:S25–30.

63. Moura FE. Influenza in the tropics. Curr Opin Infect Dis 2010;23:415–20.

64. Reed C, Chaves SS, Daily Kirley P, et al. Estimating influenza disease burden from population-based surveillance data in the United States. PLoS One 2015;10:e0118369.

65. Harper SA, Bradley JS, Englund JA, et al. Seasonal influenza in adults and children–diagnosis, treatment, chemoprophylaxis, and institutional outbreak management: clinical practice guidelines of the Infectious Diseases Society of America. Clin Infect Dis 2009;48:1003–32.

66. Shah NS, Greenberg JA, McNulty MC, et al. Severe influenza in 33 US hospitals, 2013-2014: complications and risk factors for death in 507 patients. Infect Control Hosp Epidemiol 2015;36:1251–60.

67. Bautista E, Chotpitayasunondh T, Gao Z, et al. Clinical aspects of pandemic 2009 influenza A (H1N1) virus infection. N Engl J Med 2010;362:1708–19.

68. Perez-Padilla R, de la Rosa-Zamboni D, Ponce de Leon S, et al. Pneumonia and respiratory failure from swine-origin influenza A (H1N1) in Mexico. N Engl J Med 2009;361:680–9.

69. Webb SA, Pettila V, Seppelt I, et al. Critical care services and 2009 H1N1 influenza in Australia and New Zealand. N Engl J Med 2009;361: 1925–34.

70. Shrestha SS, Swerdlow DL, Borse RH, et al. Estimating the burden of 2009 pandemic influenza A (H1N1) in the United States (April 2009-April 2010). Clin Infect Dis 2011;52(Suppl 1):S75–82.

71. Jain S, Kamimoto L, Bramley AM, et al. Hospitalized patients with 2009 H1N1 influenza in the United States, April-June 2009. N Engl J Med 2009;361:1935–44.

72. Louie JK, Acosta M, Winter K, et al. Factors associated with death or hospitalization due to pandemic 2009 influenza A(H1N1) infection in California. JAMA 2009;302:1896–902.

73. Kumar A, Zarychanski R, Pinto R, et al. Critically ill patients with 2009 influenza A(H1N1) infection in Canada. JAMA 2009;302:1872–9.

74. Kim EA, Lee KS, Primack SL, et al. Viral pneumonias in adults: radiologic and pathologic findings. Radiographics 2002;22 Spec No:S137–49.

75. Chertow DS, Memoli MJ. Bacterial coinfection in influenza: a grand rounds review. JAMA 2013; 309:275–82.

76. Rice TW, Rubinson L, Uyeki TM, et al. Critical illness from 2009 pandemic influenza A virus and bacterial coinfection in the United States. Crit Care Med 2012;40:1487–98.

77. Rothberg MB, Haessler SD. Complications of seasonal and pandemic influenza. Crit Care Med 2010;38:e91–7.

78. Noriega LM, Verdugo RJ, Araos R, et al. Pandemic influenza A (H1N1) 2009 with neurological manifestations, a case series. Influenza other Respir viruses 2010;4:117–20.

79. South East Asia Infectious Disease Clinical Research Network. Effect of double dose oseltamivir on clinical and virological outcomes in children and adults admitted to hospital with severe influenza: double blind randomised controlled trial. BMJ 2013;346:f3039.

80. Lee N, Hui DS, Zuo Z, et al. A prospective intervention study on higher-dose oseltamivir treatment in adults hospitalized with influenza A and B infections. Clin Infect Dis 2013;57:1511–9.

81. Heneghan CJ, Onakpoya I, Thompson M, et al. Zanamivir for influenza in adults and children: systematic review of clinical study reports and summary of regulatory comments. BMJ 2014;348:g2547.

82. Kiatboonsri S, Kiatboonsri C, Theerawit P. Fatal respiratory events caused by zanamivir nebulization. Clin Infect Dis 2010;50:620.

83. Gaur AH, Bagga B, Barman S, et al. Intravenous zanamivir for oseltamivir-resistant 2009 H1N1 influenza. N Engl J Med 2010;362:88–9.

84. Delaney JW, Pinto R, Long J, et al. The influence of corticosteroid treatment on the outcome of influenza A(H1N1pdm09)-related critical illness. Crit Care (London, England) 2016;20:75.

85. Han K, Ma H, An X, et al. Early use of glucocorticoids was a risk factor for critical disease and death from pH1N1 infection. Clin Infect Dis 2011; 53:326–33.

86. Choi SM, Boudreault AA, Xie H, et al. Differences in clinical outcomes after 2009 influenza A/H1N1 and seasonal influenza among hematopoietic cell transplant recipients. Blood 2011;117:5050–6.

87. de Groot RJ, Baker SC, Baric RS, et al. Middle East respiratory syndrome coronavirus (MERS-CoV): announcement of the Coronavirus Study Group. J Virol 2013;87:7790–2.

88. Zaki AM, van Boheemen S, Bestebroer TM, et al. Isolation of a novel coronavirus from a man with pneumonia in Saudi Arabia. N Engl J Med 2012; 367:1814–20.

89. Middle East respiratory syndrome (MERS). Available at: http://www.cdc.gov/coronavirus/mers/about/index.html. Accessed December 3, 2016.

90. Raj VS, Mou H, Smits SL, et al. Dipeptidyl peptidase 4 is a functional receptor for the emerging human coronavirus-EMC. Nature 2013;495:251–4.

91. Azhar EI, El-Kafrawy SA, Farraj SA, et al. Evidence for camel-to-human transmission of MERS coronavirus. N Engl J Med 2014;370:2499–505.

92. Assiri A, McGeer A, Perl TM, et al. Hospital outbreak of Middle East respiratory syndrome coronavirus. N Engl J Med 2013;369:407–16.

93. Alsolamy S. Middle East respiratory syndrome: knowledge to date. Crit Care Med 2015;43:1283–90.

94. Guery B, Poissy J, el Mansouf L, et al. Clinical features and viral diagnosis of two cases of infection with Middle East respiratory syndrome coronavirus: a report of nosocomial transmission. Lancet 2013; 381:2265–72.

95. Assiri A, Al-Tawfiq JA, Al-Rabeeah AA, et al. Epidemiological, demographic, and clinical characteristics of 47 cases of Middle East respiratory syndrome coronavirus disease from Saudi Arabia: a descriptive study. Lancet Infect Dis 2013;13: 752–61.

96. Saad M, Omrani AS, Baig K, et al. Clinical aspects and outcomes of 70 patients with Middle East respiratory syndrome coronavirus infection: a single-center experience in Saudi Arabia. Int J Infect Dis 2014;29:301–6.

97. Ajlan AM, Ahyad RA, Jamjoom LG, et al. Middle East respiratory syndrome coronavirus (MERS-CoV) infection: chest CT findings. AJR Am J Roentgenology 2014;203:782–7.

98. Centers for Disease Control and Prevention (CDC). Update: severe respiratory illness associated with Middle East respiratory syndrome coronavirus (MERS-CoV)–worldwide, 2012-2013. MMWR Morb Mortal Wkly Rep 2013;62:480–3.

99. Lee JH, Lee CS, Lee HB. An appropriate lower respiratory tract specimen is essential for diagnosis of Middle East respiratory syndrome (MERS). J Korean Med Sci 2015;30:1207–8.

100. Arabi YM, Arifi AA, Balkhy HH, et al. Clinical course and outcomes of critically ill patients with Middle East respiratory syndrome coronavirus infection. Ann Intern Med 2014;160:389–97.

101. Omrani AS, Saad MM, Baig K, et al. Ribavirin and interferon alfa-2a for severe Middle East respiratory syndrome coronavirus infection: a retrospective cohort study. Lancet Infect Dis 2014;14:1090–5.

102. Corti D, Zhao J, Pedotti M, et al. Prophylactic and postexposure efficacy of a potent human monoclonal antibody against MERS coronavirus. Proc Natl Acad Sci U S A 2015;112:10473–8.

103. Poon LL, Guan Y, Nicholls JM, et al. The aetiology, origins, and diagnosis of severe acute respiratory syndrome. Lancet Infect Dis 2004;4:663–71.

104. Christian MD, Poutanen SM, Loutfy MR, et al. Severe acute respiratory syndrome. Clin Infect Dis 2004;38:1420–7.

105. Shi Z, Hu Z. A review of studies on animal reservoirs of the SARS coronavirus. Virus Res 2008; 133:74–87.

106. Donnelly CA, Fisher MC, Fraser C, et al. Epidemiological and genetic analysis of severe acute respiratory syndrome. Lancet Infect Dis 2004;4:672–83.

107. Frieman M, Yount B, Agnihothram S, et al. Molecular determinants of severe acute respiratory syndrome coronavirus pathogenesis and virulence in young and aged mouse models of human disease. J Virol 2012;86:884–97.

108. Lau YL, Peiris JS. Pathogenesis of severe acute respiratory syndrome. Curr Opin Immunol 2005; 17:404–10.

109. Peiris JS, Lai ST, Poon LL, et al. Coronavirus as a possible cause of severe acute respiratory syndrome. Lancet 2003;361:1319–25.

110. Nicholls JM, Poon LL, Lee KC, et al. Lung pathology of fatal severe acute respiratory syndrome. Lancet 2003;361:1773–8.

111. Imai Y, Kuba K, Penninger JM. Angiotensin-converting enzyme 2 in acute respiratory distress syndrome. Cell Mol Life Sci 2007;64:2006–12.

112. Peiris JS, Chu CM, Cheng VC, et al. Clinical progression and viral load in a community outbreak of coronavirus-associated SARS pneumonia: a prospective study. Lancet 2003;361:1767–72.

113. Chan JW, Ng CK, Chan YH, et al. Short term outcome and risk factors for adverse clinical outcomes in adults with severe acute respiratory syndrome (SARS). Thorax 2003;58:686–9.

114. Ketai L, Paul NS, Wong KT. Radiology of severe acute respiratory syndrome (SARS): the emerging pathologic-radiologic correlates of an emerging disease. J Thorac Imaging 2006;21:276–83.

115. Wong KT, Antonio GE, Hui DS, et al. Severe acute respiratory syndrome: radiographic appearances

and pattern of progression in 138 patients. Radiology 2003;228:401–6.

116. Case definitions for the 4 diseases requiring notification to WHO in all circumstances under the IHR (2005). Wkly Epidemiol Rec 2009;84:52–6 [in English, French].

117. Booth CM, Stewart TE. Severe acute respiratory syndrome and critical care medicine: the Toronto experience. Crit Care Med 2005;33:S53–60.

118. Manocha S, Walley KR, Russell JA. Severe acute respiratory distress syndrome (SARS): a critical care perspective. Crit Care Med 2003;31:2684–92.

119. Stockman LJ, Bellamy R, Garner P. SARS: systematic review of treatment effects. PLoS Med 2006;3: e343.

120. Wang JT, Chang SC. Severe acute respiratory syndrome. Curr Opin Infect Dis 2004;17:143–8.

121. Graham RL, Donaldson EF, Baric RS. A decade after SARS: strategies for controlling emerging coronaviruses. Nat Rev Microbiol 2013;11:836–48.

122. Ruuskanen O, Lahti E, Jennings LC, et al. Viral pneumonia. Lancet 2011;377:1264–75.

123. Mackay IM. Human rhinoviruses: the cold wars resume. J Clin Virol 2008;42:297–320.

124. Lieberman D, Shimoni A, Shemer-Avni Y, et al. Respiratory viruses in adults with community-acquired pneumonia. Chest 2010;138:811–6.

125. Papadopoulos NG, Bates PJ, Bardin PG, et al. Rhinoviruses infect the lower airways. J Infect Dis 2000;181:1875–84.

126. Hayden FG. Rhinovirus and the lower respiratory tract. Rev Med Virol 2004;14:17–31.

127. Longtin J, Winter AL, Heng D, et al. Severe human rhinovirus outbreak associated with fatalities in a long-term care facility in Ontario, Canada. J Am Geriatr Soc 2010;58:2036–8.

128. Ghosh S, Champlin R, Couch R, et al. Rhinovirus infections in myelosuppressed adult blood and marrow transplant recipients. Clin Infect Dis 1999; 29:528–32.

129. Choi SH, Huh JW, Hong SB, et al. Clinical characteristics and outcomes of severe rhinovirus-associated pneumonia identified by bronchoscopic bronchoalveolar lavage in adults: comparison with severe influenza virus-associated pneumonia. J Clin Virol 2015;62:41–7.

130. Kraft CS, Jacob JT, Sears MH, et al. Severity of human rhinovirus infection in immunocompromised adults is similar to that of 2009 H1N1 influenza. J Clin Microbiol 2012;50:1061–3.

131. Hayden FG, Herrington DT, Coats TL, et al. Efficacy and safety of oral pleconaril for treatment of colds due to picornaviruses in adults: results of 2 double-blind, randomized, placebo-controlled trials. Clin Infect Dis 2003;36:1523–32.

132. Hayden FG, Albrecht JK, Kaiser DL, et al. Prevention of natural colds by contact prophylaxis with intranasal alpha 2-interferon. N Engl J Med 1986; 314:71–5.

133. Hayden FG, Kaiser DL, Albrecht JK. Intranasal recombinant alfa-2b interferon treatment of naturally occurring common colds. Antimicrob Agents Chemother 1988;32:224–30.

134. Walsh EE, Peterson DR, Falsey AR. Is clinical recognition of respiratory syncytial virus infection in hospitalized elderly and high-risk adults possible? J Infect Dis 2007;195:1046–51.

135. Falsey AR, Walsh EE. Respiratory syncytial virus infection in adults. Clin Microbiol Rev 2000;13:371–84.

136. Murata Y. Respiratory syncytial virus infection in adults. Curr Opin Pulm Med 2008;14:235–40.

137. Neemann K, Freifeld A. Respiratory syncytial virus in hematopoietic stem cell transplantation and solid-organ transplantation. Curr Infect Dis Rep 2015;17:490.

138. Falsey AR, Hennessey PA, Formica MA, et al. Respiratory syncytial virus infection in elderly and high-risk adults. N Engl J Med 2005;352:1749–59.

139. Hynicka LM, Ensor CR. Prophylaxis and treatment of respiratory syncytial virus in adult immunocompromised patients. Ann Pharmacother 2012;46: 558–66.

140. McColl MD, Corser RB, Bremner J, et al. Respiratory syncytial virus infection in adult BMT recipients: effective therapy with short duration nebulised ribavirin. Bone Marrow Transplant 1998; 21:423–5.

141. Waghmare A, Campbell AP, Xie H, et al. Respiratory syncytial virus lower respiratory disease in hematopoietic cell transplant recipients: viral RNA detection in blood, antiviral treatment, and clinical outcomes. Clin Infect Dis 2013;57:1731–41.

142. Pelaez A, Lyon GM, Force SD, et al. Efficacy of oral ribavirin in lung transplant patients with respiratory syncytial virus lower respiratory tract infection. J Heart Lung transplantation 2009;28:67–71.

143. Glanville AR, Scott AI, Morton JM, et al. Intravenous ribavirin is a safe and cost-effective treatment for respiratory syncytial virus infection after lung transplantation. J Heart Lung transplantation 2005;24: 2114–9.

144. Johnstone J, Majumdar SR, Fox JD, et al. Viral infection in adults hospitalized with community-acquired pneumonia: prevalence, pathogens, and presentation. Chest 2008;134:1141–8.

145. Nichols WG, Corey L, Gooley T, et al. Parainfluenza virus infections after hematopoietic stem cell transplantation: risk factors, response to antiviral therapy, and effect on transplant outcome. Blood 2001;98:573–8.

146. Gross AE, Bryson ML. Oral ribavirin for the treatment of noninfluenza respiratory viral infections: a systematic review. Ann Pharmacother 2015;49: 1125–35.

147. Moscona A, Porotto M, Palmer S, et al. A recombinant sialidase fusion protein effectively inhibits human parainfluenza viral infection in vitro and in vivo. J Infect Dis 2010;202:234–41.

148. Dhakal B, D'Souza A, Pasquini M, et al. DAS181 treatment of severe parainfluenza virus 3 pneumonia in allogeneic hematopoietic stem cell transplant recipients requiring mechanical ventilation. Case Rep Med 2016;2016:8503275.

149. van den Hoogen BG, de Jong JC, Groen J, et al. A newly discovered human pneumovirus isolated from young children with respiratory tract disease. Nat Med 2001;7:719–24.

150. Feuillet F, Lina B, Rosa-Calatrava M, et al. Ten years of human metapneumovirus research. J Clin Virol 2012;53:97–105.

151. Liao RS, Appelgate DM, Pelz RK. An outbreak of severe respiratory tract infection due to human metapneumovirus in a long-term care facility for the elderly in Oregon. J Clin Virol 2012;53:171–3.

152. Boivin G, De Serres G, Hamelin ME, et al. An outbreak of severe respiratory tract infection due to human metapneumovirus in a long-term care facility. Clin Infect Dis 2007;44:1152–8.

153. Godet C, Le Goff J, Beby-Defaux A, et al. Human metapneumovirus pneumonia in patients with hematological malignancies. J Clin Virol 2014;61: 593–6.

154. Hasvold J, Sjoding M, Pohl K, et al. The role of human metapneumovirus in the critically ill adult patient. J Crit Care 2016;31:233–7.

155. Kuiken T, van den Hoogen BG, van Riel DA, et al. Experimental human metapneumovirus infection of cynomolgus macaques (*Macaca fascicularis*) results in virus replication in ciliated epithelial cells and pneumocytes with associated lesions throughout the respiratory tract. Am J Pathol 2004;164:1893–900.

156. Schildgen V, van den Hoogen B, Fouchier R, et al. Human metapneumovirus: lessons learned over the first decade. Clin Microbiol Rev 2011;24:734–54.

157. Sumino KC, Agapov E, Pierce RA, et al. Detection of severe human metapneumovirus infection by real-time polymerase chain reaction and histopathological assessment. J Infect Dis 2005;192:1052–60.

158. Kukavica-Ibrulj I, Hamelin ME, Prince GA, et al. Infection with human metapneumovirus predisposes mice to severe pneumococcal pneumonia. J Virol 2009;83:1341–9.

159. Hamelin ME, Prince GA, Boivin G. Effect of ribavirin and glucocorticoid treatment in a mouse model of human metapneumovirus infection. Antimicrob Agents Chemother 2006;50:774–7.

160. Park SY, Baek S, Lee SO, et al. Efficacy of oral ribavirin in hematologic disease patients with paramyxovirus infection: analytic strategy using propensity scores. Antimicrob Agents Chemother 2013;57:983–9.

161. Egli A, Bucher C, Dumoulin A, et al. Human metapneumovirus infection after allogeneic hematopoietic stem cell transplantation. Infection 2012;40: 677–84.

162. Hamelin ME, Couture C, Sackett M, et al. The prophylactic administration of a monoclonal antibody against human metapneumovirus attenuates viral disease and airways hyperresponsiveness in mice. Antivir Ther 2008;13:39–46.

163. Tate JE, Bunning ML, Lott L, et al. Outbreak of severe respiratory disease associated with emergent human adenovirus serotype 14 at a US air force training facility in 2007. J Infect Dis 2009;199: 1419–26.

164. Klinger JR, Sanchez MP, Curtin LA, et al. Multiple cases of life-threatening adenovirus pneumonia in a mental health care center. Am J Respir Crit Care Med 1998;157:645–9.

165. Shields AF, Hackman RC, Fife KH, et al. Adenovirus infections in patients undergoing bone-marrow transplantation. N Engl J Med 1985;312: 529–33.

166. Ison MG. Respiratory viral infections in transplant recipients. Antivir Ther 2007;12:627–38.

167. Sun B, He H, Wang Z, et al. Emergent severe acute respiratory distress syndrome caused by adenovirus type 55 in immunocompetent adults in 2013: a prospective observational study. Crit Care 2014; 18:456.

168. Hakim FA, Tleyjeh IM. Severe adenovirus pneumonia in immunocompetent adults: a case report and review of the literature. Eur J Clin Microbiol Infect Dis 2008;27:153–8.

169. Neofytos D, Ojha A, Mookerjee B, et al. Treatment of adenovirus disease in stem cell transplant recipients with cidofovir. Biol Blood Marrow Transplant 2007;13:74–81.

170. Kim SJ, Kim K, Park SB, et al. Outcomes of early administration of cidofovir in non-immunocompromised patients with severe adenovirus pneumonia. PLoS One 2015;10:e0122642.

171. Wold WS, Toth K. New drug on the horizon for treating adenovirus. Expert Opin Pharmacother 2015; 16:2095–9.

172. Tan D, Zhu H, Fu Y, et al. Severe community-acquired pneumonia caused by human adenovirus in immunocompetent adults: a multicenter case series. PLoS One 2016;11:e0151199.

Postviral Complications

Bacterial Pneumonia

Jason E. Prasso, MD[a], Jane C. Deng, MD, MS[b],*

KEYWORDS

- Influenza • Respiratory viruses • Bacterial pneumonia • Innate immunity • Interferons

KEY POINTS

- Pneumonia remains one of the leading causes of death in the United States and worldwide.
- Influenza and other respiratory viral infections often predispose individuals to a more severe clinical course with greater morbidity and mortality than bacterial pneumonia alone.
- Postviral bacterial pneumonia is mediated by complex interactions between viruses, normal nasopharyngeal bacterial flora, and the host immune system.
- Current management strategies are largely directed toward influenza vaccination and selection of appropriate antimicrobial agents.
- Novel diagnostic tests and therapies that address the complex pathogenesis of postviral bacterial pneumonias are needed to mitigate this potentially serious complication, particularly given the ongoing threat of influenza pandemics.

BACKGROUND

Introduction

As the so-called Spanish flu raged around the world during 1918 to 1919, the burden of morbidity and mortality resulted not only from influenza infection but also from subsequent bacterial pneumonia, accounting for more than 90% of the estimated 50 million deaths caused by the pandemic.[1–4] During the 1957 and 1968 influenza pandemics, secondary bacterial infection was associated with 50% to 70% of severe infections, with the decrease attributed to the advent of antibiotics.[5–7] Coinfection was noted in approximately 30% of those infected during the H1N1 pandemic in 2009, particularly in fatal cases.[8–11] Despite substantial advances in medicine and the availability of potent antibacterial and antiviral agents, influenza and pneumonia remain among the leading causes of death in the United States and

worldwide.[12,13] The complex mechanisms underlying the pathogenesis of postviral bacterial pneumonia are incompletely understood, but involve a variety of host and microbial factors that allow secondary opportunistic bacterial infections to arise in virally infected individuals. This article reviews the current understanding of how virally infected hosts are more susceptible to bacterial pneumonia as well as the management of this important complication of viral infections.

Common Causal Organisms

Viral-bacterial coinfections are a commonly encountered clinical problem. Although the precise rates of secondary bacterial infections are difficult to quantify because of a lack of comprehensive reporting systems and the impracticality of obtaining microbiologic testing in all patients with respiratory infections, bacterial pneumonia

Disclosures: None of the authors have any financial conflicts of interest to disclose. This work was supported by NIH R01HL108949 (J.C. Deng).

[a] Division of Pulmonary and Critical Care Medicine, University of California, Los Angeles, 10833 Le Conte Avenue, CHS 37-131, Los Angeles, CA 90095, USA; [b] Division of Pulmonary and Critical Care Medicine, Veterans Affairs Healthcare System, University of Michigan, 2215 Fuller Road, 111G Pulmonary, Ann Arbor, MI 48105, USA
* Corresponding author. Division of Pulmonary Medicine, Veterans Administration Ann Arbor Healthcare System, 2215 Fuller Road, Ann Arbor, MI 48105.
E-mail address: jcdeng@med.umich.edu

Clin Chest Med 38 (2017) 127–138
http://dx.doi.org/10.1016/j.ccm.2016.11.006
0272-5231/17/Published by Elsevier Inc.

chestmed.theclinics.com

is estimated to complicate from 0.5% to 6% of influenza infections, with higher rates among hospitalized patients in intensive care units and fatal cases. Influenza is one of many viral pathogens that have been associated with bacterial coinfections.[14] Human parainfluenza virus, adenovirus, human metapneumovirus, measles, respiratory syncytial virus (RSV), human rhinovirus, and coronavirus are also commonly associated with secondary bacterial pneumonia.[15–22] Of these viruses, influenza is arguably most important given its continuously evolving virulence factors and the sheer number of individuals infected on an annual basis. Given its public health importance, as well as the fact that influenza is the most extensively studied, bacterial pneumonia following influenza infections is the primary focus of this article.

Irrespective of the offending viral organism, causal agents of secondary bacterial pneumonia largely reflect colonizing nasopharyngeal flora. This finding has fueled the theory that viral infection causes impaired mucosal and ciliary clearance of these normally nonpathogenic bacteria, which enables particular bacteria to flourish and causes invasive infections. Epidemiologically, *Streptococcus pneumoniae* and *Staphylococcus*

aureus (both methicillin-sensitive *S aureus* and methicillin-resistant *S aureus* [MRSA]) are most common, with *Streptococcus pyogenes* and *Haemophilus influenzae* less frequently isolated.[23–27] However, infections in humans are often polymicrobial, involving combinations of multiple viruses and/or bacteria. Common viral-bacterial coinfections are summarized in **Table 1**.

Clinical Presentation

The incidence of bacterial pneumonia mirrors the seasonal nature of viral infections, with increases during peak viral seasons.[19,28–31] Data from the 2009 H1N1 epidemic show that coinfection usually occurs within the first 6 days of influenza infection,[32,33] although it can develop up to 14 days after other viral infections. This delay likely represents the time needed for viral replication and the immunomodulatory effects of infection to occur.[34–36] Patients with secondary pneumonia tend to have a more severe, protracted course, with increased mortality compared with those without antecedent viral infection.[7,25,30,31,33,37–41] Although patients with comorbid conditions or at the extremes of age are at increased risk of complicated influenza infections, even previously

Table 1
Common viral-bacterial coinfections and their associated clinical infections in human hosts

Virus	Known Bacterial Coinfections	Associated Secondary Infections
Influenza	S pneumoniae S aureus S pyogenes H influenzae Moraxella catarrhalis Neisseria meningitidis	Pneumonia Otitis media Sinusitis Meningitis
Respiratory syncytial virus	S pneumoniae	Pneumonia Bronchitis/bronchiolitis
Adenovirus	S pneumoniae H influenzae M catarrhalis	Pneumonia
Coronavirus	H influenzae	Pneumonia
Human rhinovirus	S pneumoniae H influenzae S aureus M catarrhalis	Pneumonia Sinusitis Otitis media
Parainfluenza virus	S pneumoniae M catarrhalis	Pneumonia
Human metapneumovirus	S pneumoniae	Pneumonia Bronchitis
Measles virus	S pneumoniae S aureus H influenzae	Otitis media Pneumonia Tracheobronchitis

healthy patients can develop severe respiratory failure and death from bacterial pneumonias following influenza, underscoring the clinical significance of this problem.

Secondary bacterial pneumonia is one of several known infectious complications of respiratory viruses. Viral infections have also been associated with acute otitis media and bacterial sinusitis in children.[42–44] In addition, meningococcal meningitis has been reported as a complication of influenza infections.[45]

PATHOGENESIS

Several excellent reviews have been published of the current mechanistic understanding of how viral infections increase susceptibility to secondary bacterial pneumonias.[46–49] Thus, this article provides only a brief overview, with a primary focus on virally mediated effects on pulmonary host defense and subsequent impairment of bacterial clearance (**Table 2**). However, the authors acknowledge that microbiologic and epidemiologic factors can contribute to the pathogenesis of viral-bacterial coinfections.

Colonization

Colonization of the nasopharynx is generally the first step in the development of pneumonia and other bacterial infections of the upper respiratory tract, including sinusitis and otitis media.[50,51] *S pneumoniae, S aureus, H influenzae, S pyogenes,* and *Moraxella catarrhalis* are normal inhabitants of the upper respiratory tract in healthy human hosts, with the lower respiratory tract generally considered to have low abundance of bacteria.[52,53] Although these bacteria normally exist in an equilibrium governed by host, intermicrobial, and environmental factors,[54–56] under the appropriate circumstances, they can proliferate and become invasive. Studies have shown an inverse relationship between nasal carriage of *S pneumoniae* and *S aureus*.[55,57,58] Other groups have

Table 2 Known or suspected steps in the pathogenesis of secondary bacterial pneumonia	
Immune Function	Viral-mediated Effect
Nasopharyngeal colonization	• Altered host microbiota, possibly in favor of more pathogenic organisms
Direct mucosal/epithelial damage	• Breakdown of mucin by viral and bacterial neuraminidase • Destruction of epithelium and exposure of basement membrane • Impairment of ciliary function
Enhanced bacterial adherence	• Cleavage of sialic acid → exposure of receptors for bacteria on mucosal surface
Alveolar macrophage response	• Decreased number of AMs after viral infection • Downregulation of MARCO (macrophage receptor with collagenous structure) receptor resulting in impaired phagocytosis of bacteria • Reduced chemokine expression and immune cell recruitment • Desensitization of Toll-like receptors → long-term immune defects
Neutrophil response	• Possible reduced recruitment to the lung • Decreased phagocytic function • Reduced production of reactive oxygen species • Impaired NETs function
Altered cytokine milieu	• Increased type I interferons → reduced macrophage and neutrophil recruitment to the lung • Increased type II interferons → impaired macrophage phagocytic function, possible viral skewing of neutrophils • Attenuated T_H17 cell function and decreased IL-17 secretion → increased susceptibility to *S pneumoniae,* decreased production of antimicrobial peptides

Abbreviations: AMS, alveolar macrophages; IL, interleukin; NETs, neutrophil extracellular traps; T_H, T-helper.

revealed antagonistic as well as synergistic relationships between members of the normal respiratory community (eg, corynebacteria and S aureus, Corynebacterium accolens and S pneumoniae, H influenzae and S pneumoniae).[59–62]

In addition, viruses can alter bacterial composition. Our laboratory recently examined changes in the nasal microbiome following intranasal administration of live attenuated influenza vaccine. Although individual hosts had disparate microbiome profiles at baseline, after vaccination, the relative abundance of staphylococcal and Bacteroides species was significantly increased. This finding suggests that viral stimuli can alter the host microbiota, potentially by creating a suitable environment in which an otherwise nonpathogenic organism can grow and become invasive.[63,64]

Mucosal Barrier Function and Bacterial Adherence

Disruption of the mucosal barrier is an important potentiating mechanism for secondary bacterial infection. Mucin present in the respiratory tract can be partially degraded by viral and bacterial neuraminidase.[65,66] Viral neuraminidase is tropic for the sialic acid present on respiratory epithelial cells, cleavage of which may uncover receptors for bacterial ligand, thereby promoting bacterial adhesion and infection. Furthermore, the increased availability of sialic acid in the airway has been shown to promote growth and proliferation of pneumococcus, which uses this moiety as a nutrient source.[67] In murine models, higher levels of viral neuraminidase are associated with increased severity of secondary bacterial infection, whereas treatment with oseltamivir decreases bacterial adherence to epithelial cells.[68–70]

Influenza and paramyxoviruses such as RSV can also augment bacterial adhesion by augmenting expression of receptors for bacteria on the epithelial cell surface. One example is platelet-activating factor receptor (PAFR), which binds to the phosphorylcholine present in some bacterial cell walls and facilitates bacterial invasion.[71] In a mouse model of pneumococcus pneumonia, PAFR was shown to increase total lung bacterial load, bacteremia, and mortality.[72] However, blocking this receptor did not show any benefit in an influenza coinfection model, suggesting that this mechanism is not a sufficient factor for enhancing susceptibility to secondary bacterial pneumonias.[73] Other receptors involved in adhesion, such as CEACAM1 (carcinoembryonic antigen-related cell adhesion molecule 1) and ICAM-1 (intracellular adhesion molecule 1), are overly expressed on pulmonary epithelial cells after viral infection as well.[74,75]

Epithelial cell death and breakdown of tight junctions resulting from viral infection can cause increased translocation of bacteria such as H influenzae.[76,77] In addition, certain bacterial species have a known binding affinity for the basement membrane and extracellular matrix proteins,[78–81] suggesting that breakdown of the epithelium might lead to increased translocation, although this has never been proved to be a critical mechanism during infections with less cytotoxic strains of influenza in vivo. In addition, viral respiratory infections are known to negatively affect respiratory ciliary function, thereby impairing the host's ability to mechanically clear aspirated pathogens from the lung.[82,83]

Macrophage and Neutrophil Function

Resident alveolar macrophages (AMs) play an integral role in host defense against viral and bacterial pathogens alike. As the main resident innate immune cells to encounter pathogens in the resting lung, they engage in phagocytosis and killing, antigen presentation, recruitment of other cell types, and paracrine and endocrine signaling. Viral respiratory infections are known to impair macrophage phagocytic function as well as monocyte chemotaxis to the lung early after influenza infection, and this has been proposed as a potential cause for secondary bacterial infection.[49,84–89] In mouse models of sequential influenza-bacterial infection, AMs are known to be decreased in number with increased susceptibility and mortality to secondary bacterial challenge. Influenza infection has also been shown to downregulate expression of the class A scavenger receptor MARCO on AMs, which phagocytose unopsonized bacteria in the lung.[34] Augmenting AM numbers and function by exogenous granulocyte-macrophage colony-stimulating factor in animals infected with influenza improves pneumococcus clearance following secondary bacterial challenge, increases reactive oxygen species, and decreases incidence of secondary pneumonia.[90–92]

Viral infections affect the ability of AMs to attract other cell types to the lung. Neutrophils are robustly recruited following the elaboration of chemokines by AMs and epithelial cells in the setting of invasive bacterial infection. Our laboratory has shown that macrophage expression of neutrophil chemoattractants CXCL1 (C-X-C motif chemokine ligand 1) (KC) and CXCL2 (C-X-C motif chemokine ligand 2) (MIP2) is reduced after influenza infection, with consequent diminished recruitment of neutrophils to the lung.[93] Desensitization of

Toll-like receptors (TLRs) on alveolar macrophages may partially explain the decrease in neutrophil recruitment and impaired bacterial clearance. Mice infected with influenza or RSV showed decreased activation of nuclear factor kappa-B (NF-KB) and expression of KC and MIP2, resulting in decreased neutrophil recruitment to the lung after stimulation with bacterial ligands.[94] In addition, influenza infection results in an early, prolonged decrease in PMN (polymorphonuclear cell) phagocytic function and depressed reactive oxygen species production.[92,95–98] Thus, during viral infection, multiple aspects of pulmonary innate immunity are compromised, leading to impaired antibacterial host defense.

Viral Effects on the Cytokine Milieu

Viral infection elicits a robust cytokine response via activation of TLRs and retinoic acid inducible gene (RIG-I) in immune cells and downstream upregulation of NF-KB. This response results in production of type I and II interferons (IFN) as part of the host antiviral response, and these in turn alter other cytokine-mediated effects.

Type I interferons

Predominantly comprised of multiple IFN-alpha proteins and 1 IFN-beta protein, these antiviral mediators can be secreted by multiple different immune cells and help to limit viral replication.[89,99] Induction of type I IFNs is known to increase the risk of secondary bacterial infection,[34,93,99–102] despite type I IFNs also contributing to host antibacterial response.[103] Mice deficient in the type I IFN receptor are protected against subsequent bacterial challenge after influenza infection, likely because type I IFNs inhibit KC and MIP2 production and neutrophil recruitment to the lung.[93,104] Monocyte and macrophage recruitment to the upper respiratory tract is suppressed by type I IFNs via blockade of Nod2-mediated expression of CCl2 (C-C motif chemokine ligand 2; a macrophage chemoattractant), with resultant increase in carriage of S pneumoniae.[100] These studies highlight the heterogeneous effects of IFNs in the immune response to pathogens.

Type II interferon (interferon-gamma)

Viral respiratory infection also stimulates IFN-gamma production, primarily by natural killer cells but also by CD4+ T-helper (T_H) cells and CD8+ cytotoxic T cells and neutrophils. In the context of secondary bacterial pneumonia following influenza, IFN-gamma has been shown to impair phagocytosis in alveolar macrophages, partially by downregulation of the scavenger receptor MARCO.[34]

Inhibition of interleukin (IL)-10 results in increased neutrophil recruitment to the lung and improved clearance of S pneumoniae, and can salvage animals from death after sequential influenza-bacterial infection.[105,106] However, in normal hosts, exogenous administration of IL-12 results in increased levels of IFN-gamma in the lung, robust neutrophil recruitment, and improved innate pulmonary defense against S pneumoniae. In addition, in mouse models of S pneumoniae and S aureus pneumonia, IL-12–independent IFN-gamma production by neutrophils in the lung was shown to be essential to bacterial clearance, possibly because of IFN-gamma–regulated production of neutrophil extracellular traps (NETs).[107,108] These paradoxic findings in naive hosts versus hosts infected with influenza suggest that neutrophils recruited in the setting of viral respiratory infection are unable to mount antibacterial functions that would normally be activated by interferon-gamma, which may reflect distinct neutrophil phenotypes in the setting of viral versus bacterial infections. Unpublished data from our laboratory show striking transcriptional differences in neutrophils that are recruited to the lung in the setting of influenza and sequential influenza–S pneumoniae infection, compared with those recruited in the setting of S pneumoniae infection alone.

T-helper 17 cells and interleukin-17

Influenza infection is known to attenuate T_H17 cell–mediated immunity. Type I IFNs decrease production of IL-1β and IL-23, which are necessary for polarization of T_H17 cells.[109] During influenza–S aureus coinfection, there are resultant decreases in IL-17, IL-22, and monocyte chemoattractant protein-1 that correlate with reduced clearance of bacteria.[101] They also likely inhibit IL-17 secretion by gamma-delta T cells, resulting in increased susceptibility to secondary S pneumoniae infection.[109,110] In addition, influenza infection in mice was shown to suppress production of antimicrobial peptides in response to subsequent S aureus infection via a T_H17-mediated mechanism, leaving animals more susceptible to pneumonia. Exogenous administration of the antimicrobial peptide lipocalin 2 restored bacterial clearance in these animals.[111]

CLINICAL MANAGEMENT
Diagnostic Testing

Differentiating severe viral infection from viral-bacterial coinfection is a common diagnostic dilemma at the point of presentation, given the significant overlap in symptoms and laboratory markers. Microbiologic culture results take days, whereas point-of-care influenza antigen tests are insufficiently sensitive. PCR-based panels for common respiratory viral pathogens are more sensitive and can be useful, but are expensive for routine use and are not able to distinguish between colonization versus true viral infection. Furthermore, in low-volume laboratories, results may not be available for days. On radiologic imaging, lobar consolidation with or without pleural effusion is presumed to be bacterial; however, multifocal infiltrates can represent either multilobar bacterial pneumonia or acute respiratory distress syndrome from severe viral infection alone. RSV and adenovirus have some hallmark features on computed tomography scan of the chest; however, imaging studies are generally unhelpful.[112] Increased C-reactive protein level in the blood correlates with presence of pneumonia but poorly distinguishes viral from bacterial causes.[113–115] Procalcitonin (PCT), another serum biomarker, is better able to differentiate the two.[18,116–121] In one study of coinfection, low PCT level was associated with 94% negative predictive value for bacterial infection, although in patients with shock, or in malaria endemic areas, it may be less reliable.[121,122] Thus, given the absence of rapid and reliable diagnostic tests, clinicians must always consider the possibility of secondary bacterial infection in patients presenting with severe respiratory infections during influenza season and manage them accordingly.

Vaccination

Infections caused by influenza, measles, H influenzae, S pneumoniae, and some strains of adenovirus are all considered vaccine-preventable illnesses.[123] Although influenza vaccination is universally recommended, vaccination against invasive pneumococcal infection is reserved for high-risk groups, including children, the elderly, and patients with immunosuppressive or chronic lung conditions.[124,125] Although robust evidence from randomized placebo-controlled trials is lacking, data from animal models of influenza-bacterial coinfection and observational studies in patients have indicated that influenza vaccine can reduce the morbidity and mortality associated with bacterial pneumonia.[126–134] Thus, on balance, vaccination against influenza currently represents the most effective public health strategy for reducing the incidence of secondary bacterial pneumonia. However, pneumococcal vaccination did not have the same effect in a large study of elderly patients, potentially because of replacement of covered serotypes with those not included in the vaccine.[135,136] This finding mirrors data from animal models of dual infection.[137] In contrast,

vaccination against the M protein of S pyogenes seems to be protective against superinfection.[138] It is unknown whether vaccination against other pathogens affects the incidence or severity of secondary bacterial pneumonia.

Antibiotic Therapy

Antibiotic treatment of secondary bacterial pneumonia should mirror local guidelines for that of community-acquired pneumonia (ie, based on local patterns of antibiotic resistance), with the caveat that these patients are at increased risk of S aureus infection, including MRSA.[139,140] In patients with cavitation noted on imaging, severe respiratory infection requiring admission to the intensive care unit, or risk factors for hospital-acquired pathogens, treatment with either vancomycin or linezolid should be started empirically. As an aside, in a mouse model of influenza-MRSA infection, treatment with linezolid showed unique immunomodulatory effects on toxic production and lung inflammation with equivalent bacterial clearance; however, whether or not this translates to improved clinical outcomes in humans still needs to be studied.[141]

Antiviral Agents

There are 2 classes of antiviral drugs with activity against influenza: the adamantines (amantadine and rimantadine) and neuraminidase inhibitors (oseltamivir, zanamivir, and peramivir). At present, use of the adamantines has become uncommon because of high levels of drug resistance and side effects.[123,139,140,142–144] As previously mentioned, viral infection is often indistinguishable from lower respiratory tract infection. As such, during seasons of heightened influenza prevalence, empiric antiviral therapy is warranted pending the results of microbiologic testing. In ambulatory patients who have had symptoms for fewer than 48 hours, treatment with oseltamivir or zanamivir has been shown to reduce the duration of symptoms. In hospitalized patients, they may have benefit irrespective of when symptoms began.[25,145]

Given their mechanism of action, neuraminidase inhibitors should theoretically prevent or reduce the severity of secondary bacterial pneumonia. This effect has been described in animal models of disease.[69,146,147] In the pediatric population, oseltamivir use has been associated with a 44% reduction in subsequent diagnosis of otitis media.[148] Although individual trials in adult patients were not powered to detect any effect of oseltamivir on lower respiratory tract infection, a meta-analysis showed decreased incidence.[149] Inhaled ribavirin is approved for treatment of severe RSV bronchiolitis; however, the treatment is cumbersome and the drug teratogenic, which presents a problem for hospital personnel because it is aerosolized for administration. As such, it is rarely used and its effects on secondary bacterial infection are unknown.

Immunomodulatory Agents

Given the role of inflammation in viral-bacterial co-infection and the pathogenesis of secondary pneumonia, there is significant interest in the utility of immunomodulatory drugs in this setting. Corticosteroids have been studied, and although data from mouse models show some protection against secondary pneumonia, they resulted in delayed viral clearance.[150] In patients with severe influenza infection, the results of such studies show either no benefit or possible harm to patients caused by worsened infectious complications.[151–155] As such, their use is not recommended. Other agents under active investigation include statins (coenzyme A reductase inhibitors), peroxisome proliferator–activated receptor agonists, cyclooxygenase inhibitors, macrolide antibiotics, and antibody-based therapies such as intravenous immunoglobulin and experimental monoclonal antibodies, all of which are in the preclinical stages of testing.[146]

SUMMARY

Secondary bacterial pneumonia after viral respiratory infection remains a significant source of morbidity and mortality. Susceptibility is mediated by a variety of viral and bacterial factors, as well as complex interactions with the immune system of the infected host. To date, prevention and treatment strategies are limited to influenza vaccination and antibiotics/antivirals respectively. Novel approaches to identifying the individuals infected with influenza who are at increased risk for secondary bacterial pneumonias are urgently needed, given the ongoing threat of another influenza pandemic. Given the threat of further pandemics and the heightened prevalence of these viruses in general, more research into the immunologic mechanisms of this disease is warranted with the hope of discovering new potential therapies.

REFERENCES

1. Chien YW, Klugman KP, Morens DM. Bacterial pathogens and death during the 1918 influenza pandemic. N Engl J Med 2009;361(26):2582–3.
2. Morens DM, Fauci AS. The 1918 influenza pandemic: insights for the 21st century. J Infect Dis 2007;195(7):1018–28.
3. Taubenberger JK, Morens DM. 1918 influenza: the mother of all pandemics. Emerg Infect Dis 2006; 12(1):15–22.
4. Morens DM, Taubenberger JK, Fauci AS. Predominant role of bacterial pneumonia as a cause of death in pandemic influenza: implications for pandemic influenza preparedness. J Infect Dis 2008;198(7): 962–70.
5. Bisno AL, Griffin JP, Van Epps KA, et al. Pneumonia and Hong Kong influenza: a prospective study of the 1968-1969 epidemic. Am J Med Sci 1971; 261(5):251–63.
6. Oswald NC, Shooter RA, Curwen MP. Pneumonia complicating Asian influenza. Br Med J 1958; 2(5108):1305–11.
7. Louria DB, Blumenfeld HL, Ellis JT, et al. Studies on influenza in the pandemic of 1957-1958. II. Pulmonary complications of influenza. J Clin Invest 1959; 38(1 Pt 2):213–65.
8. Martin-Loeches I, Sanchez-Corral A, Diaz E, et al. Community-acquired respiratory coinfection in critically ill patients with pandemic 2009 influenza A(H1N1) virus. Chest 2011;139(3):555–62.
9. Gill JR, Sheng ZM, Ely SF, et al. Pulmonary pathologic findings of fatal 2009 pandemic influenza A/ H1N1 viral infections. Arch Pathol Lab Med 2010; 134(2):235–43.
10. Shieh WJ, Blau DM, Denison AM, et al. 2009 pandemic influenza A (H1N1): pathology and pathogenesis of 100 fatal cases in the United States. Am J Pathol 2010;177(1):166–75.
11. Cilloniz C, Ewig S, Menendez R, et al. Bacterial co-infection with H1N1 infection in patients admitted with community acquired pneumonia. J Infect 2012;65(3):223–30.
12. Heron M. Deaths: leading causes for 2013. Natl Vital Stat Rep 2016;65(2):1–95.
13. The top 10 causes of death. 2014; fact sheet. Available at: http://www.who.int/mediacentre/fact sheets/fs310/en/. Accessed June 16, 2016.
14. Metersky ML, Masterton RG, Lode H, et al. Epidemiology, microbiology, and treatment considerations for bacterial pneumonia complicating influenza. Int J Infect Dis 2012;16(5):e321–31.
15. Ballinger MN, Standiford TJ. Postinfluenza bacterial pneumonia: host defenses gone awry. J Interferon Cytokine Res 2010;30(9):643–52.
16. Simusika P, Bateman AC, Theo A, et al. Identification of viral and bacterial pathogens from hospitalized children with severe acute respiratory illness in Lusaka, Zambia, 2011-2012: a cross-sectional study. BMC Infect Dis 2015;15:52.
17. Sangil A, Calbo E, Robles A, et al. Aetiology of community-acquired pneumonia among adults in an H1N1 pandemic year: the role of respiratory viruses. Eur J Clin Microbiol Infect Dis 2012; 31(10):2765–72.

18. Falsey AR, Becker KL, Swinburne AJ, et al. Bacterial complications of respiratory tract viral illness: a comprehensive evaluation. J Infect Dis 2013; 208(3):432–41.

19. Glezen P, Denny FW. Epidemiology of acute lower respiratory disease in children. N Engl J Med 1973;288(10):498–505.

20. Louie JK, Roy-Burman A, Guardia-Labar L, et al. Rhinovirus associated with severe lower respiratory tract infections in children. Pediatr Infect Dis J 2009;28(4):337–9.

21. Echenique IA, Chan PA, Chapin KC, et al. Clinical characteristics and outcomes in hospitalized patients with respiratory viral co-infection during the 2009 H1N1 influenza pandemic. PLoS One 2013; 8(4):e60845.

22. Jennings LC, Anderson TP, Beynon KA, et al. Incidence and characteristics of viral community-acquired pneumonia in adults. Thorax 2008;63(1): 42–8.

23. Podewils LJ, Liedtke LA, McDonald LC, et al. A national survey of severe influenza-associated complications among children and adults, 2003-2004. Clin Infect Dis 2005;40(11):1693–6.

24. Centers for Disease Control and Prevention (CDC). Bacterial coinfections in lung tissue specimens from fatal cases of 2009 pandemic influenza A (H1N1) - United States, May-August 2009. MMWR Morb Mortal Wkly Rep 2009;58(38):1071–4.

25. Randolph AG, Vaughn F, Sullivan R, et al. Critically ill children during the 2009-2010 influenza pandemic in the United States. Pediatrics 2011; 128(6):e1450-8.

26. Murray RJ, Robinson JO, White JN, et al. Community-acquired pneumonia due to pandemic A(H1N1)2009 influenzavirus and methicillin resistant Staphylococcus aureus co-infection. PLoS One 2010;5(1):e8705.

27. Luchsinger V, Ruiz M, Zunino E, et al. Community-acquired pneumonia in Chile: the clinical relevance in the detection of viruses and atypical bacteria. Thorax 2013;68(11):1000–6.

28. Murphy TF, Henderson FW, Clyde WA Jr, et al. Pneumonia: an eleven-year study in a pediatric practice. Am J Epidemiol 1981;113(1):12–21.

29. Burgos J, Larrosa MN, Martinez A, et al. Impact of influenza season and environmental factors on the clinical presentation and outcome of invasive pneumococcal disease. Eur J Clin Microbiol Infect Dis 2015;34(1):177–86.

30. Investigators AI, Webb SA, Pettila V, et al. Critical care services and 2009 H1N1 influenza in Australia and New Zealand. N Engl J Med 2009;361(20): 1925–34.

31. Tyrrell DA. The pulmonary complications of influenza as seen in Sheffield in 1949. Q J Med 1952; 21(83):291–306.

32. Chertow DS, Memoli MJ. Bacterial coinfection in influenza: a grand rounds review. JAMA 2013; 309(3):275–82.

33. Rice TW, Rubinson L, Uyeki TM, et al. Critical illness from 2009 pandemic influenza a virus and bacterial coinfection in the United States. Crit Care Med 2012;40(5):1487–98.

34. Sun K, Metzger DW. Inhibition of pulmonary antibacterial defense by interferon-gamma during recovery from influenza infection. Nat Med 2008; 14(5):558–64.

35. Lee KH, Gordon A, Foxman B. The role of respiratory viruses in the etiology of bacterial pneumonia: an ecological perspective. Evol Med Public Health 2016;2016(1):95–109.

36. Belongia EA, Irving SA, Waring SC, et al. Clinical characteristics and 30-day outcomes for influenza A 2009 (H1N1), 2008-2009 (H1N1), and 2007-2008 (H3N2) infections. JAMA 2010;304(10): 1091–8.

37. Deng JC. Viral-bacterial interactions-therapeutic implications. Influenza Other Respir Viruses 2013; 7(Suppl 3):24–35.

38. Harms PW, Schmidt LA, Smith LB, et al. Autopsy findings in eight patients with fatal H1N1 influenza. Am J Clin Pathol 2010;134(1):27–35.

39. Weinberger DM, Simonsen L, Jordan R, et al. Impact of the 2009 influenza pandemic on pneumococcal pneumonia hospitalizations in the United States. J Infect Dis 2012;205(3):458–65.

40. Damasio GA, Pereira LA, Moreira SD, et al. Does virus-bacteria coinfection increase the clinical severity of acute respiratory infection? J Med Virol 2015;87(9):1456–61.

41. Viasus D, Pano-Pardo JR, Pachon J, et al. Pneumonia complicating pandemic (H1N1) 2009: risk factors, clinical features, and outcomes. Medicine (Baltimore) 2011;90(5):328–36.

42. Mina MJ, Klugman KP. The role of influenza in the severity and transmission of respiratory bacterial disease. Lancet Respir Med 2014;2(9):750–63.

43. Brealey JC, Sly PD, Young PR, et al. Viral bacterial co-infection of the respiratory tract during early childhood. FEMS Microbiol Lett 2015. [Epub ahead of print].

44. Marom T, Alvarez-Fernandez PE, Jennings K, et al. Acute bacterial sinusitis complicating viral upper respiratory tract infection in young children. Pediatr Infect Dis J 2014;33(8):803–8.

45. Cohen AL, McMorrow M, Walaza S, et al. Potential impact of co-infections and co-morbidities prevalent in Africa on influenza severity and frequency: a systematic review. PLoS One 2015; 10(6):e0128580.

46. McCullers JA. The co-pathogenesis of influenza viruses with bacteria in the lung. Nat Rev Microbiol 2014;12(4):252–62.

47. Smith AM, McCullers JA. Secondary bacterial infections in influenza virus infection pathogenesis. Curr Top Microbiol Immunol 2014;385:327–56.

48. Rynda-Apple A, Robinson KM, Alcorn JF. Influenza and bacterial superinfection: illuminating the immunologic mechanisms of disease. Infect Immun 2015;83(10):3764–70.

49. Didierlaurent A, Goulding J, Hussell T. The impact of successive infections on the lung microenvironment. Immunology 2007;122(4):457–65.

50. Bogaert D, De Groot R, Hermans PW. *Streptococcus pneumoniae* colonisation: the key to pneumococcal disease. Lancet Infect Dis 2004;4(3): 144–54.

51. Bosch AA, Biesbroek G, Trzcinski K, et al. Viral and bacterial interactions in the upper respiratory tract. PloS Pathog 2013;9(1):e1003057.

52. Morris A, Beck JM, Schloss PD, et al. Comparison of the respiratory microbiome in healthy nonsmokers and smokers. Am J Respir Crit Care Med 2013;187(10):1067–75.

53. Charlson ES, Bittinger K, Haas AR, et al. Topographical continuity of bacterial populations in the healthy human respiratory tract. Am J Respir Crit Care Med 2011;184(8):957–63.

54. Blaser MJ, Falkow S. What are the consequences of the disappearing human microbiota? Nat Rev Microbiol 2009;7(12):887–94.

55. Lewnard JA, Givon-Lavi N, Huppert A, et al. Epidemiological markers for interactions among *Streptococcus pneumoniae*, *Haemophilus influenzae*, and *Staphylococcus aureus* in upper respiratory tract carriage. J Infect Dis 2016;213(10): 1596–605.

56. Garcia-Rodriguez JA, Fresnadillo Martinez MJ. Dynamics of nasopharyngeal colonization by potential respiratory pathogens. J Antimicrob Chemother 2002;50(Suppl S2):59–73.

57. Reiss-Mandel A, Regev-Yochay G. *Staphylococcus aureus* and *Streptococcus pneumoniae* interaction and response to pneumococcal vaccination: myth or reality? Hum Vaccin Immunother 2016;12(2):351–7.

58. Regev-Yochay G, Dagan R, Raz M, et al. Association between carriage of *Streptococcus pneumoniae* and *Staphylococcus aureus* in children. JAMA 2004;292(6):716–20.

59. Margolis E, Yates A, Levin BR. The ecology of nasal colonization of *Streptococcus pneumoniae*, *Haemophilus influenzae* and *Staphylococcus aureus*: the role of competition and interactions with host's immune response. BMC Microbiol 2010;10:59.

60. Uehara Y, Nakama H, Agematsu K, et al. Bacterial interference among nasal inhabitants: eradication of *Staphylococcus aureus* from nasal cavities by artificial implantation of *Corynebacterium* sp. J Hosp Infect 2000;44(2):127–33.

61. Yan M, Pamp SJ, Fukuyama J, et al. Nasal microenvironments and interspecific interactions influence nasal microbiota complexity and *S. aureus* carriage. Not Found In Database 2013;14(6):631–40.

62. Bomar L, Brugger SD, Yost BH, et al. *Corynebacterium accolens* releases antipneumococcal free fatty acids from human nostril and skin surface triacylglycerols. MBio 2016;7(1):e01725-15.

63. Tarabichi Y, Li K, Hu S, et al. The administration of intranasal live attenuated influenza vaccine induces changes in the nasal microbiota and nasal epithelium gene expression profiles. Microbiome 2015;3:74.

64. Mina MJ, McCullers JA, Klugman KP. Live attenuated influenza vaccine enhances colonization of *Streptococcus pneumoniae* and *Staphylococcus aureus* in mice. MBio 2014;5(1):e01040–13.

65. Wheeler AH, Nungester WJ. Effect of mucin on influenza virus infection in hamsters. Science 1942;96(2482):92–3.

66. Williams OW, Sharafkhaneh A, Kim V, et al. Airway mucus: from production to secretion. Am J Respir Cell Mol Biol 2006;34(5):527–36.

67. Siegel SJ, Roche AM, Weiser JN. Influenza promotes pneumococcal growth during coinfection by providing host sialylated substrates as a nutrient source. Cell Host Microbe 2014;16(1): 55–67.

68. Peltola VT, McCullers JA. Respiratory viruses predisposing to bacterial infections: role of neuraminidase. Pediatr Infect Dis J 2004;23(Suppl 1): S87–97.

69. Peltola VT, Murti KG, McCullers JA. Influenza virus neuraminidase contributes to secondary bacterial pneumonia. J Infect Dis 2005;192(2):249–57.

70. McCullers JA, Bartmess KC. Role of neuraminidase in lethal synergism between influenza virus and *Streptococcus pneumoniae*. J Infect Dis 2003; 187(6):1000–9.

71. Cundell DR, Gerard NP, Gerard C, et al. *Streptococcus pneumoniae* anchor to activated human cells by the receptor for platelet-activating factor. Nature 1995;377(6548):435–8.

72. Rijneveld AW, Weijer S, Florquin S, et al. Improved host defense against pneumococcal pneumonia in platelet-activating factor receptor-deficient mice. J Infect Dis 2004;189(4):711–6.

73. McCullers JA, Rehg JE. Lethal synergism between influenza virus and *Streptococcus pneumoniae*: characterization of a mouse model and the role of platelet-activating factor receptor. J Infect Dis 2002;186(3):341–50.

74. Avadhanula V, Rodriguez CA, Devincenzo JP, et al. Respiratory viruses augment the adhesion of bacterial pathogens to respiratory epithelium in a viral species- and cell type-dependent manner. J Virol 2006;80(4):1629–36.

75. Swords WE, Buscher BA, Ver Steeg Ii K, et al. Non-typeable *Haemophilus influenzae* adhere to and invade human bronchial epithelial cells via an interaction of lipooligosaccharide with the PAF receptor. Mol Microbiol 2000;37(1):13–27.

76. Comstock AT, Ganesan S, Chattoraj A, et al. Rhinovirus-induced barrier dysfunction in polarized airway epithelial cells is mediated by NADPH oxidase 1. J Virol 2011;85(13):6795–808.

77. Sajjan U, Wang Q, Zhao Y, et al. Rhinovirus disrupts the barrier function of polarized airway epithelial cells. Am J Respir Crit Care Med 2008; 178(12):1271–81.

78. Tan TT, Nordstrom T, Forsgren A, et al. The respiratory pathogen *Moraxella catarrhalis* adheres to epithelial cells by interacting with fibronectin through ubiquitous surface proteins A1 and A2. J Infect Dis 2005;192(6):1029–38.

79. Heilmann C. Adhesion mechanisms of staphylococci. Adv Exp Med Biol 2011;715:105–23.

80. van der Flier M, Chhun N, Wizemann TM, et al. Adherence of *Streptococcus pneumoniae* to immobilized fibronectin. Infect Immun 1995;63(11):4317–22.

81. Plotkowski MC, Puchelle E, Beck G, et al. Adherence of type I *Streptococcus pneumoniae* to tracheal epithelium of mice infected with influenza A/PR8 virus. Am Rev Respir Dis 1986;134(5):1040–4.

82. Carson JL, Collier AM, Hu SS. Acquired ciliary defects in nasal epithelium of children with acute viral upper respiratory infections. N Engl J Med 1985; 312(8):463–8.

83. Pittet LA, Hall-Stoodley L, Rutkowski MR, et al. Influenza virus infection decreases tracheal mucociliary velocity and clearance of *Streptococcus pneumoniae*. Am J Respir Cell Mol Biol 2010; 42(4):450–60.

84. Nickerson CL, Jakab GJ. Pulmonary antibacterial defenses during mild and severe influenza virus infection. Infect Immun 1990;58(9):2809–14.

85. Astry CL, Jakab GJ. Influenza virus-induced immune complexes suppress alveolar macrophage phagocytosis. J Virol 1984;50(2):287–92.

86. Franke-Ullmann G, Pfortner C, Walter P, et al. Alteration of pulmonary macrophage function by respiratory syncytial virus infection in vitro. J Immunol 1995;154(1):268–80.

87. Jakab GJ. Immune impairment of alveolar macrophage phagocytosis during influenza virus pneumonia. Am Rev Respir Dis 1982;126(5):778–82.

88. Kleinerman ES, Daniels CA, Polisson RP, et al. Effect of virus infection on the inflammatory response. Depression of macrophage accumulation in influenza-infected mice. Am J Pathol 1976; 85(2):373–82.

89. Nicholls JM. The battle between influenza and the innate immune response in the human respiratory tract. Infect Chemother 2013;45(1):11–21.

90. Huang FF, Barnes PF, Feng Y, et al. GM-CSF in the lung protects against lethal influenza infection. Am J Respir Crit Care Med 2011;184(2):259–68.

91. Ghoneim HE, Thomas PG, McCullers JA. Depletion of alveolar macrophages during influenza infection facilitates bacterial superinfections. J Immunol 2013;191(3):1250–9.

92. Subramaniam R, Barnes PF, Fletcher K, et al. Protecting against post-influenza bacterial pneumonia by increasing phagocyte recruitment and ROS production. J Infect Dis 2014;209(11):1827–36.

93. Shahangian A, Chow EK, Tian X, et al. Type I IFNs mediate development of postinfluenza bacterial pneumonia in mice. J Clin Invest 2009;119(7): 1910–20.

94. Didierlaurent A, Goulding J, Patel S, et al. Sustained desensitization to bacterial Toll-like receptor ligands after resolution of respiratory influenza infection. J Exp Med 2008;205(2):323–9.

95. Abramson JS, Mills EL, Giebink GS, et al. Depression of monocyte and polymorphonuclear leukocyte oxidative metabolism and bactericidal capacity by influenza A virus. Infect Immun 1982; 35(1):350–5.

96. Damjanovic D, Lai R, Jeyanathan M, et al. Marked improvement of severe lung immunopathology by influenza-associated pneumococcal superinfection requires the control of both bacterial replication and host immune responses. Am J Pathol 2013; 183(3):868–80.

97. Stark JM, Stark MA, Colasurdo GN, et al. Decreased bacterial clearance from the lungs of mice following primary respiratory syncytial virus infection. J Med Virol 2006;78(6):829–38.

98. Abramson JS, Giebink GS, Mills EL, et al. Polymorphonuclear leukocyte dysfunction during influenza virus infection in chinchillas. J Infect Dis 1981; 143(6):836–45.

99. Ivashkiv LB, Donlin LT. Regulation of type I interferon responses. Nat Rev Immunol 2014;14(1): 36–49.

100. Nakamura S, Davis KM, Weiser JN. Synergistic stimulation of type I interferons during influenza virus coinfection promotes *Streptococcus pneumoniae* colonization in mice. J Clin Invest 2011; 121(9):3657–65.

101. Kudva A, Scheller EV, Robinson KM, et al. Influenza A inhibits Th17-mediated host defense against bacterial pneumonia in mice. J Immunol 2011; 186(3):1666–74.

102. Tian X, Xu F, Lung WY, et al. Poly I: C enhances susceptibility to secondary pulmonary infections by gram-positive bacteria. PLoS One 2012;7(9): e41879.

103. Boxx GM, Cheng G. The roles of type I interferon in bacterial infection. Not Found In Database 2016; 19(6):760–9.

104. Schliehe C, Flynn EK, Vilagos B, et al. The methyl-transferase Setdb2 mediates virus-induced susceptibility to bacterial superinfection. Nat Immunol 2015;16(1):67–74.

105. van der Sluijs KF, van Elden LJ, Nijhuis M, et al. IL-10 is an important mediator of the enhanced susceptibility to pneumococcal pneumonia after influenza infection. J Immunol 2004;172(12): 7603–9.

106. Penaloza HF, Nieto PA, Munoz-Durango N, et al. Interleukin-10 plays a key role in the modulation of neutrophils recruitment and lung inflammation during infection by Streptococcus pneumoniae. Immunology 2015;146(1):100–12.

107. Gomez JC, Yamada M, Martin JR, et al. Mechanisms of interferon-gamma production by neutrophils and its function during Streptococcus pneumoniae pneumonia. Am J Respir Cell Mol Biol 2015;52(3): 349–64.

108. Yamada M, Gomez JC, Chugh PE, et al. Interferon-gamma production by neutrophils during bacterial pneumonia in mice. Am J Respir Crit Care Med 2011;183(10):1391–401.

109. Zhang Z, Clarke TB, Weiser JN. Cellular effectors mediating Th17-dependent clearance of pneumococcal colonization in mice. J Clin Invest 2009; 119(7):1899–909.

110. Li W, Moltedo B, Moran TM. Type I interferon induction during influenza virus infection increases susceptibility to secondary Streptococcus pneumoniae infection by negative regulation of gamma-delta T cells. J Virol 2012;86(22):12304–12.

111. Robinson KM, McHugh KJ, Mandalapu S, et al. Influenza A virus exacerbates Staphylococcus aureus pneumonia in mice by attenuating antimicrobial peptide production. J Infect Dis 2014; 209(6):865–75.

112. Miller WT Jr, Mickus TJ, Barbosa E Jr, et al. CT of viral lower respiratory tract infections in adults: comparison among viral organisms and between viral and bacterial infections. AJR Am J Roentgenol 2011;197(5):1088–95.

113. Flanders SA, Stein J, Shochat G, et al. Performance of a bedside C-reactive protein test in the diagnosis of community-acquired pneumonia in adults with acute cough. Am J Med 2004;116(8):529–35.

114. Meili M, Kutz A, Briel M, et al. Infection biomarkers in primary care patients with acute respiratory tract infections-comparison of procalcitonin and C-reactive protein. BMC Pulm Med 2016;16:43.

115. Muller B, Harbarth S, Stolz D, et al. Diagnostic and prognostic accuracy of clinical and laboratory parameters in community-acquired pneumonia. BMC Infect Dis 2007;7:10.

116. Branche AR, Walsh EE, Vargas R, et al. Serum procalcitonin measurement and viral testing to guide antibiotic use for respiratory infections in hospitalized adults: a randomized controlled trial. J Infect Dis 2015;212(11):1692–700.

117. Li H, Luo YF, Blackwell TS, et al. Meta-analysis and systematic review of procalcitonin-guided therapy in respiratory tract infections. Antimicrob Agents Chemother 2011;55(12):5900–6.

118. Liu D, Su LX, Guan W, et al. Prognostic value of procalcitonin in pneumonia: a systematic review and meta-analysis. Respirology 2016;21(2): 280–8.

119. Timbrook T, Maxam M, Bosso J. Antibiotic discontinuation rates associated with positive respiratory viral panel and low procalcitonin results in proven or suspected respiratory infections. Infect Dis Ther 2015;4(3):297–306.

120. Schuetz P, Chiappa V, Briel M, et al. Procalcitonin algorithms for antibiotic therapy decisions: a systematic review of randomized controlled trials and recommendations for clinical algorithms. Arch Intern Med 2011;171(15):1322–31.

121. Rodriguez AH, Aviles-Jurado FX, Diaz E, et al. Procalcitonin (PCT) levels for ruling-out bacterial coinfection in ICU patients with influenza: a CHAID decision-tree analysis. J Infect 2016;72(2):143–51.

122. Diez-Padrisa N, Bassat Q, Machevo S, et al. Procalcitonin and C-reactive protein for invasive bacterial pneumonia diagnosis among children in Mozambique, a malaria-endemic area. PLoS One 2010;5(10):e13226.

123. Sanchez JL, Cooper MJ, Myers CA, et al. Respiratory infections in the U.S. military: recent experience and control. Clin Microbiol Rev 2015;28(3): 743–800.

124. Jefferson T, Di Pietrantonj C, Rivetti A, et al. Vaccines for preventing influenza in healthy adults. Cochrane Database Syst Rev 2014;3:CD001269.

125. Caldwell R, Roberts CS, An Z, et al. The health and economic impact of vaccination with 7-valent pneumococcal vaccine (PCV7) during an annual influenza epidemic and influenza pandemic in China. BMC Infect Dis 2015;15:284.

126. Tessmer A, Welte T, Schmidt-Ott R, et al. Influenza vaccination is associated with reduced severity of community-acquired pneumonia. Eur Respir J 2011;38(1):147–53.

127. Wang CS, Wang ST, Lai CT, et al. Impact of influenza vaccination on major cause-specific mortality. Vaccine 2007;25(7):1196–203.

128. Oster G, Weycker D, Edelsberg J, et al. Benefits and risks of live attenuated influenza vaccine in young children. Am J Manag Care 2010;16(9): e235-44.

129. Nichol KL, Nordin JD, Nelson DB, et al. Effectiveness of influenza vaccine in the community-dwelling elderly. N Engl J Med 2007;357(14):1373–81.

130. Spaude KA, Abrutyn E, Kirchner C, et al. Influenza vaccination and risk of mortality among adults

hospitalized with community-acquired pneumonia. Arch Intern Med 2007;167(1):53–9.

131. Voordouw BC, van der Linden PD, Simonian S, et al. Influenza vaccination in community-dwelling elderly: impact on mortality and influenza-associated morbidity. Arch Intern Med 2003;163(9):1089–94.

132. Voordouw BC, Sturkenboom MC, Dieleman JP, et al. Annual influenza vaccination in community-dwelling elderly individuals and the risk of lower respiratory tract infections or pneumonia. Arch Intern Med 2006;166(18):1980–5.

133. Voordouw BC, Sturkenboom MC, Dieleman JP, et al. Mortality benefits of influenza vaccination in elderly people. Lancet Infect Dis 2008;8(8):461–2 [author reply: 463–5].

134. Huber VC, Peltola V, Iverson AR, et al. Contribution of vaccine-induced immunity toward either the HA or the NA component of influenza viruses limits secondary bacterial complications. J Virol 2010; 84(8):4105–8.

135. Li C, Gubbins PO, Chen GJ. Prior pneumococcal and influenza vaccinations and in-hospital outcomes for community-acquired pneumonia in elderly veterans. J Hosp Med 2015;10(5):287–93.

136. Christopoulou I, Roose K, Ibanez LI, et al. Influenza vaccines to control influenza-associated bacterial infection: where do we stand? Expert Rev Vaccines 2015;14(1):55–67.

137. Mina MJ, Klugman KP, McCullers JA. Live attenuated influenza vaccine, but not pneumococcal conjugate vaccine, protects against increased density and duration of pneumococcal carriage after influenza infection in pneumococcal colonized mice. J Infect Dis 2013;208(8):1281–5.

138. Klonoski JM, Hurtig HR, Juber BA, et al. Vaccination against the M protein of *Streptococcus pyogenes* prevents death after influenza virus: *S. pyogenes* super-infection. Vaccine 2014;32(40):5241–9.

139. Lim WS, Baudouin SV, George RC, et al. BTS guidelines for the management of community acquired pneumonia in adults: update 2009. Thorax 2009;64(Suppl 3):iii1–55.

140. Mandell LA, Wunderink RG, Anzueto A, et al. Infectious Diseases Society of America/American Thoracic Society consensus guidelines on the management of community-acquired pneumonia in adults. Clin Infect Dis 2007;44(Suppl 2):S27–72.

141. Bhan U, Podsiad AB, Kovach MA, et al. Linezolid has unique immunomodulatory effects in post-influenza community acquired MRSA pneumonia. PLoS One 2015;10(1):e0114574.

142. Bright RA, Medina MJ, Xu X, et al. Incidence of adamantane resistance among influenza A (H3N2) viruses isolated worldwide from 1994 to 2005: a cause for concern. Lancet 2005;366(9492):1175–81.

143. Bright RA, Shay DK, Shu B, et al. Adamantane resistance among influenza A viruses isolated early during the 2005-2006 influenza season in the United States. JAMA 2006;295(8):891–4.

144. Rahman M, Bright RA, Kieke BA, et al. Adamantane-resistant influenza infection during the 2004-05 season. Emerg Infect Dis 2008;14(1):173–6.

145. Viasus D, Pano-Pardo JR, Pachon J, et al. Timing of oseltamivir administration and outcomes in hospitalized adults with pandemic 2009 influenza A(H1N1) virus infection. Chest 2011;140(4):1025–32.

146. McCullers JA. Preventing and treating secondary bacterial infections with antiviral agents. Antivir Ther 2011;16(2):123–35.

147. McCullers JA. Effect of antiviral treatment on the outcome of secondary bacterial pneumonia after influenza. J Infect Dis 2004;190(3):519–26.

148. Whitley RJ, Hayden FG, Reisinger KS, et al. Oral oseltamivir treatment of influenza in children. Pediatr Infect Dis J 2001;20(2):127–33.

149. Dobson J, Whitley RJ, Pocock S, et al. Oseltamivir treatment for influenza in adults: a meta-analysis of randomised controlled trials. Lancet 2015;385(9979):1729–37.

150. Ghoneim HE, McCullers JA. Adjunctive corticosteroid therapy improves lung immunopathology and survival during severe secondary pneumococcal pneumonia in mice. J Infect Dis 2014;209(9):1459–68.

151. Ramos I, Fernandez-Sesma A. Modulating the innate immune response to influenza a virus: potential therapeutic use of anti-inflammatory drugs. Front Immunol 2015;6:361.

152. Quispe-Laime AM, Bracco JD, Barberio PA, et al. H1N1 influenza A virus-associated acute lung injury: response to combination oseltamivir and prolonged corticosteroid treatment. Intensive Care Med 2010;36(1):33–41.

153. Kudo K, Takasaki J, Manabe T, et al. Systemic corticosteroids and early administration of antiviral agents for pneumonia with acute wheezing due to influenza A(H1N1)pdm09 in Japan. PLoS One 2012;7(2):e32280.

154. Kim SH, Hong SB, Yun SC, et al. Corticosteroid treatment in critically ill patients with pandemic influenza A/H1N1 2009 infection: analytic strategy using propensity scores. Am J Respir Crit Care Med 2011;183(9):1207–14.

155. Zhang Y, Sun W, Svendsen ER, et al. Do corticosteroids reduce the mortality of influenza A (H1N1) infection? A meta-analysis. Crit Care 2015;19:46.

Antiviral Treatments

Michael G. Ison, MD, MS

KEYWORDS

- Respiratory virus • Influenza • Respiratory syncytial virus (RSV) • Neuraminidase inhibitor
- Ribavirin

KEY POINTS

- All currently circulating strains of influenza are resistant to the M2 inhibitors amantadine and rimantadine.
- There are 4 approved neuraminidase inhibitors: oseltamivir, laninamivir, peramivir, and zanamivir.
- All of the neuraminidase inhibitors have the greatest clinical impact if started within 24 to 48 hours of symptom onset.
- For hospitalized adults and children, anti-influenza therapy should be initiated as soon as influenza is considered and should not wait for confirmatory testing; there is evidence of reduction in morbidity and mortality among hospitalized adults and children when started up to 5 days, and possibly longer, after symptom onset.
- Aerosol ribavirin is approved for the treatment of respiratory syncytial virus but is generally used in at-risk infants and immunocompromised adults and children.

INTRODUCTION

A wide range of viruses can affect the respiratory tract; in general, these can be divided into viruses for which the primary site of infection is the respiratory tract (classic respiratory viruses, including influenza, respiratory syncytial virus [RSV], human metapneumovirus [hMPV], parainfluenza virus [PIV], rhinovirus, and adenovirus) and viruses that can affect the respiratory tract opportunistically (ie, herpes simplex [HSV], cytomegalovirus [CMV], and measles). The focus of this article is antivirals directed at classic respiratory viruses; excellent reviews of agents for the treatment of HSV and CMV infections can be found elsewhere.[1–3] However, there is significant effort being invested in novel antivirals for respiratory viruses often directed at novel targets, combinations designed to increase potency and reduce resistance emergence, therapeutic antibodies, and immunomodulatory agents selected to mitigate immunopathologic host responses; agents in advanced clinical development are reviewed briefly here, whereas more detailed reviews may be found elsewhere.[4–6] Few antiviral drugs are currently approved for treating respiratory virus infections and most of these are specific inhibitors of influenza viruses. The emergence of new pathogens like Middle East respiratory syndrome coronavirus has also led to screening efforts to identify new therapeutics.[7,8]

M2 Inhibitors

The M2 ion channel allows hydrogen ions to flow into the viral particle and results in release of the

Disclosure Statement: M.G. Ison has received research support, paid to Northwestern University, from Alios, Astellas, Beckman Coulter, Chimerix, Gilead, Jansen/Johnson & Johnson; he has provided compensated consultation to Celltrion, Chimerix, Farmark, Genentech/Roche, Toyama/MediVector, and Shionogi, and uncompensated consultation to BioCryst, Biota, Cellex, GlaxoSmithKlein, Romark, NexBio, Theraclone, Unither Virology, and Vertex; he is also a paid member of data and safety monitor boards related to research activity conducted by Astellas, Jansen/Vertex.

Division of Infectious Diseases, Northwestern University Feinberg School of Medicine, 645 North Michigan Avenue Suite 900, Chicago, IL 60611, USA
E-mail address: mgison@northwestern.edu

Clin Chest Med 38 (2017) 139–153
http://dx.doi.org/10.1016/j.ccm.2016.11.008
0272-5231/17/

chestmed.theclinics.com

RNA segments into the infected cell. Amantadine (Symmetrel) and rimantadine (Flumadine) are symmetric tricyclic amines that specifically inhibit the replication of influenza A viruses at low concentrations (<1.0 µg/mL) by blocking the action of this M2 protein.[9–11] When used against susceptible strains, both agents are 70% to 90% effective in preventing infection and reduce duration of fever and symptoms when used for treatment.[12–14] Although this class of drugs is specifically indicated for the prevention and treatment of influenza A infections, widespread resistance to all M2 inhibitors has been documented in circulating influenza A strains, and this class of agents is not currently recommended for the prevention or treatment of influenza.[15] Cross-resistance to both agents occurs as the result of single amino acid substitutions in the transmembrane portion of the M2 protein.[11] The resistant virus seems to retain wild-type pathogenicity and causes an influenza illness indistinguishable from that caused by susceptible strains.

Both drugs achieve peak levels 3 to 5 hours after ingestion.[16–18] Amantadine and rimantadine come as 100-mg tablets and a syrup formulation (50 mg/5 mL). In adults, the usual dose for treatment or prevention of influenza A infection is 100 mg every 12 hours for both drugs. Amantadine is excreted unchanged by the kidney, whereas rimantadine undergoes extensive metabolism by the liver before being excreted by the kidney; as a result, dose adjustment with renal dysfunction is required. The most common side effects of the M2 inhibitors are minor central nervous system complaints (anxiety, difficulty concentrating, insomnia, dizziness, headache, and jitteriness) and gastrointestinal upset, which are particularly prominent in the elderly and those with renal failure.[17] Patients who receive amantadine may develop antimuscarinic effects, orthostatic hypotension, and congestive heart failure. Rates of adverse effects are lower for rimantadine than amantadine.[17,19] Given drug-drug interactions, care should be used when coadministering either agent with antihistamines or anticholinergic drugs, trimethoprim-sulfamethoxazole, triamterene-hydrochlorothiazide, quinine, quinidine, monoamine oxidase inhibitors, antidepressants, and minor tranquilizers.[20]

Neuraminidase Inhibitors

Influenza A and B viruses possess a surface glycoprotein with neuraminidase activity that cleaves terminal sialic acid residues from various glycoconjugates and destroys the receptors recognized by viral hemagglutinin. This activity is essential for release of virus from infected cells, for prevention of viral aggregates, and for viral spread within the respiratory tract.[21] Oseltamivir (Tamiflu, a prodrug of the active carboxylate), laninamivir (Inavir), peramivir (Rapiacta, Peramiflu) and zanamivir (Relenza) are sialic acid analogues that potently and specifically inhibit influenza A and B neuraminidases by competitively and reversibly interacting with the active enzyme site.[22,23] Oseltamivir and zanamivir are globally available, whereas laninamivir is approved in Japan and peramivir is approved in China, Japan, South Korea, and the United States.

Laninamivir

Laninamivir octanoate (CS-8958) is a prodrug that is converted in the airway to laninamivir (R-125489), the active neuraminidase inhibitor, and is retained at concentrations that exceed the IC_{50} (50% inhibitory concentration) for most influenza neuraminidases for at least 240 hours (10 days) after a single inhalation of 40 mg.[24] Only 15% of the drug is systemically absorbed after inhalation. Dose adjustment is not indicated for renal or hepatic insufficiency. Laninamivir octanoate (CS-8958) is currently only approved in Japan for the treatment and prevention of influenza A and B infection and is available as a 20-mg dry powder inhaler. A single inhalation of 20 mg daily for 2 days is recommended for prophylaxis, whereas a single inhalation of 40 mg for individuals greater than or equal to 10 years of age and 20 mg for children less than 10 years of age are recommended for treatment.

Laninamivir was associated with more rapid time to alleviation of influenza illness caused by infections by seasonal H1N1 virus with the H275Y substitution in children compared with a standard 5-day oseltamivir regimen, whereas studies in adults showed noninferiority versus oseltamivir in such patients.[25,26] Laninamivir shows a similar duration of fever in ambulatory children compared with patients treated with zanamivir.[27,28] Among household contacts of an index patient with influenza, 2 and 3 days of laninamivir 20 mg daily was associated with a 77% and 78% protective efficacy, respectively, compared with placebo.[29] Common side effects include nausea, vomiting, diarrhea, and dizziness.[25,26] Laninamivir was not associated with significant bronchospasm or other respiratory adverse effects in patients with chronic respiratory disease.[30]

Oseltamivir

Oral oseltamivir ethyl ester is well absorbed and rapidly cleaved by esterases in the gastrointestinal tract, liver, or blood. The bioavailability of the active metabolite, oseltamivir carboxylate, is estimated to be ~80% in previously healthy persons.[31] The plasma elimination half-life is 6 to 10 hours but is more prolonged in the elderly, although dose adjustments are not generally necessary. Administration with food seems to decrease the risk of gastrointestinal upset without decreasing bioavailability. Both the prodrug and parent are eliminated primarily unchanged through the kidney by glomerular filtration and anionic tubular secretion. The dose should be reduced by half for patients with a creatinine clearance less than 30 mL/min, and further reductions when clearance is less than 10 mL/min.[32] Distribution is not well characterized in humans, but peak bronchoalveolar lavage, middle ear fluid, and sinus fluid levels are similar to plasma levels.[31]

Oseltamivir is indicated for the prevention of influenza A and B in patients greater than or equal to 1 year old, with dosing once a day, and for the treatment of patients greater than or equal to 2 weeks of age who have influenza A and B, with twice-a-day dosing. Oseltamivir is available for oral delivery only. Oseltamivir comes as 30-mg, 45-mg, and 75-mg tablets and as a white tutti-frutti–flavored suspension (360-mg oseltamivir base for a final concentration of 6 mg/mL). The approved adult dose for treatment is 75 mg twice daily for 5 days and for prophylaxis is 75 mg once daily. Pediatric dosing is based on weight and is outlined in **Table 1**. Efficacy of prophylaxis is 84% to 92% in protecting unvaccinated patients when given for 10 days to 8 weeks.[31,33] Caution should be used with prescribing oseltamivir for prophylaxis in patients exposed to an index case because prophylaxis has been associated with emergence of resistant mutants[34]; empiric therapy or monitoring is generally recommended in these cases as a result.

Among ambulatory adults with uncomplicated influenza A or B, oseltamivir 75 mg twice daily for 5 days when started within the first 2 days of symptoms was associated with a shorter time to alleviation of uncomplicated influenza illness (29–35 hours shorter) and with reductions in severity of illness, duration of fever, time to return to normal activity, quantity of viral shedding, duration of impaired activity, and complications leading to antibiotic use, particularly bronchitis, compared with placebo in previously healthy adults.[13,15,35] Pediatric studies enrolling children as young as 2 weeks of age showed that oseltamivir is safe and is associated with significantly reduced illness duration and severity, time to resumption of full activities, and the occurrence

of complications leading to antibiotic use (particularly acute otitis media).[36–40] Most existing literature on the safety and efficacy of oseltamivir in hospitalized adults and children suggests that, among such high-risk and hospitalized individuals, there is a benefit to starting antiviral therapy through at least 5 days after symptom onset, with the greatest benefit in patients started within 48 hours after symptom onset.[41–46] All of the studies in hospitalized adults suggest that early therapy is associated with reduced incidence of lower respiratory tract complications, requirement for intensive care unit (ICU)–level care, duration of illness, duration of shedding, and mortality.[13,15,43,44,46] Duration of therapy has not been well studied but data suggest that longer duration of therapy (≥10 days) may be required, particularly in critically ill patients and those with pneumonia. Viral replication in the lower airway does not correlate with quantity or duration of replication in the upper airway. Doubling the treatment dose of oseltamivir in hospitalized patients with influenza does not seem to increase virologic efficacy, except perhaps for influenza B infections, or clinical effectiveness, although one ICU-based randomized controlled trial reported that tripling the standard dose was associated with acceleration of viral RNA clearance from the respiratory tract.[47–49] Doses of oseltamivir should be given after hemodialysis; dosing must be adjusted for renal insufficiency and renal replacement therapy (see **Table 1**). There are conflicting data about optimal dosing of oseltamivir in pregnant women, with some studies suggesting a need for higher doses (75 mg 3 times a day), whereas others suggest that no dose adjustment is needed.[50–52] Current guidelines recommend treating pregnant women with influenza infection with one of the approved neuraminidase inhibitors. The recommended pediatric dosage is listed in **Table 1**.

Oral oseltamivir is generally well tolerated and no serious end-organ toxicity has been found in controlled clinical trials. Oseltamivir is associated with nausea; abdominal discomfort; and, less often, emesis in a minority of treated patients, but this can be ameliorated by giving food with each dose. Other infrequent possible adverse events include insomnia, vertigo, and fever. Postmarketing reports suggest that oseltamivir may be associated, rarely, with skin rash, hepatic dysfunction, or thrombocytopenia. In addition, there have been reports of abnormal neurologic and behavioral symptoms that have, rarely, resulted in deaths, mostly among children; most of these reports have come from Japan. Existing

Table 1
Agents used to prevent and treat influenza

Class	Drug	Usual Adult Dosage[a]		Dose Adjustment State	Suggested Dosage
		Prophylaxis	Treatment		
M2 Inhibitor	Amantadine	100 mg q 12 h	100 mg q 12 h	Age 1–9 y	5 mg/kg to maximum of 150 mg in 2 divided doses
				CrCl 30–50 mL/min	100 mg q 24 h
				CrCl 15–30 mL/min	100 mg q 24 h
				CrCl 10–15 mL/min	100 mg q week
				CrCl 10 mL/min	100 mg q week
				Age ≥ 65 y	100 mg q 24 h
	Rimantadine	100 mg q 12 h	100 mg q 12 h	Age 1–9 y	5 mg/kg to maximum of 150 mg in 2 divided doses
				CrCl <10 mL/min	100 mg q 24 h
				Severe hepatic dysfunction	100 mg q 24 h
				Age ≥ 65 y	100 mg q 24 h
Neuraminidase Inhibitor	Laninamivir	20 mg QD × 2 d	40 mg × 1		20 mg × 1
	Oseltamivir[b]	75 mg q 24 h	75 mg q 12 h	CrCl <30 mL/min[d]	Treatment: 75 mg q 24 h
					Prophylaxis: 75 mg every other day
				Age <10 y	
				≤15 kg[e]	30 mg q 12 h (5 mL[c])
				15–23 kg[e]	45 mg q 12 h (7.5 mL[c])
				23–40 kg[e]	60 mg q 12 h (10 mL[c])
				>40 kg[e]	75 mg q 12 h (12.5 mL[c])
				Any weight, 2 wk to <1 y	3mg/kg q 12 h (0.5 mL/kg[c])

Drug			For patients with severe infection	
Peramivir	NA	300 mg once	For patients with severe infection	600 mg QD as a single-dose or multidose regimen
			Children 6–17 y	12 mg/kg QD
			Children 181 d to 5 y	10 mg/kg QD for 5 d (maximum of 600 mg QD)
			CrCl 31–49 mL/min[e]	Adult: 150 mg QD Age 6–17 y: 2.5 mg/kg QD[e] Age 180 d to 5 y: 3 mg/kg QD
			CrCl 10–30 mL/min[e]	Adult: 100 mg QD Age 6–17 y: 1.6 mg/kg QD[e] Age 180 d to 5 y: 1.9 mg/kg QD
			CrCl <10 mL/min	Adult: 100 mg on day 1 then 15 mg QD Age 6–17 y: 1.6 mg/kg on day 1 then 0.25 mg/kg QD Age 180 d to 5 y: 1.9 mg/kg on day 1 then 0.3 mg/kg
			Intermittent HD (Dose on HD days only)	≥18 y: 100 mg on day 1 then 100 mg 2 h after HD Age 6–17 y: 1.6 mg/kg on day 1 then 1.6 mg/kg 2 h after HD Age 181 d to 6 y: 1.9 mg/kg on day 1 then 1.9 mg/kg 2 h after HD
Inhaled Zanamivir[f]	2 puffs	2 puffs	No dose adjustment needed	—

Recommendations based on those provided by the Advisory Committee on Immunization Practices.[4]

Abbreviations: CrCl, creatinine clearance; HD, hemodialysis; NA, not available; q, every; QD, every day. Duration of prophylaxis depends on clinical setting.

a Duration of treatment is usually 5 days.
b Oseltamivir is indicated for prophylaxis in children 1 year old and older and for treatment in children in greater than or equal to 2 weeks of age.
c Volume of suspension.
d No treatment or prophylaxis dosing recommendations are available for patients undergoing renal dialysis.
e Initial loading dose of 600 mg or age-adjusted equivalent; maximum dosage 600 mg per day.
f Zanamivir is indicated for prophylaxis in children greater than or equal to 5 years old and for treatment in children greater than or equal to 7 years old.

Data from Fiore AE, Fry A, Shay D, et al. Antiviral agents for the treatment and chemoprophylaxis of influenza — recommendations of the Advisory Committee on Immunization Practices (ACIP). MMWR Recomm Rep 2011;60:1–24.

data suggest that these events are more likely secondary to influenza infections than oseltamivir therapy.[53,54] It is currently recommended that patients be monitored closely for behavioral abnormalities.

No clinically significant drug interactions have been recognized to date, including studies with amoxicillin, aspirin, and acetaminophen. No interactions with the cytochrome P450 enzymes occur in vitro and oseltamivir does not affect the steady-state pharmacokinetics of commonly used immunosuppressive agents.[55] However, probenecid blocks tubular secretion and doubles the half-life of oseltamivir. Protein binding is less than 10%.

Peramivir

Peramivir has low oral bioavailability and is therefore delivered intravenously. Peramivir achieves exceptionally high maximum concentrations ($\sim$45,000 ng/mL after 600-mg intravenous dose) with excellent concentrations of drug in the nasal and pharyngeal secrections.[56] Peramivir is predominately eliminated unchanged by renal excretion with a plasma terminal elimination half-life of 12 to 25 hours.[39,57] Outside the United States, peramivir is available in 150-mg and 300-mg solutions for intravenous use, whereas peramivir is available in 200-mg solutions for intravenous use in the United States. Peramivir is approved as a single-dose infusion for the treatment of previously healthy adults with uncomplicated influenza in the United States; nonetheless, it has been studied for treatment of complicated influenza in hospitalized adults and is the only intravenous therapy currently approved for the treatment of influenza. Placebo-controlled studies of a single 300-mg to 600-mg infusion of peramivir was associated with a significantly shorter time to alleviation of symptoms, significantly shorter time to resumption of patients' usual activities, and more rapid clearance of virus.[58] A single 300-mg to 600-mg infusion of peramivir was also noninferior to 5 days of oral oseltamivir 75 mg twice a day in a season when many of the viruses were resistant to oseltamivir as the result of the H275Y mutation; these data challenge the efficacy of peramivir in the management of viruses with the H275Y mutation.[59]

Peramivir has also been investigated in several studies in hospitalized adults and children but is not specifically approved for this indication. In all studies, multiple doses of peramivir were used and findings suggest that single-dose therapy is not appropriate for severely ill patients. The first study, conducted in Japan, randomized 37 high-risk patients (those with diabetes or chronic respiratory tract diseases or patients being treated with drugs that suppress immune function) to receive 300 mg or 600 mg of peramivir daily with the duration of treatment (1–5 days) based on clinical improvement, defined as resolution of fever or judgment by the principal investigator or subinvestigator that continued administration was unnecessary.[60] The median durations of influenza symptoms were 114.4 hours in the 300-mg group and 42.3 hours in the 600-mg group (hazard ratio [90% confidence interval], 0.497 [0.251–0.984]) with a similar trend in time to resolution of fever. All subsequent studies have been larger, randomized, multinational studies. In the phase 2 study, 5 days of 200 mg or 400 mg of peramivir every day was compared with oral oseltamivir 75 mg twice a day in hospitalized adults. There was a trend toward more rapid resumption of usual activities in peramivir-treated patients and greater reductions of influenza B viral titers in the nasopharynx than oseltamivir over the first 48 hours.[61] A phase 3 multidose regimen was an open-label, multinational, randomized study that was started during the 2009 A/H1N1 pandemic (October 2009 to October 2010), and was designed to compare the safety and tolerability of 2 dosing regimens of peramivir in hospitalized patients.[62] Two-hundred and thirty-four patients were randomized to receive 5 days of 300 mg of peramivir twice daily or 600 mg of peramivir once daily. The overall time to clinical resolution (TTCR) was 92 hours in the intent-to-treat infected (ITTI) group with a median time of 42 hours in the 300-mg group and 166 hours in the 600-mg group. The subjects on the 600-mg regimen ITTI analysis were noted to have higher need for supplemental oxygen at randomization, higher baseline APACHE score, and higher need for ICU admission before randomization than the subjects randomized to the 300-mg regimen, and multivariate analysis showed that the difference in TTCR between groups could be explained by differences in severity of illness before randomization. Virologic response, as measured by time-weighted change in virus titer from baseline to 48 hours, was -1.51 TCID$_{50}$ (Median Tissue Culture Infectious Dose)/mL without significant difference between the two doses ($P = .65$). In addition, no treatment differences were seen in the percentage of subjects who remained culture positive or reverse transcription polymerase chain reaction positive at 48, 72, and 96 hours postenrolment. The second phase III study was a double-blind, randomized trail conducted between September 2009 and November 2012 and enrolled 338 patients.[63] Patients were randomized to receive peramivir or standard of care in a 2:1 ratio. Only 121 patients had confirmed influenza and did not receive an NAI (neuraminidase inhibitor) as part of Standard of Care (SOC) (ITTI–non-NAI group) and were randomized to placebo (n = 43) or peramivir (n = 78) and 217 patients with confirmed influenza received NAI as part of SOC (ITTI-NAI group) and were randomized to placebo (n = 73) or peramivir (n = 144). Of note, there were important differences between the ITTI–non-NAI group and the ITTI-NAI group, namely lower mean body mass index (24.7 vs 29.1 kg/m^2) and lower influenza vaccination rate (5% vs 23%) in the ITTI–non-NAI group. In addition, the non-NAI SOC subjects had shorter symptom duration (32% vs 48% symptoms >48 hours), and were less likely to smoke (13% vs 23%), have abnormal chest radiographs at baseline (27% vs 45%), require supplemental oxygen (26% vs 36%), or have measurable virus titers at baseline (31% vs 50%). The study was terminated for futility after interim analysis. Peramivir-treated subjects in the non-NAI SOC population showed a modest, but not statically significant (P = .97), improvement in TTCR compared with subjects receiving SOC alone (42.5 vs 49.5 hours), with similar results observed in the NAI SOC population (peramivir vs placebo, 41.8 vs 48.9 hours; P = .74).

The largest pediatric study was a multicenter, open-labeled, uncontrolled study during the 2009 A/H1N1 pandemic.[64] One-hundred and six pediatric subjects, aged 125 days to 15 years, with confirmed A/H1N1 influenza received intravenous peramivir infusion at 10 mg/kg (500 mg maximum) once daily and clinical response, adverse events, and pharmacokinetics were assessed. Median time to resolution of fever was 20.6 hours, time to resolution of symptoms was 29.1 hours, and 92.9% had viral clearance by day 6 of treatment. Of note, TTCR in this pediatric study was shorter than the time noted in the adult trials. Taken together, these results suggest that intravenous peramivir likely has similar efficacy to oral oseltamivir and can be considered as an alternative to oral therapy in patients who cannot take oral therapy or in whom oral absorption is in question.

Because peramivir is renally cleared, dosing must be adjusted based on renal function (see **Table 1**).[65,66] There are limited data to guide dosing of peramivir in children, particularly among neonates.[65] No dose adjustments are needed for hepatic impairment. Recognized adverse events associated with the administration of peramivir are diarrhea, nausea, vomiting, and decreased neutrophil count; other less common adverse events observed in studies to date include dizziness, headache, somnolence, nervousness, insomnia, feeling agitated, depression, nightmares, hyperglycemia, hyperbilirubinemia, increased blood pressure, cystitis, electrocardiogram abnormalities, anorexia, and proteinuria.[67]

Zanamivir

The oral bioavailability of zanamivir is low (<5%), and most clinical trials have used intranasal or dry powder inhalation delivery. Following inhalation of the dry powder, approximately 7% to 21% is deposited in the lower respiratory tract and the remainder in the oropharynx.[68,69] Median zanamivir concentrations are more than 1000 ng/mL in induced sputum 6 hours after inhalation and remain detectable up to 24 hours. The peak plasma concentration averages 46 μg/L after a single 16-mg inhalation of zanamivir. The proprietary inhaler device for delivering zanamivir is breath actuated and requires a cooperative patient.[70]

Intravenous zanamivir displays linear dosing kinetics and the volume of distribution is approximately equivalent to that of extracellular water (16 L).[68] Intravenous zanamivir provides high peak plasma concentrations (~35,000 ng/mL after 600-mg dose in adults).[71] Ninety percent of the drug is excreted unchanged in the urine with an elimination half-life of approximately 2 hours. Intravenous zanamivir clearance is highly correlated with renal function.[72] Zanamivir is approved for the prevention and treatment of acute, uncomplicated influenza in ambulatory adults and children and is delivered by inhalation with a proprietary breath-activated device (Diskhaler). The usual adult treatment dose is 2 inhalations (10 mg) twice a day for 5 days and once a day for 10 days for prophylaxis. Intravenous zanamivir is currently only available by compassionate use.

Once-daily inhaled zanamivir for 10 days to 4 weeks is between 79% and 84% effective in preventing laboratory-confirmed symptomatic influenza.[69] Zanamivir is indicated for the treatment of uncomplicated acute illness caused by influenza A and B viruses in adults and pediatric patients 7 years of age and older who have been symptomatic for no more than 2 days.[15] Inhaled zanamivir in adults has consistently shown at least 1 less day of disabling influenza symptoms, and most studies have found a reduction in the number of nights of disturbed sleep, in time to resumption of normal activities, and in the use of symptom relief medications.[13,15] Similar therapeutic benefits have also been shown in children aged 5 to 12 years.[73] Zanamivir has also been associated with a 40% reduction in lower respiratory tract complications of influenza leading to antibiotics, particularly bronchitis and pneumonia.[74] Zanamivir seems generally well tolerated and effective in treating influenza in patients with mild to moderate asthma or, less often, chronic obstructive pulmonary disease.[74,75]

Intravenous zanamivir is in advanced clinical development and has been used in seriously ill patients with influenza, especially those with suspected oseltamivir-resistant variants. Most of the emergency investigational new drug uses of intravenous zanamivir were in patients who were clinically failing other antiviral therapy, with at least 25% of patients having proven or clinically suspected resistance to oseltamivir; 10.5% of patients died.[76] A phase 2 study in critically ill patients with pandemic 2009 H1N1 found that treatment was associated with significant antiviral effects, even though therapy was initiated a median of 4.5 days after symptom onset. Of patients with influenza detected on initial sample, 2 days of therapy were associated with a median 1.42 $\log_{10}$ copies per milliliter decline in viral load.[71] There were no drug-related trends in safety parameters identified. The 14-day and 28-day all-cause mortalities were 13% and 17%, respectively.[71] A phase 3 study comparing intravenous zanamivir and oral oseltamivir in hospitalized adults was recently completed but results are not available at the time of the writing.

Dose adjustment is not necessary for renal or hepatic dysfunction. Certain populations, particularly very young, frail, or cognitively impaired patients, may have difficulty using the drug delivery system.[70] Intravenous zanamivir requires dose adjustment for renal insufficiency. All patients should receive an initial 600-mg loading dose. The maintenance dose and dosing interval are reduced with worsening renal function and it should be dosed according to updated guidance provided with the compassionate use drug.[71,72]

Topically applied zanamivir is generally well tolerated in controlled studies, including those involving patients with asthma and chronic obstructive pulmonary disease.[75] Postmarketing reports indicate that bronchospasm may be an uncommon but potentially severe problem, particularly in patients with acute influenza and underlying reactive airway disease.[15] Anecdotal reports of hospitalization and fatality indicate that inhaled zanamivir should be used cautiously in such patients.[15] The currently available inhaled formulation cannot be used in patients on ventilators because obstruction of filters and death of patients has been reported. One randomized controlled trial in ambulatory adults found that the combination of inhaled zanamivir and oral oseltamivir was less effective than oseltamivir monotherapy.[77] Zanamivir is not associated with teratogenic effects in preclinical studies (US

Food and Drug Administration pregnancy category C) and should be considered as an option in pregnant women with proven influenza.[15]

Ribavirin

Ribavirin (Virazole, Rebetol) is a guanosine analogue with a wide range of antiviral activity, including influenza viruses, RSV, and parainfluenza viruses. Ribavirin is rapidly phosphorylated by intracellular enzymes and the triphosphate inhibits influenza virus RNA polymerase activity and competitively inhibits the guanosine triphosphate–dependent 5′ capping of influenza viral messenger RNA. In addition, ribavirin depletes cellular guanine pools[78,79] and may inhibit virus replication by lethal mutagenesis. Oral ribavirin has a bioavailability of 33% to 45% in adults and children and achieves peak plasma concentration of 0.6 µg/mL 1 to 2 hours after ingestion of a 400-mg dose in adults. Ribavirin has a short initial (0.3–0.7 hour) and a long terminal (18–36 hours) phase half-life and is eliminated by hepatic metabolism and renal clearance.[80] After aerosol administration, plasma levels increase with exposure and range from 0.2 to 1 µg/mL. Respiratory secretions have levels up to 1000 µg/mL, which decline with a half-life of 1.4 to 2.5 hours.

Ribavirin is available in 3 formulations: oral (approved for combined use in hepatitis C), intravenous (investigational in the United States), and aerosol. Ribavirin for aerosolization is available as a solution of 6 g/100 mL, which is diluted to a final concentration of 20 mg/mL and delivered by small particle aerosol for 12 to 18 hours with a proprietary device (SPAG-2 nebulizer). A higher concentration of aerosol solution (60 mg/mL) has been given over 2 hours 3 times daily in some studies and seems well tolerated.[81] Ribavirin also comes in 200-mg tablets and sterile solution for injection.

Ribavirin aerosol is currently indicated for the treatment of severe RSV in children. Trials of aerosolized ribavirin for the treatment of severe RSV infection in infants have shown no consistent effect on duration of hospitalization time, mortality, or pulmonary functions.[13] Current guidelines recommend that aerosolized ribavirin be considered in the treatment of high-risk infants and young children, as defined by congenital heart disease, chronic lung disease, immunodeficiency states, prematurity, and age less than 6 weeks, as well as for those hospitalized with severe illness.[13] Aerosolized ribavirin has shown minimal efficacy in treating influenza in hospitalized children.[82]

Ribavirin has also been studied for the treatment of RSV and parainfluenza virus infections in mmunocompromised patients. Intravenous ribavirin seems to be ineffective in reducing RSV-associated mortality in hematopoietic stem cell transplant (HSCT) patients with RSV pneumonia; here may be benefit among lung transplant recipents.[83] Aerosolized ribavirin may provide benefit n selected patient groups with less severe RSV disease. Survival was improved when treatment vas started before respiratory failure or when nfection was limited to the upper respiratory ract.[84] Observational studies suggest that combination therapy with antibodies (either intravenous mmunoglobulin, RespiGam, or palivizumab) seems more effective, particularly when started before severe respiratory distress.[84] Oral ribavirin has been tried in the management of RSV with varable success.[85] In the management of parainfluenza virus in bone marrow transplant recipients, 2 case series found that aerosolized ribavirin failed to improve 30-day mortality or reduce the duration of viral replication relative to no treatment.[86] Ribavirin has not been clearly shown to have consistent clinical activity for the treatment of adenovirus infections and is not recommended for this indication.[87]

Systemic ribavirin is contraindicated in patients with creatinine clearance less than 50 mL/min and the dose should be reduced by one-third for patients less than 10 years of age. Dose adjustment is needed if there is a substantial decline in hematocrit and the drug should be discontinued if the hemoglobin level decreases to less than 8.5 g/dL. Systemic ribavirin can cause a dose-related extravascular hemolytic anemia and, at higher doses, suppression of bone marrow release of erythroid elements. Aerosolized ribavirin can cause bronchospasm, mild conjunctival irritation, rash, psychological distress if administered in an oxygen tent, and (rarely) acute water intoxication. Bolus intravenous administration may cause rigors. Antagonism of both drugs may occur when ribavirin is combined with zidovudine. Ribavirin is contraindicated in pregnant women and in male partners of women who are pregnant because of teratogenicity of the drug. Pregnancy should be avoided during therapy and for 6 months after completion of therapy in both female patients and in female partners of male patients taking ribavirin (pregnancy category X).

Nitazoxanide

Nitazoxanide is an antiparasitic agent with apparent antiviral activities, including influenza virus and norovirus.[88,89] The mechanism of action of nitazoxanide against influenza viruses is through blockage of maturation of the viral hemagglutinin

at the posttranslational stage.[89] Nitazoxanide reduced symptom duration in phase 2b/3 trials in adults and adolescents with uncomplicated influenza[90]; a phase 3 trial is underway.[91] The drug also showed clinical efficacy in a small randomized trial of viral gastroenteritis.[92,93]

Cidofovir

No antiviral agents are specifically approved for the treatment of adenovirus. Cidofovir, which is a potent inhibitor of adenovirus in cell culture, has been used (either 5 mg/kg weekly for 2 weeks then every other week or 1 mg/kg 3 times a week), but data suggest that its efficacy/toxicity (predominantly nephrotoxicity) ratio is narrow. As a result, its use is limited generally to patients with significant evidence of disseminated adenovirus disease, preemptive treatment in pediatric HSCT patients with persistent replication. Earlier onset of therapy generally is associated with the best results and failure to develop a significant (1 log or greater) reduction in adenovirus load within 2 weeks of initiation of therapy is generally associated with poor outcomes.[87,94]

Combination Therapy

Combination therapy has been studied using a variety of combinations of antivirals and adjunctive therapies with the hope of improving antiviral activity, improving clinical outcomes, and reducing the risk of development of antiviral resistance for influenza.[95] There is evidence of in vitro synergy or additive effects with oseltamivir and amantadine; oseltamivir and favipiravir; peramivir and rimantadine; peramivir and oseltamivir; and a triple combination of amantadine, ribavirin, and oseltamivir.[95–99] In a study of oral rimantadine and nebulized zanamivir in an era with virus susceptible to M2 inhibitors, the combination was associated with trends toward faster cough resolution and lesser risk of adamantane resistance emergence.[100] The combination of oseltamivir and either convalescent plasma or hyperimmune globulin is associated with reduced mortality compared with patients treated with oseltamivir alone.[95,101] A study of oseltamivir, sirolimus, and corticosteroids was likewise associated with reduced mortality among critically ill patients.[102] The triple combination of amantadine, ribavirin, and oseltamivir was found to have similar PKs (pharmacokinetics) to each individual antiviral during monotherapy following a single dose and can be administered safely in immunocompromised patients; additional clinical studies of this triple combination are currently underway (NCT01227967). Likewise, the combination of oseltamivir and nitazoxanide has been studied; at the time of writing, the study is complete but results have not been made public (NCT01610245). Despite their theoretic benefits, the optimal use of combination therapy is still under investigation.[95] Similarly, combinations of therapy, typically ribavirin plus antibody preparations, have also been studied for the treatment of RSV and parainfluenza virus in immunocompromised patients. For RSV, the lowest rate of progression to lower tract disease and lowest mortality has been observed with the combination of aerosolized ribavirin and an antibody preparation (either RSV immunoglobulin, intravenous immunoglobulin, or palivizumab).[84]

Investigational Agents

Favipiravir (T-705)

Favipiravir is a broad antiviral that seems to inhibit RNA-dependent RNA polymerase but not mammalian RNA or DNA synthesis. It is approved in Japan for treatment of influenza in selected circumstances and phase 3 studies from ex-Japan for the treatment of acute uncomplicated influenza have recently been completed but results are pending.[103] The antiviral has in vitro activity against several RNA viruses, including West Nile virus, dengue virus, yellow fever virus, and Ebola.

FluDase (DAS181)

DAS181 is a recombinant fusion protein that cleaves sialic acid residues from respiratory epithelial cell surfaces, and prevents influenza and parainfluenza viral infection.[104–107] A phase 2 trial showed reduction in influenza viral load in healthy adults but had a more limited impact on symptoms.[108] DAS181 has also been used to treat several immunocompromised patients with PIV infection with a complete or partial response shown in 81% of patients.[109–113] A phase 2 randomized trial of DAS181 in immunocompromised hosts with PIV lower respiratory tract infection is ongoing.

Presatovir (GS-5806)

GS-5806 is an oral RSV entry inhibitor that showed reductions in viral load and clinical severity in phase 1 studies.[114–116] Phase 2 trials are underway in hospitalized patients and adult HSCT and lung transplant recipients.[117–120]

ALS-8176

ALS-8176, a nucleoside analogue targeting RSV polymerase, showed reduction of viral load and decreased disease severity in a human challenge model.[121] Studies in hospitalized infants are ongoing.[122]

ALN-RSV01

ALN-RSV01, a small interfering RNA, was effective in a challenge model[123] and reduced cumulative daily symptom scores and incidence of progressive bronchiolitis obliterans syndrome in lung transplant recipients.[124,125] There is currently no ongoing clinical development.

REFERENCES

1. Limaye AP, Boeckh M. CMV in critically ill patients: pathogen or bystander? Rev Med Virol 2010;20: 372–9.
2. Luyt CE, Combes A, Trouillet JL, et al. Virus-induced acute respiratory distress syndrome: epidemiology, management and outcome. Presse Med 2011;40:e561–8.
3. Travi G, Pergam SA. Cytomegalovirus pneumonia in hematopoietic stem cell recipients. J Intensive Care Med 2014;29:200–12.
4. Hayden FG. Newer influenza antivirals, biotherapeutics and combinations. Influenza Other Respir Viruses 2013;7(Suppl 1):63–75.
5. Hurt AC, Hui DS, Hay A, et al. Overview of the 3rd isirv-Antiviral Group Conference–advances in clinical management. Influenza Other Respir Viruses 2015;9:20–31.
6. McKimm-Breschkin JL, Fry AM. Meeting report: 4th ISIRV antiviral group conference: novel antiviral therapies for influenza and other respiratory viruses. Antiviral Res 2016;129:21–38.
7. Chan JF, Chan KH, Kao RY, et al. Broad-spectrum antivirals for the emerging Middle East respiratory syndrome coronavirus. J Infect 2013;67:606–16.
8. de Wilde AH, Jochmans D, Posthuma CC, et al. Screening of an FDA-approved compound library identifies four small-molecule inhibitors of Middle East respiratory syndrome coronavirus replication in cell culture. Antimicrobial Agents Chemother 2014;58:4875–84.
9. Hay AJ, Wolstenholme AJ, Skehel JJ, et al. The molecular basis of the specific anti-influenza action of amantadine. EMBO J 1985;4:3021–4.
10. Pinto LH, Holsinger LJ, Lamb RA. Influenza virus M2 protein has ion channel activity. Cell 1992;69: 517–28.
11. Hay AJ, Zambon MC, Wolstenholme AJ, et al. Molecular basis of resistance of influenza A viruses to amantadine. J Antimicrob Chemother 1986; 18(Suppl B):19–29.
12. Alves Galvao MG, Rocha Crispino Santos MA, Alves da Cunha AJ. Amantadine and rimantadine for influenza A in children and the elderly. Cochrane Database Syst Rev 2012;(1):CD002745.
13. Hsu J, Santesso N, Mustafa R, et al. Antivirals for treatment of influenza: a systematic review and meta-analysis of observational studies. Ann Intern Med 2012;156:512–24.
14. Kaiser L, Hayden FG. Hospitalizing influenza in adults. In: Swartz MN, editor. Current clinical topics

in infectious diseases. Malden (MA): Blackwell Science; 1999. p. 112–34.

15. Fiore AE, Fry A, Shay D, et al. Antiviral agents for the treatment and chemoprophylaxis of influenza -- recommendations of the Advisory Committee on Immunization Practices (ACIP). MMWR Recomm Rep 2011;60:1–24.

16. Aoki FY, Sitar DS. Clinical pharmacokinetics of amantadine hydrochloride. Clin Pharmacokinet 1988;14:35–51.

17. Hayden FG, Aoki FY. Amantadine, rimantadine and related agents. In: Barriere SL, editor. Antimicrobial therapy and vaccines. Baltimore (MD): Williams and Wilkins; 1999. p. 1344–65.

18. Hayden FG, Minocha A, Spyker DA, et al. Comparative single-dose pharmacokinetics of amantadine hydrochloride and rimantadine hydrochloride in young and elderly adults. Antimicrobial Agents Chemother 1985;28:216–21.

19. Keyser LA, Karl M, Nafziger AN, et al. Comparison of central nervous system adverse effects of amantadine and rimantadine used as sequential prophylaxis of influenza A in elderly nursing home patients. Arch Intern Med 2000;160:1485–8.

20. Wills RJ. Update on rimatadine's clinical pharmacokinetics. J Respir Dis 1989;10:s20–5.

21. Colman PM. Influenza virus neuraminidase: structure, antibodies, and inhibitors. Protein Sci 1994;3:1687–96.

22. Moscona A. Neuraminidase inhibitors for influenza. N Engl J Med 2005;353:1363–73.

23. Kamali A, Holodniy M. Influenza treatment and prophylaxis with neuraminidase inhibitors: a review. Infect Drug Resist 2013;6:187–98.

24. Yamashita M. Laninamivir and its prodrug, CS-8958: long-acting neuraminidase inhibitors for the treatment of influenza. Antivir Chem Chemother 2010;21:71–84.

25. Watanabe A, Chang SC, Kim MJ, et al. Long-acting neuraminidase inhibitor laninamivir octanoate versus oseltamivir for treatment of influenza: a double-blind, randomized, noninferiority clinical trial. Clin Infect Dis 2010;51:1167–75.

26. Sugaya N, Ohashi Y. Long-acting neuraminidase inhibitor laninamivir octanoate (CS-8958) versus oseltamivir as treatment for children with influenza virus infection. Antimicrobial Agents Chemother 2010;54:2575–82.

27. Koseki N, Kaiho M, Kikuta H, et al. Comparison of the clinical effectiveness of zanamivir and laninamivir octanoate for children with influenza A(H3N2) and B in the 2011-2012 season. Influenza Other Respir Viruses 2014;8:151–8.

28. Katsumi Y, Otabe O, Matsui F, et al. Effect of a single inhalation of laninamivir octanoate in children with influenza. Pediatrics 2012;129:e1431–6.

29. Kashiwagi S, Watanabe A, Ikematsu H, et al. Laninamivir octanoate for post-exposure prophylaxis of influenza in household contacts: a randomized double blind placebo controlled trial. J Infect Chemother 2013;19:740–9.

30. Watanabe A. A randomized double-blind controlled study of laninamivir compared with oseltamivir for the treatment of influenza in patients with chronic respiratory diseases. J Infect Chemother 2013;19:89–97.

31. McClellan K, Perry CM. Oseltamivir: a review of its use in influenza. Drugs 2001;61:263–83.

32. He G, Massarella J, Ward P. Clinical pharmacokinetics of the prodrug oseltamivir and its active metabolite Ro 64-0802. Clin Pharmacokinet 1999; 37:471–84.

33. Ison MG, Szakaly P, Shapira MY, et al. Efficacy and safety of oral oseltamivir for influenza prophylaxis in transplant recipients. Antivir Ther 2012;17:955–64.

34. Baz M, Abed Y, Papenburg J, et al. Emergence of oseltamivir-resistant pandemic H1N1 virus during prophylaxis. N Engl J Med 2009;361:2296–7.

35. Kaiser L, Wat C, Mills T, et al. Impact of oseltamivir treatment on influenza-related lower respiratory tract complications and hospitalizations. Arch Intern Med 2003;163:1667–72.

36. Acosta EP, Jester P, Gal P, et al. Oseltamivir dosing for influenza infection in premature neonates. J Infect Dis 2010;202:563–6.

37. Kamal MA, Acosta EP, Kimberlin DW, et al. The posology of oseltamivir in infants with influenza infection using a population pharmacokinetic approach. Clin Pharmacol Ther 2014;96(3):380–9.

38. Kimberlin DW, Acosta EP, Prichard MN, et al. Oseltamivir pharmacokinetics, dosing, and resistance among children aged <2 years with influenza. J Infect Dis 2013;207:709–20.

39. Whitley RJ, Hayden FG, Reisinger KS, et al. Oral oseltamivir treatment of influenza in children. Pediatr Infect Dis J 2001;20:127–33.

40. Piedra PA, Schulman KL, Blumentals WA. Effects of oseltamivir on influenza-related complications in children with chronic medical conditions. Pediatrics 2009;124:170–8.

41. Kumar D, Michaels MG, Morris MI, et al. Outcomes from pandemic influenza A H1N1 infection in recipients of solid-organ transplants: a multicentre cohort study. Lancet Infect Dis 2010;10:521–6.

42. Reid G, Huprikar S, Patel G, et al. A multicenter evaluation of pandemic influenza A/H1N1 in hematopoietic stem cell transplant recipients. Transpl Infect Dis 2013;15:487–92.

43. Lee N, Ison MG. Diagnosis, management and outcomes of adults hospitalized with influenza. Antivir Ther 2012;17:143–57.

44. Lee N, Ison MG. Editorial commentary. "Late" treatment with neuraminidase inhibitors for severely ill patients with influenza: better late than never? Clin Infect Dis 2012;55:1205–8.

45. Louie JK, Yang S, Acosta M, et al. Treatment with neuraminidase inhibitors for critically ill patients with influenza A (H1N1)pdm09. Clin Infect Dis 2012;55:1198–204.

46. Muthuri SG, Venkatesan S, Myles PR, et al. Effectiveness of neuraminidase inhibitors in reducing mortality in patients admitted to hospital with influenza A H1N1pdm09 virus infection: a meta-analysis of individual participant data. Lancet Respir Med 2014;2:395–404.

47. Lee N, Hui DS, Zuo Z, et al. A prospective intervention study on higher-dose oseltamivir treatment in adults hospitalized with influenza a and B infections. Clin Infect Dis 2013;57:1511–9.

48. South East Asia Infectious Disease Clinical Research Network. Effect of double dose oseltamivir on clinical and virological outcomes in children and adults admitted to hospital with severe influenza: double blind randomised controlled trial. BMJ 2013;346:f3039.

49. Kumar A. Viral clearance with standard or triple dose oseltamivir therapy in critically ill patients with pandemic (H1N1) 2009 influenza. Denver (CO): ICAAC; 2013. p. B-1470.

50. Beigi RH, Han K, Venkataramanan R, et al. Pharmacokinetics of oseltamivir among pregnant and nonpregnant women. Am J Obstet Gynecol 2011; 204:S84–8.

51. Greer LG, Leff RD, Rogers VL, et al. Pharmacokinetics of oseltamivir according to trimester of pregnancy. Am J Obstet Gynecol 2011;204:S89–93.

52. Greer LG, Leff RD, Rogers VL, et al. Pharmacokinetics of oseltamivir in breast milk and maternal plasma. Am J Obstet Gynecol 2011;204:524.e1-4.

53. Toovey S, Prinssen EP, Rayner CR, et al. Post-marketing assessment of neuropsychiatric adverse events in influenza patients treated with oseltamivir: an updated review. Adv Ther 2012;29:826–48.

54. Hoffman KB, Demakas A, Erdman CB, et al. Neuropsychiatric adverse effects of oseltamivir in the FDA adverse event reporting system, 1999-2012. BMJ 2013;347:f4656.

55. Lam H, Jeffery J, Sitar DS, et al. Oseltamivir, an influenza neuraminidase inhibitor drug, does not affect the steady-state pharmacokinetic characteristics of cyclosporine, mycophenolate, or tacrolimus in adult renal transplant patients. Ther Drug Monit 2011;33:699–704.

56. Boltz DA, Aldridge JR Jr, Webster RG, et al. Drugs in development for influenza. Drugs 2010;70:1349–62.

57. Chairat K, Tarning J, White NJ, et al. Pharmacokinetic properties of anti-influenza neuraminidase inhibitors. J Clin Pharmacol 2012;53(2):119–39.

58. Kohno S, Kida H, Mizuguchi M, et al. Efficacy and safety of intravenous peramivir for treatment of seasonal influenza virus infection. Antimicrobial Agents Chemother 2010;54:4568–74.

59. Kohno S, Yen MY, Cheong HJ, et al. Phase III randomized, double-blind study comparing single-dose intravenous peramivir with oral oseltamivir in patients with seasonal influenza virus infection. Antimicrobial Agents Chemother 2011;55:5267–76.

60. Kohno S, Kida H, Mizuguchi M, et al. Intravenous peramivir for treatment of influenza A and B virus infection in high-risk patients. Antimicrobial Agents Chemother 2011;55:2803–12.

61. Ison MG, Hui DS, Clezy K, et al. A clinical trial of intravenous peramivir compared with oral oseltamivir for the treatment of seasonal influenza in hospitalized adults. Antivir Ther 2013;18:651–61.

62. Ison MG, Fraiz J, Heller B, et al. Intravenous peramivir for treatment of influenza in hospitalized patients. Antivir Ther 2014;19:349–61.

63. de Jong MD, Ison MG, Monto AS, et al. Evaluation of intravenous peramivir for treatment of influenza in hospitalized patients. Clin Infect Dis 2014;59: e172–85.

64. Sugaya N, Kohno S, Ishibashi T, et al. Efficacy, safety, and pharmacokinetics of intravenous peramivir in children with 2009 pandemic H1N1 influenza A virus infection. Antimicrobial Agents Chemother 2012;56:369–77.

65. Arya V, Carter WW, Robertson SM. The role of clinical pharmacology in supporting the emergency use authorization of an unapproved anti-influenza drug, peramivir. Clin Pharmacol Ther 2010;88: 587–9.

66. Thomas B, Hollister AS, Muczynski KA. Peramivir clearance in continuous renal replacement therapy. Hemodialysis Int 2010;14:339–40.

67. Centers for Disease Control and Prevention. Emergency use authorization of Peramivir IV: fact sheet for health care providers. 2009.

68. Cass LM, Efthymiopoulos C, Bye A. Pharmacokinetics of zanamivir after intravenous, oral, inhaled or intranasal administration to healthy volunteers. Clin Pharmacokinet 1999;36(Suppl 1):1–11.

69. Dunn CJ, Goa KL. Zanamivir: a review of its use in influenza. Drugs 1999;58:761–84.

70. Diggory P, Fernandez C, Humphrey A, et al. Comparison of elderly people's technique in using two dry powder inhalers to deliver zanamivir: randomised controlled trial. BMJ 2001;322:577–9.

71. Marty FM, Man CY, van der Horst C, et al. Safety and pharmacokinetics of intravenous zanamivir treatment in hospitalized adults with influenza: an open-label, multicenter, single-arm, phase II study. J Infect Dis 2014;209:542–50.

72. Weller S, Jones LS, Lou Y, et al. Pharmacokinetics of zanamivir following intravenous administration to subjects with and without renal impairment. Antimicrobial Agents Chemother 2013;57:2967–71.

73. Hedrick JA, Barzilai A, Behre U, et al. Zanamivir for treatment of symptomatic influenza A and B

infection in children five to twelve years of age: a randomized controlled trial. Pediatr Infect Dis J 2000;19:410–7.

74. Lalezari J, Campion K, Keene O, et al. Zanamivir for the treatment of influenza A and B infection in high-risk patients - a pooled analysis of randomized controlled trials. Arch Intern Med 2001;161: 212–7.

75. Murphy KR, Eivindson A, Pauksens K, et al. Efficacy and safety of inhaled zanamivir for the treatment of influenza in patients with asthma or chronic obstructive pulmonary disease - a double-blind, randomised, placebo-controlled, multicentre study. Clin Drug Invest 2000;20: 337–49.

76. Chan-Tack KM, Gao A, Himaya AC, et al. Clinical experience with intravenous zanamivir under an emergency investigational new drug program in the United States. J Infect Dis 2013;207:196–8.

77. Duval X, van der Werf S, Blanchon T, et al. Efficacy of oseltamivir-zanamivir combination compared to each monotherapy for seasonal influenza: a randomized placebo-controlled trial. PLoS Med 2010;7:e1000362.

78. Wray SK, Gilbert BE, Knight V. Effect of ribavirin triphosphate on primer generation and elongation during influenza virus transcription in vitro. Antiviral Res 1985;5:39–48.

79. Wray SK, Gilbert BE, Noall MW, et al. Mode of action of ribavirin: effect of nucleotide pool alterations on influenza virus ribonucleoprotein synthesis. Antiviral Res 1985;5:29–37.

80. Paroni R, Del Puppo M, Borghi C, et al. Pharmacokinetics of ribavirin and urinary excretion of the major metabolite 1,2,4-triazole-3-carboxamide in normal volunteers. Int J Clin Pharmacol Ther Toxicol 1989;27:302–7.

81. Chemaly RF, Torres HA, Munsell MF, et al. An adaptive randomized trial of an intermittent dosing schedule of aerosolized ribavirin in patients with cancer and respiratory syncytial virus infection. J Infect Dis 2012;206:1367–71.

82. Rodriguez WJ, Hall CB, Welliver R, et al. Efficacy and safety of aerosolized ribavirin in young children hospitalized with influenza: a double-blind, multicenter, placebo-controlled trial. J Pediatr 1994;125:129–35.

83. Glanville AR, Scott AI, Morton JM, et al. Intravenous ribavirin is a safe and cost-effective treatment for respiratory syncytial virus infection after lung transplantation. J Heart Lung Transplant 2005;24:2114–9.

84. Shah JN, Chemaly RF. Management of RSV infections in adult recipients of hematopoietic stem cell transplantation. Blood 2011;117:2755–63.

85. Marcelin JR, Wilson JW, Razonable RR, Mayo Clinic Hematology/Oncology and Transplant Infectious Diseases Services. Oral ribavirin therapy for respiratory syncytial virus infections in moderately to severely immunocompromised patients. Transpl Infect Dis 2014;16:242–50.

86. Ison MG. Respiratory viral infections in transplant recipients. Antivir Ther 2007;12:627–38.

87. Ison MG. Adenovirus infections in transplant recipients. Clin Infect Dis 2006;43:331–9.

88. Rossignol JF. Nitazoxanide: a first-in-class broad-spectrum antiviral agent. Antiviral Res 2014;110: 94–103.

89. Rossignol JF, La Frazia S, Chiappa L, et al. Thiazolides, a new class of anti-influenza molecules targeting viral hemagglutinin at the post-translational level. J Biol Chem 2009;284:29798–808.

90. Haffizulla J, Hartman A, Hoppers M, et al. Effect of nitazoxanide in adults and adolescents with acute uncomplicated influenza: a double-blind, randomised, placebo-controlled, phase 2b/3 trial. Lancet Infect Dis 2014;14:609–18.

91. Romark Laboratories. A phase III randomized double-blind placebo controlled trial to evaluate the efficacy and safety of nitazoxanide in the treatment of acute uncomplicated influenza. In: ClinicalTrials.gov [Internet]. Bethesda (MD): National Library of Medicine (US); 2015 [cited 22 Dec 2015].

92. Rossignol JF, Abu-Zekry M, Hussein A, et al. Effect of nitazoxanide for treatment of severe rotavirus diarrhoea: randomised double-blind placebo-controlled trial. Lancet 2006;368:124–9.

93. Rossignol JF, El-Gohary YM. Nitazoxanide in the treatment of viral gastroenteritis: a randomized double-blind placebo-controlled clinical trial. Aliment Pharmacol Ther 2006;24:1423–30.

94. Ison MG, Green M. Practice ASTIDCo. Adenovirus in solid organ transplant recipients. Am J Transplant 2009;9(Suppl 4):S161–5.

95. Dunning J, Baillie JK, Cao B, et al, International Severe Acute Respiratory and Emerging Infection Consortium (ISARIC). Antiviral combinations for severe influenza. Lancet Infect Dis 2014;14: 1259–70.

96. Atiee G, Lasseter K, Baughman S, et al. Absence of pharmacokinetic interaction between intravenous peramivir and oral oseltamivir or rimantadine in humans. J Clin Pharmacol 2012;52: 1410–9.

97. Pukrittayakamee S, Jittamala P, Stepniewska K, et al. An open-label crossover study to evaluate potential pharmacokinetic interactions between oral oseltamivir and intravenous zanamivir in healthy Thai adults. Antimicrobial Agents Chemother 2011;55:4050–7.

98. Nguyen JT, Hoopes JD, Le MH, et al. Triple combination of amantadine, ribavirin, and oseltamivir is highly active and synergistic against drug resistant

influenza virus strains in vitro. PLoS One 2010;5:
e9332.

99. Seo S, Englund JA, Nguyen JT, et al. Combination
therapy with amantadine, oseltamivir and ribavirin
for influenza A infection: safety and pharmacokinetics. Antivir Ther 2013;18:377–86.

100. Ison MG, Gnann JW Jr, Nagy-Agren S, et al. Safety
and efficacy of nebulized zanamivir in hospitalized
patients with serious influenza. Antivir Ther 2003;8:
183–90.

101. Hung IF, To KK, Lee CK, et al. Convalescent
plasma treatment reduced mortality in patients
with severe pandemic influenza A (H1N1) 2009 virus infection. Clin Infect Dis 2011;52:447–56.

102. Wang CH, Chung FT, Lin SM, et al. Adjuvant treatment with a mammalian target of rapamycin inhibitor, sirolimus, and steroids improves
outcomes in patients with severe H1N1 pneumonia and acute respiratory failure. Crit Care
Med 2014;42:313–21.

103. MDVI, LLC. Phase 3 efficacy and safety study of favipiravir for treatment of uncomplicated influenza in
adults. In: ClinicalTrials.gov [Internet]. Bethesda
(MD): National Library of Medicine (US); 2015
[cited 21 Dec 2015].

104. Malakhov MP, Aschenbrenner LM, Smee DF,
et al. Sialidase fusion protein as a novel
broad-spectrum inhibitor of influenza virus
infection. Antimicrobial Agents Chemother
2006;50:1470–9.

105. Belser JA, Lu X, Szretter KJ, et al. DAS181, a novel
sialidase fusion protein, protects mice from lethal
avian influenza H5N1 virus infection. J Infect Dis
2007;196:1493–9.

106. Triana-Baltzer GB, Gubareva LV, Klimov AI, et al.
Inhibition of neuraminidase inhibitor-resistant influenza virus by DAS181, a novel sialidase fusion protein. PLoS One 2009;4:e7838.

107. Triana-Baltzer GB, Gubareva LV, Nicholls JM, et al.
Novel pandemic influenza A(H1N1) viruses are
potently inhibited by DAS181, a sialidase fusion
protein. PLoS One 2009;4:e7788.

108. Moss RB, Hansen C, Sanders RL, et al. A phase II
study of DAS181, a novel host directed antiviral for
the treatment of influenza infection. J Infect Dis
2012;206:1844–51.

109. Waghmare A, Wagner T, Andrews R, et al. Successful treatment of parainfluenza virus respiratory
tract infection with DAS181 in 4 immunocompromised children. J Pediatr Infect Dis Soc 2015;4:
114–8.

110. Chalkias S, Mackenzie MR, Gay C, et al. DAS181
treatment of hematopoietic stem cell transplant patients with parainfluenza virus lung disease
requiring mechanical ventilation. Transpl Infect
Dis 2014;16:141–4.

111. Drozd DR, Limaye AP, Moss RB, et al. DAS181
treatment of severe parainfluenza type 3 pneumonia in a lung transplant recipient. Transpl Infect
Dis 2013;15:E28–32.

112. Guzman-Suarez BB, Buckley MW, Gilmore ET, et al.
Clinical potential of DAS181 for treatment of
parainfluenza-3 infections in transplant recipients.
Transpl Infect Dis 2012;14:427–33.

113. Salvatore M, Satlin MJ, Jacobs SE, et al. DAS181
for the treatment of parainfluenza virus infections
in 16 hematopoietic stem cell transplant recipients
at a single center. Biol Blood Marrow Transplant
2016;22(5):965–70.

114. DeVincenzo JP, Whitley RJ, Mackman RL, et al. Oral
GS-5806 activity in a respiratory syncytial virus challenge study. N Engl J Med 2014;371:711–22.

115. Mackman RL, Sangi M, Sperandio D, et al. Discovery of an oral respiratory syncytial virus (RSV)
fusion inhibitor (GS-5806) and clinical proof of
concept in a human RSV challenge study. J Med
Chem 2015;58:1630–43.

116. Samuel D, Xing W, Niedziela-Majka A, et al. GS-5806
inhibits pre- to postfusion conformational changes of
the respiratory syncytial virus fusion protein. Antimicrobial Agents Chemother 2015;59:7109–12.

117. Gilead Sciences. Efficacy, pharmacokinetics,
and safety of GS-5806 in hospitalized adults
with respiratory syncytial virus (RSV) infection.
In: ClinicalTrials.gov [Internet]. Bethesda (MD):
National Library of Medicine (US); 2015 [cited
2015 Nov 24].

118. Gilead Sciences. GS-5806 in lung transplant (LT)
recipients with respiratory syncytial virus (RSV)
infection. In: ClinicalTrials.gov [Internet]. Bethesda
(MD): National Library of Medicine (US); 2015
[cited 2015 Nov 24].

119. Tylden GD, Hirsch HH, Rinaldo CH. Brincidofovir
(CMX001) inhibits BK polyomavirus replication in
primary human urothelial cells. Antimicrobial
Agents Chemother 2015;59:3306–16.

120. Gilead Sciences. GS-5806 in hematopoietic cell
transplant recipients with respiratory syncytial virus
(RSV) infection of the lower respiratory tract. In:
ClinicalTrials.gov [Internet]. Bethesda (MD): Na-
tional Library of Medicine (US); 2015 [cited 2015
Nov 24].

121. DeVincenzo JP, McClure MW, Symons JA, et al. Activity of oral ALS-008176 in a respiratory syncytial
virus challenge study. N Engl J Med 2015;373:
2048–58.

122. Parker S, Crump R, Foster S, et al. Co-administra-
tion of the broad-spectrum antiviral, brincidofovir
(CMX001), with smallpox vaccine does not
compromise vaccine protection in mice chal-
lenged with ectromelia virus. Antiviral Res 2014;
111:42–52.

123. DeVincenzo J, Lambkin-Williams R, Wilkinson T, et al. A randomized, double-blind, placebo-controlled study of an RNAi-based therapy directed against respiratory syncytial virus. Proc Natl Acad Sci U S A 2010;107:8800–5.

124. Zamora MR, Budev M, Rolfe M, et al. RNA interference therapy in lung transplant patients infected with respiratory syncytial virus. Am J Respir Crit Care Med 2011;183:531–8.

125. Gottlieb J, Zamora MR, Hodges T, et al. ALN-RSV01 for prevention of bronchiolitis obliterans syndrome after respiratory syncytial virus infection in lung transplant recipients. J Heart Lung Transplant 2016;35(2):213–21.

Vaccines in the Prevention of Viral Pneumonia

Clementine S. Fraser, BMBS, BSc, MRCP,
Akhilesh Jha, MBBS, BSc, MRCP,
Peter J.M. Openshaw, MBBS, BSc, PhD, FRCP, FMedSci*

KEYWORDS

- Influenza • Vaccination • Respiratory syncytial virus (RSV) • Parainfluenza • Adenovirus
- Lower respiratory tract infection (LRTI) • Viral pneumonia

KEY POINTS

- Viral pneumonias are a major cause of disease and death across the globe.
- Vaccination is a most effective way of preventing infection, but is only available for a limited (but expanding) number of respiratory pathogens.
- Current seasonal influenza vaccines confer insufficient protection, especially in some high-risk populations (eg, older adults).
- Research into correlates of protection has identified new ways to develop universal influenza vaccines that induce broad and long-lasting humoral and cell-mediated responses.
- Respiratory syncytial virus is a common cause of viral pneumonia and a largely unrecognized killer of frail elderly persons. Many promising vaccines are under development and there are high hopes of effective vaccines in the near future.

INTRODUCTION

Pneumonia is of huge global public health concern. Viral and bacterial pneumonias are major and leading causes of global mortality, the impact being greatest in children, the elderly and the immunodeficient, and those with comorbidities.[1–3] In 2015, pneumonia was estimated to cause 41.7 deaths per 100,000 population.[4] In 2010, it is thought that there were approximately 15 million hospital admissions for severe acute lower respiratory infections (ALRI) in children less than 5 years old, and that 265,000 of these resulted in death. However only 62% of children with ALRI are admitted to hospital, with most deaths happening in the community (81%).[5]

The introduction of molecular (polymerase chain reaction–based) diagnostics enabled pathogens to be identified in many patients with community-acquired pneumonia, but in many cases the initiating infection remains unidentified. Respiratory viruses are implicated in about 45% of pneumonia cases requiring hospitalization in children[6] but some viruses (rhinovirus and adenovirus in particular) are found both in symptomatic and asymptomatic individuals.[7]

The relative importance of viral infections as a cause of pneumonia has increased not only because of improved diagnostics but also because of the introduction of bacterial vaccines such as the Hib conjugate (*Haemophilus influenzae* type B conjugate vaccine) and pneumococcal

Disclosure: P.J.M. Openshaw holds a Wellcome Trust grant (WP108516) supporting vaccine testing with Mucosis BV, and collaborates with GlaxoSmithKline on RSV disease.
Respiratory Sciences, National Heart and Lung Institute, Imperial College London (St Mary's Campus), Norfolk Place, Paddington, London W2 1PG, UK
* Corresponding author.
E-mail address: p.openshaw@imperial.ac.uk

conjugate vaccines.[8] Vaccination is also available for influenza and vaccination against varicella zoster, rubella, and measles helps to prevent additional cases of viral pneumonia and its complications.

The burden of ALRI caused by viral pathogens indicates clearly that additional effective, durable, and affordable vaccines are urgently needed.

VIRAL VACCINES

Current licensed vaccines include inactivated, subunit, vectored, and live attenuated preparations. Inactivated vaccines may be made up of whole virus, split virus, subunit, or viruslike particles. Whole virus is grown in culture and then inactivated using a variety of methods, including chemical or heat treatments, to render them nonpathogenic. Vaccines containing whole killed organisms are generally cheaper to produce but may have a disadvantageous safety (reactogenicity) or immunogenicity profile. Spilt virus vaccines are a type of inactivated vaccine, split using organic solvents or detergents. Subunit vaccines comprise isolated or biosynthetic viral proteins that are selected to stimulate appropriate protective immune response while avoiding adverse host reactions.

Some vaccines, especially those that are highly purified and refined, may need to be combined with adjuvants and/or require the inoculation of multiple doses to be immunogenic. Adjuvants augment the host's immune response to vaccination, normally by providing a collateral danger signal via the innate immune system and thus boosting the protective acquired immune response. They enhance immunologic memory, allowing greater optimized antigen presentation.[9] Examples of adjuvants include alum (aluminum salts), virosomes, MP59, and AS03.

EXPERIMENTAL VACCINES

There are many different innovative vaccine approaches that are currently in clinical development and for the most part these focus on directing pathogen genomic material to the target host immune cell (**Fig. 1**). DNA vaccines involve the injection of DNA encoding specific antigens into muscle leading to de novo antigen expression and the stimulation of both B and T cells. A major advantage of DNA vaccines is the stability,

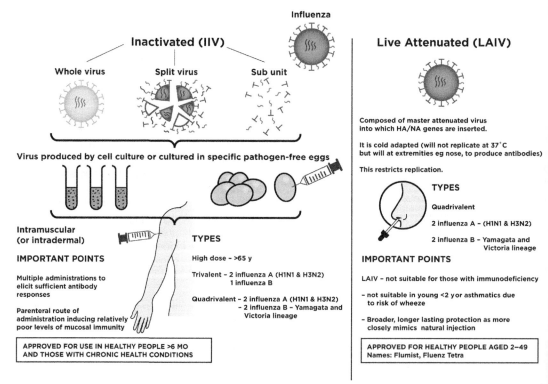

Fig. 1. Influenza vaccines. HA, hemagglutinin; IIV, inactivated influenza vaccine; LAIV, live attenuated influenza vaccine; NA, neuraminidase.

the absence of any infectious material, and the possibility of rapid scale-up. Drawbacks include the difficulty of translating apparent benefits from animal models into humans and the need for repeated and large volume injections. Most ongoing trials are in the treatment of human immunodeficiency virus (HIV) and certain cancers, but there are some studies of DNA vaccines for influenza.[10,11]

Recombinant vector vaccines are designed to introduce microbial DNA from an attenuated virus or bacterium using another pathogenic virus or bacterium to deliver genetic material to the appropriate host immune cell. Therefore, this closely mimics natural infection and triggers a corresponding immune response. Dendritic cell vaccines work in a similar way but exploit the immune system's own antigen-presenting cells to present pathogenic DNA. These vaccines are mostly being investigated in the context of HIV infection and cancer.[12]

CHALLENGE MODELS AND VACCINE DEVELOPMENT

Animal models are useful preliminary models for analyses of immune biology and identification of potential vaccine candidates. However, animals and humans can differ in their immune responses and correlates of protection,[13] confounded by the fact that those who experience the most severe viral disease are not typically those studied in challenge models (infants, pregnant women, and the elderly).[14]

Some of the common causes of viral pneumonia, current vaccination programs, their efficacy, and potential vaccine strategies for the future, including influenza, respiratory syncytial virus (RSV), parainfluenza virus (PIV), and adenovirus, are discussed later.

INFLUENZA

Influenza virus is the commonest cause of viral pneumonia in adults and the only virus that has an established global vaccination program. Epidemics have been estimated to cause 2 million to 5 million cases of severe illness and 250,000 to 500,000 deaths per year across the globe. Annual infection rates are estimated to be 5% to 10% in adults and 20% to 30% in children. Those at increased risk of severe disease are infants, the elderly, pregnant women, and those with major comorbidities.[15] Vaccination against influenza virus has been available since the 1940s and remains the most effective way of preventing disease.

There are 3 types of influenza: A, B, and C (A and B causing most human disease). Influenza B is more genetically stable than influenza A, with less antigenic drift and consequent immunologic variation.[16] Influenza vaccines have to be reformulated because of the constantly evolving nature of influenza viruses caused by antigenic shift and drift in response to immunologic pressure and reassortment events. Mutations in surface proteins hemagglutinin (HA) and neuraminidase (NA) accumulate under a variety of influences: an error-prone RNA polymerase, host immune pressures, and coinfection of a host with multiple strains can lead to gene reassortment.

Seasonal influenza vaccines vary depending on geographic region and are tailored to the circulating strains. Each year in February and September the World Health Organization (WHO) recommends viruses for inclusion in seasonal influenza vaccines in the southern and northern hemispheres, using information from classic reassortment and reverse genetics techniques.[17]

In 2010, the United States Advisory Committee on Immunization Practices expanded the recommendation for influenza vaccination to include all individuals 6 months of age and older.[18] However, globally, because of limited resources, this is not always possible and therefore high-risk groups are prioritized (**Box 1**). Live attenuated vaccination is currently being introduced to protect children in the United Kingdom.

Types of Influenza Vaccines

Licensed influenza vaccines are inactivated (whole virus, split virus, or subunit) or live attenuated (**Table 1**). Inactivated influenza vaccines (IIVs) are generally produced from highly purified, egg-grown influenza viruses and delivered intramuscularly or intradermally. A trivalent IIV has been available since 1978. In 2003 in the United States and in 2011 in Europe a live attenuated influenza vaccine (LAIV) for intranasal use was approved for use in healthy adults and children.

Trivalent or quadrivalent?

Trivalent vaccines contain antigens from 2 A strains and 1 B strain from a single lineage. Historically, several examples of mismatch between the vaccine and the circulating B strain have occurred. In the years 2001 to 2011, the predominant circulating influenza B lineage was different from that contained in the trivalent vaccine in 5 out of 10 seasons.[19] It is now generally recommended that quadrivalent influenza vaccines should be used containing 2 influenza A strains (H1N1 and H3N2 subtypes) and 2 influenza B strains (Victoria and Yamagata lineages).

Box 1
Populations to prioritize for influenza vaccination

High-risk groups prioritized for vaccination[a]

- Children (not recommended in all European countries[b])
- More than 65 years old (most of Europe[c])
- Chronic comorbidities:
  - Pulmonary (eg, chronic obstructive pulmonary disease, asthma)
  - Chronic cardiovascular disease (except hypertension)
  - Renal, hepatic, hematological disorders (including sickle cell disease)
  - Metabolic disorders (including diabetes mellitus)
  - Neurologic disorders (including neuromuscular/neurodevelopmental)
- Immunosuppressed (by medication, genetic or acquired/HIV)
- Pregnancy
- Six months through 18 years of age and receiving long-term aspirin (Reyes syndrome triggered by influenza)
- Morbid obesity (body mass index [BMI] $\geq$40 for adults or BMI >2.33 standard deviations greater than the mean for children)

Environment

- Nursing home residents
- Patients in long-term care facilities
- Health care personnel
- Military personnel
- Household contacts or caregivers of children less than 5 years old or adults 50 years of age or older
- Contacts/caregivers of those at increased risk

[a]Universal vaccination is recommended in the United States and Estonia.
[b]Austria, Estonia, Finland, Latvia, Malta, Poland, Slovakia, Slovenia, and the United Kingdom recommend vaccination in healthy children; age preferences differ.
[c]Most European countries recommend vaccination in people more than 65 years old. Austria, Belgium, and Ireland recommend vaccination in people more than 50 years old. Malta and Poland recommend vaccination in people more than 55 years old; Germany, Greece, Iceland, The Netherlands, and Slovakia recommend vaccination in people more than 59/60 years old.

Table 1
Snapshot of current RSV vaccines

	Preclinical	Phase I	Phase II	Phase III	Market Approved
Live attenuated	7	5	0	0	0
Inactivated	1	0	0	0	0
Particle	12	1	1	2	0
Subunit	10	2	2	0	0
RNA/DNA	4	0	0	0	0
Vector	8	3	0	0	0
Other (including antibody)	2	1	0	0	1
Total n = 62	44	12	3	2	1

From PATH. Vaccine development – Vaccine Development Global Program. Available at: http://sites.path.org/vaccine development/respiratory-syncytial-virus-rsv/vaccine-development/. Accessed May 19, 2016.

Vaccine Efficacy

The effectiveness of influenza vaccines is related to the age and immune competence of the recipient, as well as the antigenic matching of vaccine to circulating strains. A recent Cochrane Review of inactivated seasonal influenza vaccination in healthy adults showed an overall efficacy in preventing confirmed influenza of 60% (a number needed to vaccinate of 719).[20] It was concluded that vaccination did not have a demonstrable effect on hospital admissions or working days lost.[20] In years with poor vaccine matching, benefit is much lower, although the vaccine can still provide protection against severe outcomes.[21] A case-control study showed that previous vaccinees achieved mortality reduction rates of up to 75% (95% confidence interval [CI], 31%–91%), but only a 9% (95% CI, 0%–59%) reduction in mortality was seen in those who had never received a vaccination.[22]

Efficacy for the LAIV in healthy adults is similar to that of inactivated vaccine,[20] but depends on the take of the vaccine on the mucosal surface. LAIV given intranasally as a large-particle spray seems superior to inactivated trivalent influenza vaccine (TIV) with respect to protection against influenza strains that diverge from the vaccine strain,[23] indicating a degree of heterosubtypic protection.

INFLUENZA VACCINATION IN AT-RISK POPULATIONS

For a list of vaccination recommendations for at-risk populations, see **Box 1**.[24–26]

Pregnant Women

It is recommended that, if vaccination is in short supply, the first population group targeted should be pregnant mothers,[25] because influenza may be more severe in pregnancy, and it increases perinatal infant mortality, prematurity, and smaller birth size and weight.[27] Maternal vaccination may also benefit newborn children.[28]

The use of the IIV is recommended in pregnancy. It has been shown that vaccination reduces risk to both mother and infant (via passive immunity). An Indian study of 340 women showed a 63% reduction of proven influenza illness in infants up to 6 months of age and prevention of approximately a third of febrile respiratory illnesses in mothers and young infants.[29] In addition, maternal immunization results in the presence of antibody titers against influenza A vaccine subtypes in a significant proportion of mothers and their infants. Hemagglutination-inhibition antibody levels for influenza A subtypes are greater in infants of vaccinated mothers up to 20 weeks of age; however, the immunogenicity varies depending on the strain[30,31].

Children

LAIV is now the vaccine of choice for healthy children aged 2 to 18 years, because of the significant weight of evidence suggesting vaccine effectiveness.[32] A meta-analysis of 9 randomized controlled trials that compared LAIV with placebo showed a relative efficacy of 77% against antigenically similar strains and 72% efficacy regardless of antigenic similarity, whereas comparison with TIV showed that 46% fewer children experienced influenza illness.[33] Other studies have also shown LAIV to consistently provide a higher level of protection in children compared with inactivated vaccines or placebo.[34–36] Regarding other vaccine types, a Cochrane Review in children aged 6 months to 2 years showed that inactivated TIV is not significantly more efficacious than placebo.[34] However a 2011 randomized controlled trial involving 4707 children aged 6 to 72 months (1941 vaccinated) showed that the adjuvant influenza vaccine (MF59 adjuvant trivalent vaccine) was significantly more effective than control or lone trivalent vaccine at preventing influenzalike illness[37] When given to children (aged 6–15 years) the TIV vaccine has been associated with an increase in the rates of noninfluenza respiratory virus infection.[38] This study was performed in the pandemic season, 2008 to 2009; however, these data have not been replicated in different age groups (<5 years and >50 years).[39]

Older Adults

Most deaths associated with influenza occur in frail elderly persons,[18,40] therefore influenza vaccination is generally recommended for all those more than 65 years of age.[18] This recommendation is particularly important for patients with comorbidities, such as chronic lung disease, heart failure, or diabetes. Effectiveness of vaccination at preventing influenza in the elderly is a matter of ongoing debate, with a great degree of heterogeneity in published studies.[41] A robust randomized controlled trial in this age group showing significant benefit of vaccine in older adults is lacking.[42]

Comprehensive reviews come to differing conclusions depending on study design, methodology, inclusion criteria, and varying approaches to the correction of season-to-season variation of vaccine matching.[35,43,44] Two large meta-analyses assessing the same body of evidence have come to differing conclusions. One group concluded that there was insufficient evidence with respect to older adults,[42] and the other concluded that, when virus was circulating, vaccination reduced influenza-related and nonfatal complications by 28% and confirmed cases of influenza by 5%.[45] These differences highlight the importance of taking into account the large number of factors that affect the estimation of influenza vaccine effectiveness and the importance of careful and thorough evaluation. Failure to find an effect may be caused as much by methodological shortcomings as by lack of efficacy.

To improve vaccine immunogenicity in older age groups, higher-dose vaccines have been trialed, resulting in significantly greater antibody responses.[46] Promising data have also been seen with the use of adjuvanted vaccines.[47] LAIV is mostly ineffective in older adults because of previous immunity hindering local mucosal infection and therefore vaccine-induced immune response.[48]

Asthmatics

Globally, asthma is considered a priority group for vaccination,[24,49] and clear guidelines can result in greatly increased uptake in vaccination.[32] However, there are inconsistent reports of vaccine effectiveness in persons with asthma, largely because of differences in patient subgroups, research methodology, and variability in the definition of asthma.

LAIV has been shown to cause a 35% relative risk (RR) reduction in culture-confirmed influenza compared with TIV in a large trial (n = 2229) of asthmatic children aged 6 to 17 years with no increase in exacerbations of their underlying asthma.[50] A study of younger children aged 6 to 59 months concluded that LAIV reduced proven influenza cases by 55% compared with TIV but the youngest children (aged 6–11 months) experienced a higher hospitalization rate after LAIV compared with TIV (6.1% vs 2.6%).[36] Because of the small but significant potential for LAIV to cause wheeze and increased hospital admissions, the Centers for Disease Control and Prevention (CDC) recommend avoiding its use in children aged 2 to 4 years who have had an episode of wheeze in the preceding 12 months.[24]

A Cochrane systematic review concluded that vaccination with IIV did not result in a significant reduction in the number, duration, or severity of influenza-related asthma exacerbations but did improve symptoms, and also noted that there was no evidence that LAIV vaccine causes asthma exacerbations.[51]

Reports of low effectiveness can adversely affect uptake of vaccination among patients, and a health care worker recommendation to vaccinate is highly predictive of adherence.[52]

Pandemic Influenza Vaccines

Rapid deployment of vaccines as part of the response to pandemic threats is often problematic, largely because of the delay in production of new vaccines and the speed of spread of novel influenza strains. Three influenza pandemics occurred last century: 1918, 1957, and 1968, with a total mortality of 50 million to 100 million people.[53] In 2009 an influenza pandemic was declared by the WHO (caused by the influenza A H1N1 virus). The emergence of a new and genetically very different influenza strain caused a pandemic with significant mortality even in persons with no comorbidities[54] because of a lack of herd immunity and vaccinations not being matched to the novel influenza strain.

Seasonal vaccines generally offer little or no protection against novel pandemic strains, although there are hints that weak heterosubtypic protection may occur with LAIV. Developing a novel influenza vaccine requires safety and immunogenicity testing, but generally not field trials of efficacy. Even with expedited testing, production inevitably lags behind the timeline required for novel pandemic strains. A new vaccine typically takes 4 to 6 months to make, by which time the pandemic peak may be passed. Second, antigens from some novel influenza strains (eg, avian H5N1) are poorly immunogenic, making effective induction of immunity with vaccination difficult even with the use of adjuvants and multiple doses.[55] Ideally, a universal influenza vaccine that provides broadly cross-reactive protection through the induction of antibodies and/or T cells to the conserved regions of the virus need to be developed to counter future epidemic and pandemic threats.[53]

Correlates of Protection: Influenza Vaccination

Influenza vaccination induces antibodies, primarily against the major surface glycoproteins HA and NA. Antibodies directed against HA are the most widely accepted correlate of protection.[56] HA is the viral receptor-binding protein and antibodies that are directed to epitopes located in or near to this can prevent binding of the virus to its receptor and thus its infectivity. Titers of 1:40 HA inhibition antibody or greater have been shown to provide a 50% level of protection in healthy adults and this concentration of vaccine-induced antibody is used as a benchmark during vaccine development.[57] This is not necessarily the case for LAIV, for which secretory immunoglobulin A (IgA) is a better correlate of mucosal protection.[58]

T cells are abundant in the lung mucosa and have the ability to recognize conserved internal viral proteins. Although not preventing infection, higher peripheral CD4+ T-cell counts are associated with less virus shedding and less severe influenza illness, even in the absence of specific antibodies.[59] Presence of cross-reactive CD8+ T cells has also been associated with a reduced symptom burden as well as higher levels of interferon (IFN) gamma and interleukin (IL)-2 in influenza infection.[60] Because T lymphocytes (CD4+ or CD8+) preferentially recognize the more conserved internal proteins, this creates great potential for broad responses.[61]

As already mentioned, frail elderly persons do not mount as good an immune response as younger people. T-cell senescence is well described, particularly in studies of cytotoxic T cells. In a study of noninstitutionalized elderly persons, prevaccination IFN-γ levels were 10 times lower, IL-10 levels were 3 times greater, and the Th1/Th2 ratio was lower in those who developed influenza in the weeks following vaccination.[62]

The Future of Influenza Vaccines

Given the increasing emergence of influenza strains that are resistant to varying antiviral therapies (adamantaines,[63] rimantadine, zanamivir, and oseltamivir[64]), and that classic influenza vaccines must be updated regularly to match the new strains, prevention of disease using novel vaccine platforms should be given urgent priority.

Cell culture technology offers the potential to produce large quantities of vaccine antigen, and adjuvants allowing less viral antigen to be used. MF59 and AS03 have both been shown to be safe and effective and are now licensed adjuvant vaccines.[65] Recently, 2 synthetic Toll-like receptor adjuvants (IZ105 and IV270) have shown promise in murine challenge studies.[66]

The most promising universal influenza vaccines are those that induce cross-reactive humoral and cell-mediated responses. Universally conserved antigens with some promise include the extracellular domain of M2,[67] but this locus is poorly immunogenic.[68] The stalk portion of HA (HA2) is an attractive target because it contains several epitopes that are highly conserved.[69]

The nonstructural NS1 protein deletion blocks viral replication and stimulates an antibody and cellular immune response. Intranasal delivery of a live NS1 vaccine has been shown to be safe and immunogenic.[70] Vaccines that induce CD8 T-cell responses targeting viral nucleoprotein (NP), matrix protein 1 (M1), and polymerase basic 1 offer the prospect of universal influenza vaccines that might additionally accelerate viral clearance[71] (**Box 2**).

RESPIRATORY SYNCYTIAL VIRUS
Burden of Disease and Early Attempts at Vaccination

As recently reviewed,[72] respiratory syncytial virus (RSV) is responsible for more than 30 million episodes of acute respiratory tract infection globally. With up to 20% of infants less than 1 year of age requiring medical attention because of RSV disease, the need for an effective vaccination that can elicit durable protection in at-risk groups is clear.[73,74]

Although other common respiratory pathogens, such as influenza virus and _H influenzae_, have established immunization programs, a vaccine against RSV remains elusive, in part because of studies in the 1960s that showed that alumprecipitated formalin-inactivated RSV vaccine

---

Box 2
Current issues in influenza vaccinology

Improving traditional approaches

   How can durability of protection be enhanced?

   How might adjuvants be best used?

   How can vaccines be targeted to appropriate risk groups?

   Better influenza strain prediction

Future vaccine development

   Development of universal vaccines against all existing and emerging strains

   Evaluation of cross-reactive stalk/stem antibodies

   Overcoming weak immunogenicity of some influenza antigens

   Optimization of vaccine delivery methods

Improving manufacturing

   Acceleration of production techniques

   Manufacture of new vaccines to meet emerging/zoonotic strains

   Improved stability and convenient formulation

can augment subsequent disease.[75,76] Such vaccines not only fail to prevent infection but dramatically increase hospitalization rates in young children during natural infection. This effect seems to be associated with an induction of poorly neutralizing antibody, skewing toward the production of Th2 cytokines[77,78] and a local deficit in regulatory T cells.[79] These events hampered efforts in vaccine discovery, but in recent years academics, vaccine manufacturers, and international organizations such as WHO have made development of safe and effective vaccines a realistic prospect.[80]

Antigenic Targets for Prophylaxis and Vaccination

RSV is a negative-sense, single-stranded RNA virus consisting of 10 genes that encode 11 proteins; the surface glycoproteins F and G are responsible for fusion and attachment to the host cell membrane respectively. F and G are both targets for neutralizing antibody and are the key vaccine antigens.[81]

F protein is crucial in facilitating the fusion of the virus and cell membrane, thereby permitting cellular infection (and cell fusion into syncytia). Before fusion, (pre-F) protein has a metastable conformation and forms trimeric structures extending 11 nm from the surface. On fusion with the host cell membrane the structure extends to 16 nm and assumes a new postfusion conformation that is highly stable. Both pre-F and post-F forms can be found on the viral surface and share 2 major sites for antibody binding; however, neutralizing antibody is predominantly against the less stable prefusion form of F, which is now the generally preferred component of RSV vaccine candidates.[82]

The G protein can be either membrane bound or secretory. The soluble form may act as a decoy to assist in viral evasion,[83] but G (in either form) also engages the CX3CR1 fractalkine (CX3CL1) receptor, shown to impair IFN production by epithelial and dendritic cells in vitro.[84] The CX3C motif is located within the central conserved domain of G, flanked by mucinlike serine-threonine–rich domains that are heavily O-glycosylated.

Vaccination with layer-by-layer nanoparticles carrying the G protein CX3C motif has recently been shown to induce blocking antibodies and attenuate RSV pathogenesis in mice.[85] However, given the degree of glycosylation and variability of G protein, coupled with recent advancements in structural biology techniques, F protein has been identified as the most promising target for vaccination.[86]

Although antibody induction is the major goal of vaccination against RSV disease, the recent demonstration that local mucosal CD8 T cells play a part in controlling viral load offers the prospect that T-cell induction by vaccines might also be beneficial.[87–89]

Respiratory Syncytial Virus Prophylaxis

Palivizumab is a humanized monoclonal antibody against F protein. It targets antigenic site II on the viral protein and works prophylactically (but not therapeutically) to reduce hospitalization rates in infants with RSV bronchiolitis.[81] It is licensed for use in selected high-risk infants less than 1 year of age, and is given as 5 monthly doses by intramuscular injection. In some cases, it can be given in the second year of life,[90] but it finds little use outside these indications. Disadvantages include prohibitive cost and the lack of efficacy in patients with established disease. Most failures of prophylaxis reflect delay in onset of prophylaxis or in the administration or scheduling of monthly injections. The seasonality is variable depending on geographic location.[72,91]

Recent evidence suggests that palivizumab also reduces the prevalence of wheeze in the first year of life, presumably by delaying RSV infection beyond the critical first few months of life. This effect occurs after the end of treatment, lending strength to the argument that wheeze is a delayed effect of bronchiolitis in premature infants.[82]

Another monoclonal antibody, motavizumab, was developed with greater affinity to site II; this showed an 87% relative reduction (RR, 0·13; 95% CI, 0·08 to 0·21) in the proportion of healthy, term infants admitted to hospital with RSV compared with placebo but has subsequently been discontinued because of nonsuperiority to palivizumab and side effects related to skin reactions. In native American (Navajo) infants born at 36 weeks' gestational age, motavizumab is ineffective at preventing post-RSV wheeze.[92]

Respiratory Syncytial Virus Vaccine Development

Because of the requirement of vaccines for diverse target populations (young infants, older infants, pregnant women, and the elderly), multiple strategies may be required. These strategies include live attenuated, particle-based, subunit, and vector-based vaccine approaches. For example, young RSV-naive infants might benefit from live attenuated vaccines, whereas adults (who have experienced multiple infections) or immunosenescent older individuals may require different approaches.

An RSV F nanoparticle vaccine (Novavax Inc, Rockville, MD) is currently the most advanced vaccine in clinical trials for the protection of older adults (≥60 years of age), having been shown to be well tolerated and immunogenic in healthy adults. However, a phase 3 clinical trial in 11,856 older adults failed to meet its primary objective of preventing RSV-associated lower respiratory tract disease or its secondary objective of reducing all symptomatic respiratory disease due to RSV [NCT02608502]. The reasons for this failure of efficacy are yet to be established but a milder RSV season was noted during the study and the vaccine was tolerated safely. A related study in women in their third trimester of pregnancy is being carried out with the aim of reducing RSV lower respiratory infection in their infants up to 3 months of age [NCT02624947].

A promising live attenuated vaccine, MEDI-559 MedImmune/National Institute of Allergy and Infectious Diseases, Bethesda, MD) induces a substantial immune response in 59% of children aged 5 to 24 months.[93] A range of other candidate vaccines are progressing from the preclinical testing stage to clinical trials, including a mucosal vaccine based on bacterialike particles coated in F (Mucosis BV, NL). The RSV vaccines in different phases of development are shown in Table 1.

Overcoming Hurdles for Respiratory Syncytial Virus Vaccine Development

The ideal RSV vaccine would elicit long-lasting upper and lower respiratory tract protection, be well tolerated in infants and adults, and be free of risk of subsequent disease augmentation. Natural infection causes only partial protection against reinfection despite the low rates of antigenic variability, which indicates that an effective vaccine needs to surpass natural infection but avoid causing excessive T cell–mediated host immune disease. This issue is especially important in infants with an immature immune system.[94] These young infants are especially at risk of severe RSV infection, and may benefit from maternal immunization[95] to induce protective antibody that will be transferred to the child via the placenta and breast milk, but accurate correlates of protection and an understanding of the optimal route and timing of maternal vaccination are lacking. Vaccine effectiveness is typically assessed by the level of induced systemic RSV-specific neutralizing antibodies but this may not be an accurate predictor of durable immunity, with a human challenge model of RSV infection suggesting that the presence of mucosal RSV-specific IgA may provide a better correlate of protection.[96] A nonprofit organization, PATH, is developing an international RSV antibody reference standard to permit greater comparability between research studies.[97] These wide-ranging and intensive efforts to develop a range of suitable vaccines raise the hope of successfully combating RSV-mediated disease in the near future.

PARAINFLUENZA VACCINATION

Parainfluenza viruses (PIVs) are single-stranded RNA viruses that, like RSV, are members of the Paramyxoviridae family and cause an approximately similar spectrum of symptoms. There are 4 major serotypes of PIV (PIV1–PIV4), with PIV1 and PIV2 being associated with croup, PIV3 with pneumonia, and PIV4 with upper respiratory tract infection.[98]

The usual course of infection results in a mild self-limiting illness but susceptible individuals, particularly those who are immunocompromised, can experience a more serious, protracted illness marked by severe pneumonia and prolonged viral shedding.[99,100] Most children by the age of 5 years, and virtually all adults, have antibodies to PIV with multiple reinfections common but usually characterized by only mild disease limited to the nose and pharynx.[101,102] Because PIV3 is the most common serotype, and has the ability to cause bronchiolitis in infants, most vaccine efforts have been directed toward it.

The virus contains 6 proteins that are common across serotypes. Two of them (fusion glycoprotein F and hemagglutinin-neuraminidase glycoprotein [HN]) are present on the viral surface and are the main targets for neutralizing antibodies. There is as yet no vaccine to prevent PIV infection despite nearly 60 years of research and development. Current strategies include the use of nasally delivered live attenuated vaccines, the use of reverse genetics, bovine/human chimeras, and subunit vaccines that express F and HN proteins.[103]

The live attenuated vaccine HPIVcp45 is derived from a live strain of HPIV3 that has undergone cold passage 45 times. The accumulation of 15 attenuating mutations has rendered it nonpathogenic, and it is undergoing phase 1 trials in both adults and infants. It is reported to have a 94% infectivity rate and lacks transmissibility.[104–106] A larger phase II study with a population size of 380 children aged 6 to 18 months, including 226 seronegative children, showed that it generated adequate antibody response in 84% of seronegative recipients with no significant difference in adverse events compared with placebo.[107]

In other trials, a recombinant form of the vaccine (rHPIV3cp45), rederived from complementary DNA, showed a shorter passage time and reduced the risk of contamination or reversion.[108] It has been used in a phase 1 study of 40 seronegative children between 6 and 35 months old and generates virus-specific antibodies with a tolerable safety profile.[109] Another trial using rHPIV3cp45 in healthy young seronegative infants between 6 and 12 months old showed strong immunogenicity. These studies involved the delivery of multiple doses of vaccine with appropriate intervals, which is necessary to sustain durable immune responses, and children in particular are likely to benefit from the nasal route of administration because of the ability to generate protective mucosal and systemic immunity.[108]

An antigenically similar bovine PIV3 vaccine has been developed either alone or as a chimeric recombinant virus with human PIV3 (rB/HPIV3). rB/HPIV3 was highly restricted in replication in adults and seropositive children but caused significant infectivity among seronegative children.[110–112]

HPIV1 and HPIV2 vaccines are in development but are at a less advanced stage, with only 3 trials that have undergone human clinical trial testing at present (identifiers: NCT00641017, NCT00186927, NCT01139437). Results from a recent live attenuated HPIV1 vaccine trial suggested that it is appropriately restricted in adults and seropositive children but inadequately infectious in seronegative children, highlighting the challenges faced in developing novel vaccines that are safely tolerated but also have the ability to cause sufficient immunogenicity in their target populations.[113]

Delivery to young infants of combined vaccines that target PIV and RSV to elicit broad protective immunity may also be a feasible prospect in this age group and, if successful, could reduce the significant burden of disease caused by these common respiratory pathogens.[114,115]

ADENOVIRUS

Adenoviruses were first discovered in 1953.[116] They display diverse respiratory manifestations, from simple upper respiratory tract infections to severe fatal pneumonia.[117] Those most at risk are children less than 5 years old, the immunocompromised (most notably those who have received bone marrow transplants),[118] and those living in crowded conditions, such as the military. Most acute respiratory infections among US military trainees are attributable to adenovirus.[119]

The introduction of an adenovirus vaccine has greatly reduced military respiratory infection morbidity since its introduction in the 1970s. However, in 1995 the sole manufacturer ceased production of this vaccine. Over a 2-year period in the 1990s, when adenovirus vaccines were diminishing, 3413 throat cultures were taken from trainees with acute respiratory illnesses, with 1814 (53.1%) being positive for adenovirus. Trainees who were unvaccinated (n = 2322) were more likely to yield a positive adenovirus culture (odds ratio [OR], 13.2) especially for serotypes 4 or 7 (OR, 28.1). During this period there were also several epidemics of adenovirus in these military bases, affecting thousands of trainees.[120]

In 2011 a live vaccine against adenovirus type 4 and 7 (oral) was licensed in the United States and administered within the military in that year. The phase 3 trial revealed a vaccine efficacy rate of 99.3% (with only 1 episode of febrile respiratory illness in the vaccinated group); 73% of vaccine recipients seroconverted to ADV-4, whereas 63% seroconverted to ADV-7 by day 28.[121] After reintroduction of the vaccine, episodes of febrile respiratory illness reduced dramatically.[122]

THE FUTURE OF VIRAL VACCINATION

Vaccination is one of the most successful disease prevention strategies of the last century. However, vaccines against some important respiratory viruses are lacking; with the exception of influenza and adenovirus, there are no licensed vaccines against common causes of viral pneumonia. One of the major issues it to better understand the ways in which viruses evade immune protection, and how this information can be used to induce long-lasting, robust, and nonpathogenic immunity at the mucosal surface. It is possible that vaccines

---

Box 3
Research gaps and open questions

Questions

 How can optimal mucosal immunity be induced?

 Does T-cell immunity reduce severity or enhance recovery?

 How can universal vaccination be best achieved?

Risks

 Might novel vaccines enhance disease?

 Will viral resistance emerge?

 What are the drawbacks of adjuvants?

might be designed that would prevent symptomatic disease, while allowing infection (and possibly onward transmission) to occur. Such a vaccine would have the disadvantage of having a lesser impact on community circulation, thereby protecting the vaccine recipient but not others at risk. It is to be hoped that a new generation of vaccines will be developed that induce a balanced protective cell-mediated and antibody response and confer durable cross-protection against novel viral strains. With advances in virology, immunology, and vaccinology, it is hoped that these new vaccines will be developed soon (**Box 3**).

REFERENCES

1. Rudan I, O'Brien KL, Nair H, et al. Epidemiology and etiology of childhood pneumonia in 2010: estimates of incidence, severe morbidity, mortality, underlying risk factors and causative pathogens for 192 countries. J Glob Health 2013;3(1):010401.

2. Joos L, Chhajed PN, Wallner J, et al. Pulmonary infections diagnosed by BAL: a 12-year experience in 1066 immunocompromised patients. Respir Med 2007;101(1):93–7.

3. Falsey AR, Walsh EE. Viral pneumonia in older adults. Clin Infect Dis 2006;42(4):518–24.

4. Naghavi M, Wang H, Lozano R, et al. Global, regional, and national age–sex specific all-cause and cause-specific mortality for 240 causes of death, 1990–2013: a systematic analysis for the Global Burden of Disease Study 2013. Lancet 2015;385(9963):117–71.

5. Nair H, Simoes EAF, Rudan I, et al. Global and regional burden of hospital admissions for severe acute lower respiratory infections in young children in 2010: a systematic analysis. Lancet 2013; 381(9875):1380–90.

6. Michelow IC, Olsen K, Lozano J, et al. Epidemiology and clinical characteristics of community-acquired pneumonia in hospitalized children. Pediatrics 2004;113(4):701–7.

7. Homaira N, Luby S, Hossain K, et al. Respiratory viruses associated hospitalization among children aged <5 years in Bangladesh: 2010-2014. PLoS One 2016;11(2):e0147982.

8. Moberley S, Holden J, Tatham DP, et al. Vaccines for preventing pneumococcal infection in adults. Cochrane Database Syst Rev 2013;(1):CD000422.

9. Jalilian B, Christiansen SH, Einarsson HB, et al. Properties and prospects of adjuvants in influenza vaccination - messy precipitates or blessed opportunities? Mol Cell Ther 2013;1(1):2.

10. Zhang H, El Zowalaty ME. DNA-based influenza vaccines as immunoprophylactic agents toward universality. Future Microbiol 2015;11(1):153–64.

11. Bicho D, Queiroz JA, Tomaz CT. Influenza plasmid DNA vaccines: progress and prospects. Curr Gene Ther 2015;15(6):541–9.

12. Palucka K, Banchereau J. Dendritic-cell-based therapeutic cancer vaccines. Immunity 2013; 39(1):38–48.

13. Shultz LD, Brehm MA, Garcia-Martinez JV, et al. Humanized mice for immune system investigation: progress, promise and challenges. Nat Rev Immunol 2012;12(11):786–98.

14. Pollard A, Savulescu J, Oxford J, et al. Human microbial challenge: the ultimate animal model. Lancet Infect Dis 2012;12(12):903–5.

15. WHO. WHO seasonal influenza. Bulletin of the World Health Organization. Available at: http://www.who.int/mediacentre/factsheets/fs211/en/. Accessed May 24, 2016.

16. Centers for Disease Control and Prevention. Epidemiology and prevention of vaccine-preventable diseases. CDC Pink Book. Available at: http://www.cdc.gov/vaccines/pubs/pinkbook/flu.html. Accessed May 24, 2016.

17. WHO. Recommended composition of influenza virus vaccines for use in the 2016-2017 northern hemisphere influenza season. Available at: http://www.who.int/influenza/vaccines/virus/recommendations/201602_recommendation.pdf?ua=1. Accessed May 24, 2016.

18. Centers for Disease Control and Prevention. Prevention and control of influenza with vaccines: recommendations of the Advisory Committee on Immunization Practices (ACIP), 2010. MMWR Recomm Rep 2010;59(RR-8):1–62. Available at: http://www.cdc.gov/mmwr/preview/mmwrhtml/rr5908a1.htm. Accessed May 24, 2016.

19. Ambrose CS, Levin MJ. The rationale for quadrivalent influenza vaccines. Hum Vaccin Immunother 2012;8(1):81–8.

20. Demicheli V, Jefferson T, La A, et al. Vaccines for preventing influenza in healthy adults (Review). Cochrane Database Syst Rev 2014;(3):CD001269.

21. Tessmer A, Welte T, Schmidt-Ott R, et al. Influenza vaccination is associated with reduced severity of community-acquired pneumonia. Eur Respir J 2011;38(1):147–53.

22. Ahmed AH, Nicholson KG, Nguyen-Van-Tam JS. Reduction in mortality associated with influenza vaccine during 1989-90 epidemic. Lancet 1995; 346(8975):591–5.

23. Belshe R, Lee M-S, Walker RE, et al. Safety, immunogenicity and efficacy of intranasal, live attenuated influenza vaccine. Expert Rev Vaccines 2004;3(6):643–54.

24. Centre for Disease Control and Prevention. Prevention and control of seasonal influenza with vaccines. Recommendations of the Advisory Committee on Immunization Practices–United States, 2013-2014.

MMWR Recomm Rep 2013;62(RR-07):1–43. Available at: http://www.cdc.gov/mmwr/preview/mmwr html/rr6207a1.htm. Accessed June 1, 2016.

25. WHO. Vaccines against influenza WHO position paper - November 2012. Weekly epidemiological record. Available at: http://www.who.int/wer/2012/wer8747.pdf?ua=1. Accessed May 24, 2016.

26. The Department of Health, Public Health England. The Department Health/Pubic Health England: The National Flu Immunisation Programme 2015/16. Available at: https://www.gov.uk/government/up loads/system/uploads/attachment_data/file/5261 44/Annual_flu_letter_24_03_15superseded.pdf. Accessed May 27, 2016.

27. Pierce M, Kurinczuk JJ, Spark P, et al. Perinatal outcomes after maternal 2009/H1N1 infection: national cohort study. BMJ 2011;342:d3214.

28. Phadke VK, Omer SB. Maternal vaccination for the prevention of influenza: current status and hopes for the future. Expert Rev Vaccines 2016;15(10): 1255–80.

29. Zaman K, Roy E, Arifeen SE, et al. Effectiveness of maternal influenza immunization in mothers and infants. N Engl J Med 2008;359(15):1555–64.

30. Steinhoff MC, MacDonald N, Pfeifer D, et al. Influenza vaccine in pregnancy: policy and research strategies. Lancet 2014;383(9929):1611–3.

31. Steinhoff MC, Omer SB, Roy E, et al. Influenza immunization in pregnancy–antibody responses in mothers and infants. N Engl J Med 2010;362(17): 1644–6.

32. Centers for Disease Control and Prevention. Vaccination coverage among persons with asthma – United States, 2010-2011 influenza season. Morbidity and mortality weekly report. Available at: http://www.cdc.gov/mmwr/preview/mmwrhtml/mm 6248a1.htm. Accessed May 24, 2016.

33. Rhorer J, Ambrose CS, Dickinson S, et al. Efficacy of live attenuated influenza vaccine in children: a meta-analysis of nine randomized clinical trials. Vaccine 2009;27(7):1101–10.

34. Jefferson T, Rivetti A, Harnden A, et al. Vaccines for preventing influenza in healthy children. Cochrane Database Syst Rev 2012;(8):CD004879.

35. Osterholm MT, Kelley NS, Sommer A, et al. Efficacy and effectiveness of influenza vaccines: a systematic review and meta-analysis. Lancet Infect Dis 2012;12(1):36–44.

36. Belshe RB, Edwards KM, Vesikari T, et al. Live attenuated versus inactivated influenza vaccine in infants and young children. N Engl J Med 2007; 356(7):685–96.

37. Vesikari T, Knuf M, Wutzler P, et al. Oil-in-water emulsion adjuvant with influenza vaccine in young children. N Engl J Med 2011;365(15):1406–16.

38. Cowling BJ, Fang VJ, Nishiura H, et al. Increased risk of noninfluenza respiratory virus infections associated with receipt of inactivated influenza vaccine. Clin Infect Dis 2012;54(12): 1778–83.

39. Sundaram ME, McClure DL, Vanwormer JJ, et al. Influenza vaccination is not associated with detection of noninfluenza respiratory viruses in seasonal studies of influenza vaccine effectiveness. Clin Infect Dis 2013;57(6):789–93.

40. Simonsen L, Reichert TA, Viboud C, et al. Impact of influenza vaccination on seasonal mortality in the US elderly population. Arch Intern Med 2005; 165(3):265–72.

41. Simonsen L, Taylor RJ, Viboud C, et al. Mortality benefits of influenza vaccination in elderly people: an ongoing controversy. Lancet Infect Dis 2007; 7(10):658–66.

42. Jefferson T, Di Pietrantonj C, Al-ansary L, et al. Vaccines for preventing influenza in the elderly. Cochrane Database Syst 2010;2:1–32.

43. Darvishian M, Bijlsma MJ, Hak E, et al. Effectiveness of seasonal influenza vaccine in community-dwelling elderly people: a meta-analysis of test-negative design case-control studies. Lancet Infect Dis 2014;14(12):1228–39.

44. Lang PO, Mendes A, Socquet J, et al. Effectiveness of influenza vaccine in aging and older adults: comprehensive analysis of the evidence. Clin Interv Aging 2012;7:55–64.

45. Beyer WEP, McElhaney J, Smith DJ, et al. Cochrane re-arranged: support for policies to vaccinate elderly people against influenza. Vaccine 2013;31(50):6030–3.

46. DiazGranados CA, Dunning AJ, Kimmel M, et al. Efficacy of high-dose versus standard-dose influenza vaccine in older adults. N Engl J Med 2014; 371(7):635–45.

47. McElhaney JE, Coler RN, Baldwin SL. Immunologic correlates of protection and potential role for adjuvants to improve influenza vaccines in older adults. Expert Rev Vaccines 2013;12(7):759–66.

48. Belshe RB, Gruber WC, Mendelman PM, et al. Correlates of immune protection induced by live, attenuated, cold-adapted, trivalent, intranasal influenza virus vaccine. J Infect Dis 2000;181(3):1133–7.

49. O'Flanagan D, Cotter S, Mereckiene J. Seasonal influenza vaccination in EU / EEA, influenza season 2011-12, Vaccine European New Integrated Collaboration (VENICE) II Consortium September 2012- February 2013. Available at: http://venice. cineca.org/VENICE_Seasonal_Influenza_2011-12_ 1.0v.pdf. Accessed June 1, 2016.

50. Fleming DM, Crovari P, Wahn U, et al. Comparison of the efficacy and safety of live attenuated cold-adapted influenza vaccine, trivalent, with trivalent inactivated influenza virus vaccine in children and adolescents with asthma. Pediatr Infect Dis J 2006;25(10):860–9.

51. Cates CJ, Jefferson TO, Rowe BH. Vaccines for preventing influenza in people with asthma. Cochrane Database Syst Rev 2008;(2):CD000364.

52. Lyn-Cook R, Halm EA, Wisnivesky JP. Determinants of adherence to influenza vaccination among inner-city adults with persistent asthma. Prim Care Respir J 2007;16(4):229–35.

53. Lambert LC, Fauci AS. Influenza vaccines for the future. N Engl J Med 2010;363(21):2036–44.

54. Dunning J, Openshaw PJM. Impact of the 2009 influenza pandemic. Thorax 2010;65(6):471–2.

55. Treanor JJ, Campbell JD, Zangwill KM, et al. Safety and immunogenicity of an inactivated subvirion influenza A (H5N1) vaccine. N Engl J Med 2006; 354:1343–51.

56. McCullers JA, Huber VC. Correlates of vaccine protection from influenza and its complications. Hum Vaccin Immunother 2012;8(1):34–44.

57. Trombetta C, Perini D, Mather S, et al. Overview of serological techniques for influenza vaccine evaluation: past, present and future. Vaccines 2014;2(4): 707–34.

58. Barria MI, Garrido JL, Stein C, et al. Localized mucosal response to intranasal live attenuated influenza vaccine in adults. J Infect Dis 2013; 207(1):115–24.

59. Wilkinson TM, Li CK, Chui CSC, et al. Preexisting influenza-specific CD4+ T cells correlate with disease protection against influenza challenge in humans. Nat Med 2012;18(2):276–82.

60. Sridhar S, Begom S, Bermingham A, et al. Cellular immune correlates of protection against symptomatic pandemic influenza. Nat Med 2013;19(10): 1305–12.

61. Thomas PG, Keating R, Hulse-Post DJ, et al. Cell-mediated protection in influenza infection. Emerg Infect Dis 2006;12(1):48–54.

62. McElhaney JE, Xie D, Hager WD, et al. T cell responses are better correlates of vaccine protection in the elderly. J Immunol 2006;176(10):6333–9.

63. Bright RA, Medina MJ, Xu X, et al. Incidence of adamantane resistance among influenza A (H3N2) viruses isolated worldwide from 1994 to 2005: a cause for concern. Lancet 2005;366(9492): 1175–81.

64. Dharan NJ, Gubareva LV, Meyer JJ, et al. Infections with oseltamivir-resistant influenza A(H1N1) virus in the United States. JAMA 2009;301(10):1034–41.

65. Tetsutani K, Ishii KJ. Adjuvants in influenza vaccines. Vaccine 2012;30(52):7658–61.

66. Goff PH, Hayashi T, Martínez-Gil L, et al. Synthetic toll like receptor 4 (TLR4) and TLR7 ligands as influenza virus vaccine adjuvants induce rapid, sustained, and broadly protective responses. J Virol 2015;89(6):3221–35.

67. Jegerlehner A, Schmitz N, Storni T, et al. Influenza A vaccine based on the extracellular domain of M2:

68. El Bakkouri K, Descamps F, De Filette M, et al. Universal vaccine based on ectodomain of matrix protein 2 of influenza A: Fc receptors and alveolar macrophages mediate protection. J Immunol 2011;186(2):1022–31.

69. Staneková Z, Varečková E. Conserved epitopes of influenza A virus inducing protective immunity and their prospects for universal vaccine development. Virol J 2010;7:351.

70. Wacheck V, Egorov A, Groiss F, et al. A novel type of influenza vaccine: safety and immunogenicity of replication-deficient influenza virus created by deletion of the interferon antagonist NS1. J Infect Dis 2010;201(3):354–62.

71. Xiang K, Ying G, Yan Z, et al. Progress on adenovirus-vectored universal influenza vaccines. Hum Vaccin Immunother 2015;11(5):1209–22.

72. Jha A, Jarvis H, Fraser C, et al. Respiratory syncytial virus. Eur Respir Soc Monogr 2016;72:84–109.

73. Nair H, Nokes DJ, Gessner BD, et al. Global burden of acute lower respiratory infections due to respiratory syncytial virus in young children: a systematic review and meta-analysis. Lancet 2010;375(9725):1545–55.

74. Meissner HC, Ingelfinger JR, Meissner HC. Viral bronchiolitis in children. N Engl J Med 2016; 374(1):62–72.

75. Kim HW, Canchola JG, Brandt CD, et al. Respiratory syncytial virus disease in infants despite prior administration of antigenic inactivated vaccine. Am J Epidemiol 1969;89(4):422–34.

76. Fulginiti VA, Eller JJ, Joyner JW, et al. Respiratory virus immunization. Am J Epidemiol 1969;89(4): 435–48.

77. De Swart RL, Kuiken T, Timmerman HH, et al. Immunization of macaques with formalin-inactivated respiratory syncytial virus (RSV) induces interleukin-13-associated hypersensitivity to subsequent RSV infection. J Virol 2002;76(22):11561–9.

78. Acosta P, Caballero M, Polacka P. Brief history and characterization of enhanced respiratory syncytial. Clin Vaccine Immunol 2016;23(3):189–95.

79. Loebbermann J, Durant L, Thornton H, et al. Defective immunoregulation in RSV vaccine-augmented viral lung disease restored by selective chemoattraction of regulatory T cells. Proc Natl Acad Sci U S A 2013;110(8):2987–92.

80. Guvenel AK, Chiu C, Openshaw PJ. Current concepts and progress in RSV vaccine development. Expert Rev Vaccines 2014;13(3):333–44.

81. Connors M, Collins PL, Firestone CY, et al. Respiratory syncytial virus (RSV) F, G, M2 (22K), and N proteins each induce resistance to RSV challenge, but resistance induced by M2 and N proteins is relatively short-lived. J Virol 1991;65(3):1634–7.

82. McLellan JS, Chen M, Leung S, et al. Structure of RSV fusion·glycoprotein trimer bound to a prefusion-specific neutralizing antibody. Science 2013;340(6136):1113–7.

83. Bukreyev A, Yang L, Fricke J, et al. The secreted form of respiratory syncytial virus G glycoprotein helps the virus evade antibody-mediated restriction of replication by acting as an antigen decoy and through effects on Fc receptor-bearing leukocytes. J Virol 2008;82(24):12191–204.

84. Chirkova T, Boyoglu-Barnum S, Gaston KA, et al. Respiratory syncytial virus G protein CX3C motif impairs human airway epithelial and immune cell responses. J Virol 2013;87(24):13466–79.

85. Jorquera P, Oakley K, Powell T, et al. Layer-by-layer nanoparticle vaccines carrying the G Protein CX3C motif protect against RSV infection and disease. Vaccines 2015;3(4):829–49.

86. McLellan JS, Chen M, Joyce MG, et al. Structure-based design of a fusion glycoprotein vaccine for respiratory syncytial virus. Science 2013;342(6158):592–8.

87. Jozwik A, Habibi MS, Paras A, et al. RSV-specific airway resident memory CD8+ T cells and differential disease severity after experimental human infection. Nat Commun 2015;6:10224.

88. The IMpact-RSV Study Group. Palivizumab, a humanized respiratory syncytial virus monoclonal antibody, reduces hospitalization from respiratory syncytial virus infection in high-risk infants. Pediatrics 1998;102(3 Pt 1):531–7.

89. Blanken MO, Rovers MM, Molenaar JM, et al. Respiratory syncytial virus and recurrent wheeze in healthy preterm infants. N Engl J Med 2013;368(19):1791–9.

90. Committee on Infectious Diseases and Bronchiolitis Guidelines. Updated guidance for palivizumab prophylaxis among infants and young children at increased risk of hospitalization for respiratory syncytial virus infection. Pediatrics 2014;134(2):415–20.

91. Ralston S, Lieberthal A, Meissner H, et al. Clinical practice guideline: the diagnosis, management, and prevention of bronchiolitis. Pediatrics 2014;134:e1474–502.

92. O'Brien KL, Chandran A, Weatherholtz R, et al. Efficacy of motavizumab for the prevention of respiratory syncytial virus disease in healthy Native American infants: a phase 3 randomised double-blind placebo-controlled trial. Lancet Infect Dis 2015;15(12):1398–408.

93. Malkin E, Yogev R, Abughali N, et al. Safety and immunogenicity of a live attenuated RSV vaccine in healthy RSV-seronegative children 5 to 24 months of age. PLoS One 2013;8(10):e77104.

94. Polack FP. The changing landscape of respiratory syncytial virus. Vaccine 2015;33(47):6473–8.

95. Saso A, Kampmann B. Vaccination against respiratory syncytial virus in pregnancy: a suitable tool to combat global infant morbidity and mortality? Lancet Infect Dis 2016;16:e153–63.

96. Habibi MS, Jozwik A, Makris S, et al. Impaired antibody-mediated protection and defective IgA B-cell memory in experimental infection of adults with respiratory syncytial virus. Am J Respir Crit Care Med 2015;191(9):1040–9.

97. PATH. Vaccine development – Vaccine Development Global Program. Available at: http://sites.path.org/vaccinedevelopment/respiratory-syncytial-virus-rsv/vaccine-development/. Accessed May 19, 2016.

98. Munoz FM. Parainfluenza viruses in children. UpToDate. Available at: https://www.uptodate.com/contents/parainfluenza-viruses-in-children.Accessed May 20, 2016.

99. Lehners N, Tabatabai J, Prifert C, et al. Long-term shedding of influenza virus, parainfluenza virus, respiratory syncytial virus and nosocomial epidemiology in patients with hematological disorders. PLoS One 2016;11(2):e0148258.

100. Cohen AL, Sahr PK, Treurnicht F, et al. Parainfluenza virus infection among human immunodeficiency virus (HIV)-infected and HIV-uninfected children and adults hospitalized for severe acute respiratory illness in South Africa, 2009–2014. Open Forum Infect Dis 2015;2(4):ofv139.

101. Parrott R, Vargosko A, Kim H, et al. Acute respiratory diseases of viral etiology. III. parainfluenza. Myxoviruses. Am J Public Health Nations Health 1962;52:907–17.

102. Glezen WP, Frank AL, Taber LH, et al. Parainfluenza virus type 3: seasonality and risk of infection and reinfection in young children. J Infect Dis 1984;150(6):851–7.

103. Schmidt A. Progress in respiratory virus vaccine development. Semin Respir Crit Care Med 2011;32(04):527–40.

104. Karron RA, Belshe RB, Wright PF, et al. A live human parainfluenza type 3 virus vaccine is attenuated and immunogenic in young infants. Pediatr Infect Dis J 2003;22(5):394–405.

105. Karron RA, Wright PF, Newman FK, et al. A live human parainfluenza type 3 virus vaccine is attenuated and immunogenic in healthy infants and children. J Infect Dis 1995;172(6):1445–50.

106. Madhi SA, Cutland C, Zhu Y, et al. Transmissibility, infectivity and immunogenicity of a live human parainfluenza type 3 virus vaccine (HPIV3cp45) among susceptible infants and toddlers. Vaccine 2006;24(13):2432–9.

107. Belshe RB, Newman FK, Tsai TF, et al. Phase 2 evaluation of parainfluenza type 3 cold passage mutant 45 live attenuated vaccine in healthy children 6-18 months old. J Infect Dis 2004;189(3):462–70.

108. Schmidt AC, Schaap-Nutt A, Bartlett EJ, et al. Progress in the development of human parainfluenza virus vaccines. Expert Rev Respir Med 2011;5(4):515–26.

109. Englund JA, Karron RA, Cunningham CK, et al. Safety and infectivity of two doses of live-attenuated recombinant cold-passaged human parainfluenza type 3 virus vaccine rHPIV3cp45 in HPIV3-seronegative young children. Vaccine 2013;31(48):5706–12.

110. van Wyke Coelingh KL, Winter CC, Tierney EL, et al. Attenuation of bovine parainfluenza virus type 3 in nonhuman primates and its ability to confer immunity to human parainfluenza virus type 3 challenge. J Infect Dis 1988;157(4):655–62.

111. Greenberg DP, Walker RE, Lee M-S, et al. A bovine parainfluenza virus type 3 vaccine is safe and immunogenic in early infancy. J Infect Dis 2005; 191(7):1116–22.

112. Karron RA, Thumar B, Schappell E, et al. Evaluation of two chimeric bovine-human parainfluenza virus type 3 vaccines in infants and young children. Vaccine 2012;30(26):3975–81.

113. Karron RA, San Mateo J, Thumar B, et al. Evaluation of a live-attenuated human parainfluenza type 1 vaccine in adults and children. J Pediatr Infect Dis Soc 2015;4(4):143–6.

114. Schmidt AC, Auliffe JMMC, Murphy BR, et al. Recombinant bovine/human parainfluenza virus type 3 (B/HPIV3) expressing the respiratory syncytial virus (RSV) G and F proteins can be used to achieve simultaneous mucosal immunization against RSV and HPIV3. J Virol 2001;75(10):4594–603.

115. Bernstein DI, Malkin E, Abughali N, et al. Phase 1 study of the safety and immunogenicity of a live, attenuated respiratory syncytial virus and parainfluenza virus type 3 vaccine in seronegative children. Pediatr Infect Dis J 2012;31(2):109–14.

116. Rowe WP, Huebner RJ, Gilmore LK, et al. Isolation of a cytopathogenic agent from human adenoids undergoing spontaneous degeneration in tissue culture. Proc Soc Exp Biol Med 1953;84(3):570–3.

117. Potter RN, Cantrell JA, Mallak CT, et al. Adenovirus-associated deaths in US military during postvaccination period, 1999–2010. Emerg Infect Dis 2012; 18(3):507–9.

118. Echavarría M. Adenoviruses in immunocompromised hosts. Clin Microbiol Rev 2008;21(4): 704–15.

119. Hilleman MR, Gauld RL, Butler RL, et al. Appraisal of occurrence of adenovirus-caused respiratory illness in military populations. Am J Hyg 1957; 66(1):29–41.

120. Gray G, Goswami P, Malasig M, et al. Adult adenovirus infections: loss of orphaned vaccines precipitates military respiratory disease epidemics. Clin Infect Dis 2000;31(3):663–70.

121. Kuschner RA, Russell KL, Abuja M, et al. A phase 3, randomized, double-blind, placebo-controlled study of the safety and efficacy of the live, oral adenovirus type 4 and type 7 vaccine, in U.S. military recruits. Vaccine 2013;31(28):2963–71.

122. Hoke CH, Hawksworth A, Snyder CE. Initial assessment of impact of adenovirus type 4 and type 7 vaccine on febrile respiratory illness and virus transmission in military basic trainees, March 2012. MSMR 2012;19(3):2–5.

Index

Note: Page numbers of article titles are in **boldface** type.

Moving?

Make sure your subscription moves with you!

To notify us of your new address, find your **Clinics Account Number** (located on your mailing label above your name), and contact customer service at:

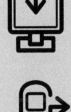

Email: journalscustomerservice-usa@elsevier.com

800-654-2452 (subscribers in the U.S. & Canada)
314-447-8871 (subscribers outside of the U.S. & Canada)

Fax number: 314-447-8029

Elsevier Health Sciences Division
Subscription Customer Service
3251 Riverport Lane
Maryland Heights, MO 63043

*To ensure uninterrupted delivery of your subscription, please notify us at least 4 weeks in advance of move.

Printed and bound by CPI Group (UK) Ltd, Croydon, CR0 4YY

08/05/2025

01864696-0014